Active Bodies

Active Bodies

A HISTORY OF WOMEN'S PHYSICAL EDUCATION IN TWENTIETH-CENTURY AMERICA

Martha H. Verbrugge

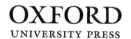
OXFORD
UNIVERSITY PRESS

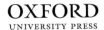

OXFORD
UNIVERSITY PRESS

Oxford University Press is a department of the University of Oxford. It furthers
the University's objective of excellence in research, scholarship, and education
by publishing worldwide. Oxford is a registered trade mark of Oxford University
Press in the UK and certain other countries.

Published in the United States of America by Oxford University Press
198 Madison Avenue, New York, NY 10016, United States of America.

© Oxford University Press 2012

First issued as an Oxford University Press paperback, 2017

Library of Congress Cataloging-in-Publication Data
Verbrugge, Martha H.
Active bodies : a history of women's physical education in twentieth-century
America / Martha H. Verbrugge.
p. cm.
Includes bibliographical references and index.
ISBN 978-0-19-516879-2 (hardcover : alk. paper); 978-0-19-084413-4 (paperback : alk. paper)
1. Women physical education teachers—United States.
2. Physical education teachers—United States. 3. Physical education for women—United States.
4. Discrimination in sports—United States. 5. Women—Education—United States.
6. Educational equalization—United States. I. Title.
GV362.V47   2012
613.7082—dc23   2011030958

To my siblings

Anne, Lois, and Robert

{ CONTENTS }

Acknowledgments   ix

Introduction: Body, Science, and Difference in the Gym   **3**

1. **"Who is that woman?": Female Physical Educators, 1890s–1940s**   **14**

2. **Active Womanhood and the Science of Sex Differences,**
   1890s–1940s   **47**

3. **Gym Periods and Monthly Periods, 1900–1940**   **63**

4. **Gender, Race, and Equity: Howard University and the University of**
   Nebraska   **77**

5. **"The joy of hard play": Competitive Activities for College Women,**
   1920s–1950s   **102**

6. **Separate and Unequal: The Public Schools of Washington, D.C.,**
   1890s–1950s   **153**

7. **"It's just the gym": Female Physical Educators, 1950–2005**   **174**

8. **Physical Fairness: Science, Feminism, and Sex Differences,**
   1950–2005   **201**

9. **Exercising Caution: Physical Activity and Reproductive Health,**
   1940–2005   **232**

Conclusion: Justice in the Gym   **253**

Endnote Abbreviations   259
Notes   261
Select Bibliography   339
Index   379

{ ACKNOWLEDGMENTS }

While finishing this book, I thought about the common expression "the journey is the destination." To be sure, this project has been an exciting intellectual journey. I studied a full century of American history, visited libraries and archives across the country, interacted with scholars from diverse fields, and navigated the twists and turns that appear during any long trip. The destination, though, is equally gratifying. Besides enjoying the completion of a major project, I welcome the chance to acknowledge the many individuals who helped along the way.

This book would have been impossible without the assistance of knowledge-able archivists and librarians. Although some have retired or moved on to new positions, a number deserve special thanks for their keen interest and resource-fulness: Nancy Dosch and Mike Everman at the Archives of the American Alliance for Health, Physical Education, Recreation and Dance (formerly located in Reston, Virginia); Jeffrey Monseau, archivist at Springfield College; Margery Sly of the Smith College Archives; Joellen ElBashir of the Moorland-Spingarn Research Center at Howard University; Hayden Wetzel and Judy Capurso of the Charles Sumner School Museum and Archives, Washington, D.C.; Ginny Daley (Special Collections) and Tom Harkins (Archives) at Duke University; Ken Grossi of the Oberlin College Archives; Bernard Schermetzler and Vicki Tobias of the Archives at the University of Wisconsin, Madison; Susan Rishworth, formerly at the American College of Obstetricians and Gynecologists; Renee McKinney at the Spelman College Archives; and Wilma R. Slaight and Jean N. Berry of the Wellesley College Archives. In many cases, librarians helped arrange interviews with active or retired physical educators; I am grateful to the many teachers and coaches who shared their life stories and professional experiences with me.

Shortly after starting this project, I began attending the annual meetings of the North American Society for Sport History (NASSH). A more hospitable community of scholars cannot be found. I have benefited enormously from their knowledge, insights, enthusiasm, and friendship. I am especially indebted to Roberta J. Park, Patricia A. Vertinsky, and Nancy Bouchier. Thanks also go to Mel Adelman, Nancy Bardwell, Susan Birrell, Allen Guttmann, Joan Hult, Rita Liberti, Patrick Miller, Catriona Parratt, Maureen Smith, Ron Smith, Alison Wrynn, and Susan Zieff. Even small moments had a big impact; Bruce Kidd's question after my John R. Betts Honor Lecture in 2005, for example, inspired me to redesign chapter 8.

I conceived of this project as an examination of American physical education through the lens of the history of science. My long-standing ties to historians of

science and medicine proved invaluable as I refashioned some familiar topics—
such as the relationship between biomedical knowledge and everyday life, the
marginalization of female experts, and the problematic history of the science
of sex differences—and applied these issues to the story of a health-related
profession outside our field's usual purview. Rima D. Apple deserves a special
salute; with the perceptiveness (and fortitude) of a first-rate scholar, she read an
early draft of the entire manuscript and offered crucial advice. I also am grateful
to Naomi Rogers, Margaret Marsh, Susan Reverby, Liz Watkins, Lara Freidenfelds, and other historians of medicine for their ongoing interest and cogent
questions about my work.

The support of my home institution was vital. My colleagues in the History
Department at Bucknell University provided astute feedback on various
sections of the book. Professional staff members of the Writing Center, the
Interlibrary Loan Department of Bertrand Library, and Debra Cook-Balducci,
an instructional technologist, gave indispensable assistance and advice. Several
undergraduates, especially Laura Leviski and Amanda Tamm, worked diligently
on research assignments, large and small. In addition to several summer grants,
the university's award of a Presidential Professorship provided crucial funds
and release time during the final stages of the project.

Two awards from the National Endowment for the Humanities—a Travel
to Collections grant and a Fellowship for College and University Teachers
(FB-28294-91)—enabled me to launch the project. A stipend from the Small
Research Grants Program of the Spencer Foundation supported my residency
at the Five College Women's Studies Research Center at Mount Holyoke College
in 1995–96. As the 1998 History Research Fellow of the American College of
Obstetricians and Gynecologists and Ortho Pharmaceuticals, I had access to
ACOG's extensive resources and library. An award from the National Institutes
of Health (NLM Grant for Scholarly Works in Biomedicine and Health 1G13
LM008926-01) enabled me to write a first draft of the manuscript in 2006–08.
The book's contents are solely my responsibility and do not necessarily repre-
sent the views of these agencies or institutions.

Portions of chapters 2, 3, 8, and 9, in somewhat different form, appeared
in the following publications: "Recreating the Body: Women's Physical Educa-
tion and the Science of Sex Differences in America, 1900–1940," *Bulletin of the
History of Medicine* 71, no. 2 (Summer 1997): 273–304, © 1997 by The Johns
Hopkins University Press, and reprinted by permission of the publisher; "Gym
Periods and Monthly Periods: Concepts of Menstruation in American Physical
Education, 1900–1940," in Mary M. Lay et al., eds., *Body Talk: Rhetoric,
Technology, Reproduction,* © 2000 by the Board of Regents of the University
of Wisconsin System, and reprinted courtesy of the University of Wisconsin
Press; and "Gender, Science, and Fitness: Perspectives on Women's Exercise in
the United States in the Twentieth Century," *Health and History* 4, no. 1 (2002):
57–72, and reprinted by permission of the Australian and New Zealand Society

of the History of Medicine. I am grateful to the publishers for permission to include the above materials in this book.

Several individuals at Oxford University Press helped bring this book to fruition. As my acquisitions editor, Jeffrey House shepherded the prospectus through the approval process and honed the project's central issues. Upon retirement, Jeffrey handed the project over to Susan Ferber, whose editorial acumen and hands-on approach reduced the manuscript's clutter and enabled its unique content and interpretations to stand out. I also appreciated the able assistance of Rick Stinson, my production editor, and Mary Sutherland, my copy editor. Mary's keen eye for detail and her patient help and good cheer were invaluable during the final stages.

I have saved the most heartfelt thanks for last. My best friends coaxed me away from the office for "recess" and other adventures, respected my work-related absences from "Fun 101," and were by my side during difficult times. Memories of my parents surfaced throughout the project. Mom fostered my devotion to books, lucid prose, and meticulous research. Her well-used copy of the 14th edition of *The Chicago Manual of Style* was always close at hand. Dad inspired my passion for science and sports. He bought me a chemistry set and my first baseball glove, took me to research labs and football games at the University of Minnesota, and found time to explain tough physics problems as well as play basketball with me. Having worked at various universities, my brother, sisters, and brothers-in-law understand the joys and rigor of academic life. For their steadfast love and support, I dedicate this book to my siblings, Anne, Lois, and Robert.

Active Bodies

{Introduction}

Body, Science, and Difference in the Gym

"Gym class." For many Americans—young and old, male and female—this phrase evokes strong images. Among teenagers, it brings to mind fitness tests, coed soccer, multicultural games, and group showers. Older generations might think back to dodge ball, sit-ups, social dance, and the humiliation of wearing ill-fitting gym suits. Regardless of age, few people forget the satisfaction of mastering a difficult skill in "PE" or the pain of being picked last for a team.

The vividness of these memories speaks to the resonance of physical education in American culture. Lessons in physical activity take place not only in schools and colleges but also in community centers, retirement homes, social service agencies, and commercial gyms and fitness clubs. Instruction can entail basic exercise, proficiency tests, recreational and competitive games, and information about health, hygiene, physiology, and sex. Physical education also conveys indelible lessons about the body and the self; it teaches discipline and spontaneity, competition and cooperation, self-esteem and embarrassment, confidence and alienation. Most Americans understand these meanings at a visceral level; other school lessons—from parsing a sentence to solving quadratic equations—are long forgotten, but we still remember how gym class both empowered and demoralized us. This paradox seems intrinsic to everyone's experience of physical education.

Other features, however, vary by social address. Age, gender, race, ethnicity, sexual orientation, socio-economic status, and locality have always affected people's experiences in gym class. During the early decades of the twentieth century, physical education gained a foothold in America's public schools. Prior to 1915, only three states required physical education for school-aged youth; shortly after World War I the number grew to twenty-eight; in 1929 the total was forty-six.[1] Young boys and girls typically exercised together in racially segregated primary schools. In secondary schools, white boys participated in military drills and sports, while white girls practiced calisthenics; the same held true for black pupils in upper grades. At boarding schools for Native Americans, boys competed in baseball and football, and girls learned calisthenics, recreational games, and good posture. In some rural and urban areas, white and black girls had access to more vigorous activities, both in and out of school. Physical training at colleges and universities also varied by gender, race, and class in the early 1900s. At white institutions, physical educators taught group exercise, social recreation, and low-key intramural sports to the daughters of elite and middle-class families; occasionally, gym class evolved into competitive athletics. Similar programs developed for young women at some historically black institutions, both coed and female-only. Activities for male undergraduates were strikingly different. In coed and all-male institutions, white and black, men's physical education usually took a backseat to burgeoning programs in varsity sports.

Supervised activity also occurred outside educational institutions. Under the watchful eye of recreation leaders, visitors to municipal playgrounds participated in gender-coded activities in areas divided by age and sex. The boys' section often had a jungle gym and facilities for basketball, baseball, handball, and track and field; girls played on swings and seesaws and practiced basketball, croquet, and tennis.[2] Voluntary organizations and settlement homes in urban neighborhoods also sponsored recreation classes. The Young Women's Hebrew Association and the racially segregated centers of the Young Women's Christian Association taught hygiene, exercise, and sports to groups organized by age, marital status, and socio-economic class.[3]

Physical education changed dramatically during the interwar years and even more so after mid-century. In 1954, the Supreme Court's landmark ruling in *Brown v. Board of Education of Topeka* directed school districts to desegregate their dual systems, including physical education and athletics. Title IX of the Educational Amendments Act of 1972 was equally transformative. Although its impact on varsity athletics is well-known, Title IX also applies to physical education, recreation, and intramural sports.[4] To achieve gender equity, many secondary schools replaced sex-segregated instruction with coed gym class. Section 504 of the Rehabilitation Act of 1973 mandated that schools receiving federal assistance provide individuals with disabilities "equal opportunities for comparable participation" in physical education and athletics.[5] During the 1980s and 1990s, concern over diversity and inclusion increased; some physical educators advocated new multicultural curricula to "create a learning environment . . . that reflects and embraces the diversity of the world in which we live."[6]

Despite these sea changes, people's experiences in gym class did not become uniform or equitable after mid-century; a participant's age, gender, race, ethnicity, religion, and sexual orientation still mattered. A partial explanation might be the disparate requirements for school-based physical education. Although most states currently mandate activity classes to some extent, fewer than 10 percent of the country's schools provide daily instruction for pupils in all grades throughout the academic year. Only one-half of pupils in grades K–12 have physical education every day, including just one-third of high school students. Exemptions are liberal, from playing in the marching band to serving as hall monitor.[7]

Even universal requirements, however, would not erase the impact of social variables on participation rates, attitudes, or experiences. Regardless of curricula and regulations, gender remains a powerful factor in physical education. Active girls and women, even proficient ones, often feel embarrassed and incompetent, especially if judgmental males are present. Young girls report that boys are "'rough'" and "'bossy'" during coed games. Many boys "'think girls are just plain failures. . . . [They] always try to make the girls feel bad some way.'"[8] Fitness tests reinforce the assumption of sex-based ability. In middle schools, boys demonstrate upper-body strength by performing as many pull-ups as they can; by contrast, instructors measure girls' hang times while their flexed arms keep their chins above the pull-up bar, after being lifted into position. This format depicts boys who "underperform" and girls who can execute "real" pull-ups as gender anomalies.[9]

Experiences also vary by race, ethnicity, religion, and sexual orientation. When researchers in the early 1990s asked urban teenagers why they liked gym class, 75 percent of Anglo-Americans identified "being with friends" as their primary reason, while nearly three-quarters of Hispanic Americans answered "becoming more fit." Activity preferences also differed; 17 percent of Asian Americans and 12 percent of Anglo-Americans disliked basketball, whereas no African Americans did.[10] Sometimes, a youngster reports that he or she does not participate in gym class "'because my religion says I shouldn't.'"[11] Gay and lesbian youth still face painful discrimination in gym class, from jokes and slurs to physical harassment, despite teachers' belief that their gym is a "safe space."[12]

Economic circumstances also affect pupils' opportunities. In affluent schools, physical education now looks "more like Cirque du Soleil than an Army boot camp."[13] Suburban districts have transformed their dreary old gymnasia into high-tech health clubs, where pupils, with heart rate monitors strapped to their chests, aim for their personalized fitness zones on treadmills and stationary bikes.[14] Nearly one-quarter of states permit online, self-directed physical education; after working out in any manner and at any time they choose, students transmit data from their school-issued heart rate monitors to their instructors via e-mail.[15] Poor districts have no such advantages. In New York City, more than one-half of elementary schools have no playground, and 18 percent of all schools lack a gymnasium. Squeezed by annual equipment budgets as small as $200, teachers conduct gym class in cafeterias, hallways, and lobbies.[16] Along with gender, race, and sexual orientation, socio-economic class confers privileges or burdens in the gym.

The factors governing students' experiences have affected teachers' status as well. Throughout the profession's development during the twentieth century, physical educators' gender, race, and sexual orientation influenced their circumstances. In the early 1900s, the division of gym class by participants' age, sex, and race also configured instructors' duties: women did "women's work" and blacks did "race work." White females supervised white girls and women and, sometimes, black females and young white boys. African American men and women taught only black youngsters and adults. Although this arrangement guaranteed jobs for white and black women alike, they worked primarily with individuals whom society deemed unskilled and unworthy. Moreover, despite the common belief that teaching was a respectable occupation for women, many Americans were suspicious of those who helped other females play, sweat, and compete.

Training programs for prospective teachers, male and female, increased during the early decades of the twentieth century, but opportunities were more plentiful for young whites than young blacks. Once employed, female personnel faced discrimination. In many coeducational colleges and universities, men's departments (usually synonymous with varsity athletics) had more visibility and clout than did women's separate programs of general instruction and intramural games. Before mid-century, segregation and racism limited the resources of black staff at African American schools, YWCAs, and other institutions. Although professional societies for white teachers usually welcomed female members, white women formed many independent organizations to better serve their unique interests. Because white groups typically excluded African Americans or, at best, marginalized them, black physical educators established their own professional societies, both single-sex and mixed. Overall, male instructors, coaches, administrators, and professional leaders—especially white men—benefited in the early 1900s from the field's partitioning by sex and race. Although female professionals objected to second-class treatment in a male-dominated field, they welcomed the authority that sex segregation seemed to confer. In this respect, the work of women physical educators, white and black, was simultaneously constrained and empowered.

The transformation of American physical education during the second half of the twentieth century had far-reaching implications for teachers. Higher professional standards made formal training a necessity. Women's share of undergraduate degrees in physical education almost doubled between 1950 and 1974 and then stabilized.[17] The scarcity of African Americans earning undergraduate and advanced degrees, however, raised the prospect that black physical educators were an "endangered species."[18] Job discrimination heightened this concern. When dual school systems desegregated in the 1950s and 1960s, many white-dominated districts demoted or fired their black male coaches, gym teachers, and administrators, while retaining white employees, irrespective of ability or seniority.[19] In the decades following the passage of Title IX, professional opportunities for white and black women fell sharply, even as female participation in recreation and athletics soared. When the number of school-based gym teachers plunged between the late 1970s and early 1990s, the teaching corps in grades K–12 became increasingly male, especially in high schools.[20] The number of female head coaches, sports officials, athletic trainers, equipment managers, and athletic administrators in secondary schools also shrank.[21] At the collegiate level, women bore the brunt of the consolidation of men's and women's departments in coed institutions as well as the shift from mandatory physical education to recreational services and varsity athletics. Increasingly, female personnel, especially African Americans, were concentrated in the lower echelons of college programs and underrepresented in high-status administrative and coaching positions.[22] Whatever their rank, women contended with pervasive heterosexism in their field and American society. Every female physical educator and coach, regardless of sexual orientation, lived under a cloud of suspicion that could sidetrack, even terminate her career.[23] Male/female, white/black, and straight/gay constituted hierarchical relationships that privileged some teachers and disadvantaged others.

Binary structures also dominated teachers' ideas about physical activity in the twentieth century. The logic seemed simple: Bodies differ, people differ, therefore activities must differ. From skill training and fitness tests to recreation and sports, the argument ran, activities should suit an individual's physical and personal makeup, present and future. Accepting age, sex, and race as meaningful, even self-evident categories in biology and society, many physical educators believed that male/female and other presumed dualities were free of ambiguity or overlap. Considerations of age emerged early in the field's history. Which activities, teachers asked, are appropriate and beneficial for various age groups, especially children and older youth? Concepts of sex differences proved especially durable.[24] Whenever teachers devised instructional methods, in-class activities, or fitness tests, many confidently assumed that boys differed from girls as did men from women. Physical educators whose interests lay more in research than teaching also took sex differences for granted; investigations of physical activity in relation to biomechanics, physiology, or psychology typically featured only one sex or contrasted male and female characteristics.

Until the late twentieth century, however, few physical educators, white or black, openly discussed how sexual orientation and gym class might intersect. Instead, most teachers used well-understood codes to stigmatize homosexuality— from favoring "feminine" sports before mid-century to tolerating pupils' homophobia in recent decades.[25] Although white instructors were equally silent on racial issues, classroom activities loudly proclaimed their prejudice. During the interwar years, for example, white female teachers organized historical pageants and clog dances that romanticized daily life on slave plantations, where supposedly happy, innately rhythmic blacks enjoyed singing and dancing after working in the fields.[26] Research studies also naturalized racial difference by claiming that being black or white affected motor skill and development.[27]

Teachers' interpretations of biology and behavior reflected those of modern science and culture. Between the sixteenth and twentieth centuries, Western scientists formulated a distinctive paradigm of difference. It represented the human body as a stable mechanism whose innate properties transcended time and place. It posited that nature's tidy dualities mapped directly onto everyday life and society. Applied to sex and gender, the standard view asserted a biological binary of male and female, male superiority and female deficiency, and an automatic linkage between female (sex) and femininity (gender).[28] Similar discourses developed around race, sexuality, and other presumed dualities.[29]

Adopting this system of binaries, physical educators taught twentieth-century Americans how "to do" masculinity or femininity, whiteness or blackness, and other identities that biology supposedly encoded. Rehearsing difference in the gym, however, entailed more than socialization into prescribed roles or the transmission of a hidden curriculum of accepted values, attitudes, and behaviors. By privileging some groups and marginalizing others, physical education helped constitute and maintain social inequities.[30] When a schoolboy in the early 1900s participated in military drills and his sister practiced calisthenics, both performed a gender system that associated power and status with manhood. When white-dominated school districts showered resources on white pupils and shortchanged black programs, physical educators and their pupils experienced racial privilege and subordination. In contemporary gyms, pupils' jokes about "picking the 'faggot' last" as a team member and teachers' failure to cite gay role models represent homosexuals as inept and gay athletes as nonexistent. These practices reward heterosexual males and marginalize gay and lesbian youth as well as any skilled girl or unskilled boy.[31]

Physical education's complicity in discrimination may seem unremarkable—comprising simply one more site where social hierarchies were produced in twentieth-century America. The "fleshing out" of difference also occurred in workplaces, hospitals, stores, churches, and private homes.[32] The articulation between gym class and social inequity, though, was significant for two reasons: Physical education located difference directly in the body, and it privileged scientific discourse.

There is nothing abstract about gym class; the quality of one's performance seems concrete and incontrovertible. Fitness tests, supervised workouts, and athletic contests reveal, often quantitatively, the body's supposedly native abilities and deficiencies. Speed and distance can be measured; aerobic power and body composition tested; laps and pull-ups counted; scores kept and winners announced. Numbers alone seem to express "how good we are"—a phrase that conflates skill and self-worth. *Who* we are seems equally apparent in the gym. Imagine that the final score of an intercollegiate basketball game was 41–40. If the players were male, most spectators would call the "close contest" a "tight defensive game." If the players were female, fans might "attribute the low score to poor playing skills."[33] Although this example comes from 1981, the explanations might still sound credible. Some Americans continue to believe that sex and race determine skill and, conversely, that performance gaps reveal innate differences rather than inequities in opportunities and resources. This naturalization of difference becomes self-perpetuating; once displayed for all to see, apparent disparities are then inscribed directly on the body. By practicing difference in the gym, people embody powerful lessons of body, self, and inequity—in literal as well as symbolic ways.[34]

Such lessons are even more compelling when buttressed by science. During the twentieth century, some leading physical educators urged their colleagues to produce original knowledge about the human body. Most teachers replied that the goals of training good instructors and refining classroom methods were more important. Despite the continual tension between research and pedagogy in American physical education, no one doubted that enlisting science would benefit the field.[35]

When physical education developed in the late nineteenth and early twentieth centuries, it faced problems common to all nascent professions.[36] Some aims were practical: secure an occupational niche, build an infrastructure, and train practitioners. More broadly, leaders had to unite the field around a cohesive identity, articulate its purpose, and earn respect. Physical education's credibility gap was large, since many citizens and academic leaders wondered if training the body was as critical as training the mind. These challenges occupied physical educators for decades, prompting one leader to diagnose the field "a hapless neurotic" beset by insecurity.[37] To solidify the profession, physical educators associated their work with up-to-date pedagogical theories and methods, aligned gym class with popular notions of health, morality, and citizenship, and borrowed concepts and prestige from scientific disciplines.

Given science's rising cultural authority, physical education legitimized its core ideas and practices (and still does) by drawing on expert knowledge of the human body. Although gym teachers have always been concerned with the cognitive and psychosocial aspects of activity, their work necessarily begins and ends with the material body—its structure and movement, limits and potential, problems and improvement. Effective instruction is essentially applied science: based on available theories and research, which individuals can engage in which activities and for what purpose?

Physical educators tapped many scientific fields. At the turn of the twentieth century, professional leaders and rank-and-file teachers thought about health and fitness in both mechanistic and moral terms. Focusing on structure and performance, they adopted anthropometry (which assessed people's size and strength) as well as physiological principles related to health and personal development.[38] Between the 1910s and 1930s, the field's emphasis on educating the whole individual—body, mind, and spirit—through physical activity made the social sciences seem increasingly relevant; nevertheless, teachers did not abandon biomechanical and physiological perspectives.[39] During the second half of the century, America's preoccupation with fitness steadily pulled physical education toward biomedicine and public health. Amid these broad changes, however, two premises remained constant in American physical education: the centrality of difference and the reliability of scientific knowledge.

Standing at the crossroads of science, culture, and daily life, physical education offers a unique lens for analyzing debates over difference and equity in twentieth-century America. Across the decades, gym class affected how ordinary people understood and experienced gender, race, and sexuality. Physical education's complicated messages about identity and physicality slid quietly into people's lives, becoming embodied in routine attitudes and habits. Conversely, social and intellectual context informed physical educators' perspectives on active bodies. As gender politics, race relations, discourses of sexuality, and the science of the body changed during the twentieth century, teachers revisited and often disagreed over how difference and equity should be practiced in the gym. The history of physical education has not been examined, comprehensively and critically, against America's distinctive political and social backdrop.[40] Analyzing physical education brings into new focus the tension between the nation's egalitarian ideals and record of discrimination as well as the complex interactions between gender, race, and sexuality in American life. Such a study also sheds light on ongoing disputes among experts and the public about active female bodies—their abilities and limits as delineated by biology and culture.

This book examines the history of physical education for girls and women in the United States during the twentieth century—from the early years of organized instruction in schools and other settings through the revolution in physical activity during the latter part of the century. Although women's athletics grabbed the public spotlight after mid-century, physical education remained a vital conduit for females interested in sports as an avocation or career. Accordingly, competitive athletics appear in this book as a byproduct of or alternative to instructional programs.[41]

The analysis focuses on the work and ideas of women who taught gym class, rather than their students' experiences. Because women teachers worked primarily with females—the ostensibly inferior sex—such a study underscores the core issues of body, difference, and equity in American physical education. Despite their students' secondary status, women instructors regarded themselves as stewards of active female bodies and agents of fairness for the "fair sex." Concepts of difference helped teachers articulate their ideas about female health and physicality, justify instructional programs and policies, resolve disputes over female exercise and sports, launch or impede new activities, and prescribe racialized models of femininity and sexuality. Female physical educators also deployed notions of difference to consolidate their monopoly over programs for girls and women as well as protest inequities that both they and their students suffered.

As American culture, politics, and education changed during the twentieth century, women gym teachers modified their ideas, instructional programs, and professional strategies. Their perspectives also depended on their own personal backgrounds. This study focuses on white and black women because American physical education itself invoked this schema in the twentieth century, even though racial identities encompassed a broader spectrum.[42] Although black and white physical educators worked in many venues, this book examines the most common sites, including public schools and undergraduate institutions. Besides teaching gym class, physical educators often supervised clubs, ran intramural events, coached teams, and advised girls and young women. A substantial number also served as mid- or high-level administrators, while a select group became prominent leaders and authors who represented their profession on national and international stages. This book emphasizes rank-and-file female teachers along with well-known administrators and leaders; research-oriented physical educators appear more prominently toward the end of the narrative.

The book opens with a historical overview of American physical education as an instructional field and quasi-scientific profession between the late 1800s and mid-1900s. Chapter 1 profiles the women who trained and worked as physical educators during this period. The next two chapters explore teachers' ideas about the female body between 1900 and 1940. Chapter 2 examines how female physical educators, primarily white teachers, interpreted sex differences and active womanhood. Did they regard the female body as resilient or frail? Did they accentuate or minimize the physical and psychosocial differences between men and women? Did they attribute women's qualities to nature or nurture, to biology or culture? Teachers regarded reproductive functions as the most important item on their list of sex differences. Since many female instructors worked with pubescent girls and young adults, they were particularly concerned with how exercise affected menstruation and whether girls should participate in gym class or sports during menses. Chapter 3 analyzes teachers' changing views of menstruation and their policies about gym periods and monthly periods before mid-century.

Physical educators adapted their philosophies and programs to the particularities of where and whom they taught. In the early decades of the twentieth century, public schools enrolled youngsters of diverse races and socio-economic backgrounds, while colleges tended to be reserved for young adults from the middle and upper classes. The case studies in chapters 4 and 5 explore this relationship between ideas, curricula, and context, focusing on collegiate environments between the 1920s and 1950s. Chapter 4 compares two prominent university teachers, Mabel Lee and Maryrose Reeves Allen, who worked at coeducational institutions dominated by men and preoccupied with men's sports. Lee, a white woman, was a teacher and administrator at the University of Nebraska for three decades; in 1931 she became the first female president of the American Physical Education Association. Allen, an African American, directed the women's program at Howard University for more than forty years and was an influential mentor and leader among black physical educators. Deploying notions of sex differences, both of these women advocated feminine, noncompetitive activities for their female students and a separate department

for their female staff, while also objecting to disparities between women's physical education and men's athletics. Whereas Lee envisaged all women as white,
middle-class, and heterosexual, Allen interrogated race and bigotry.

Lee and Allen represented two distinguished examples on the broad continuum of college-level teachers before mid-century. Chapter 5 looks at physical education and sports for female students at colleges and universities across
the country between the 1920s and 1950s. The sample includes large and small
institutions, public and private, elite and middle-tier, coed and female-only,
predominantly white and historically black. Each school's unique character
affected teachers' attitudes about active womanhood and their decisions about
sports for female undergraduates. The process was complex, as students, faculty members, administrators, alumni, trustees, and donors tried to influence
whether and how women at their institution would compete.

Disagreements over active female bodies also broke out in noncollegiate settings before mid-century. Chapter 6 examines the public schools of Washington, D.C., where pupils' diversity by age, race, and class complicated teachers'
deliberations over curricular and extracurricular programs. Tracing physical
education and sports for boys and girls in the white and black divisions of
the city's public schools from the introduction of formal physical training in
1889 through racial desegregation in 1954, the chapter shows how white school
officials systematically privileged or marginalized different bodies in the gym
based on gender and race, while teachers, pupils, parents, and other constituencies challenged their decisions. Among the most forceful critics were black
administrators and instructors who subverted notions of racial difference to
assert power and agency.

As the fight for civil rights expanded across the country after mid-century,
arguments over active bodies became increasingly divisive. The Supreme
Court's 1954 decision in *Brown v. Board of Education of Topeka* focused the
nation's attention on racial disparities in education. Energized by the civil
rights movement, other struggles for social justice arose, including feminism,
gay rights, and disability rights. These campaigns destabilized familiar dualities
such as man/woman and sparked new disputes about the meaning of difference
and equity in a modern democratic society. Supporters of women's rights debated whether to pursue gender equality (grounded in the liberal premise that
people's potential did not depend on their sex) or gender equity (the political
correlate of a belief in sex differences). Adding to the controversy, federal legislation banning discrimination based on sex, race, and disability in various
settings sent mixed signals about equality versus equity.

These broad developments forced physical educators to reevaluate what
fairness meant for their students and themselves. Set against the backdrop
of legal, social, and political upheavals after mid-century, the final chapters
correspond to the first three. Chapter 7 analyzes women's professional status
as gym teachers, coaches, and administrators between 1950 and 2005. Despite

new opportunities, most female personnel lost ground; white and black women waged new battles over departmental structure and resources as well as their professional rights and autonomy. While pursuing parity for themselves, teachers and coaches also redefined fairness for their students and athletes. Chapter 8 analyzes how female teachers and coaches conceptualized sex differences and active womanhood in the late twentieth century. Grappling with the same questions as feminists did between the 1960s and 1990s, physical educators wondered if they should work toward equality or equity for their diverse students. Should difference—by gender, race, ethnicity, or sexuality—be ignored, accommodated, or transformed? Some physical educators listened intently as comparable disputes over difference flared up among natural and social scientists; research-based teachers, in particular, entertained new ideas about human dualities, their physical markers, and the biological versus cultural roots of women's behavior.

Teachers' toughest decisions still related to reproductive physiology, especially menstruation. Chapter 9 analyzes recent developments in the debate over female exercise and reproductive health. At mid-century, most biomedical experts concluded that exercise and sports did not compromise the monthly cycle, and many women physical educators agreed. During the 1970s and 1980s, however, specialists reported cases of "exercise-induced amenorrhea" in dedicated young athletes. In the early 1990s, experts postulated that reproductive dysfunction, eating disorders, and premature osteoporosis could arise simultaneously in female athletes and might affect any girl or woman who exercised. As concern escalated over the well-being of active females, rank-and-file gym teachers and coaches monitored their students' health in new ways.

Although the world of female physical educators—their ideas, work, and status—changed profoundly in some respects during the twentieth century, their field remains distinctly gendered, hierarchical, and insecure. They must still decipher the female body and decide how to accommodate its "nature" in the gym. Debates continue over the meaning of active womanhood, difference, and fairness. Focusing on how women physical educators at diverse institutions interpreted and applied scientific information, this book examines teachers' constructs of body, difference, and equity in relation to American science, law, education, politics, and culture. It critiques physical education's preoccupation with "difference" and elucidates the many factors—social, intellectual, and professional—that constrained white and black female teachers. It also shows how these very conditions engendered disagreement, resistance, and innovation. Despite the heavy burden of difference and inequity in their field's history, some female physical educators believed that active bodies both deserved and promoted justice.

"Who is that woman?"

FEMALE PHYSICAL EDUCATORS, 1890s–1940s

In the late 1940s, Winifred Van Hagen, a prominent physical educator in California, attended "Family Fun Night" at a small public school in the state. Watching her, a local resident exclaimed to his friends, "Who is that woman? She has the strength of a man, the refinement of a lady, and plays like a kid."[1] For many Americans, female gym teachers probably did seem odd. Although supervising children was suitably maternal and teaching had long been an accepted vocation, joining youngsters in their fun and games apparently breached mature womanhood. By earning a living in the gym, Van Hagen also seemed both masculine and feminine. Her physical energy indicated manliness, but her demeanor was graceful. No wonder the observer at "Family Fun Night" was bewildered.

The jobs that Van Hagen held between the 1910s and 1940s did not exist in the United States a century earlier. Through most of the 1800s, physical education was not a recognized occupation. Americans referred to structured exercise, whether private or supervised, as physical culture. Its advocates were an eclectic group of men and women who shared general interests rather than a uniform philosophy or unique qualifications. Doctors recommended physical activity for disease prevention and therapy. Educators and health reformers championed exercise for mental and physical improvement. Among them were Catharine Beecher and Dioclesian Lewis, whose systems of calisthenics rivaled European schemes. Public and private schools usually depended on regular instructors to handle physical culture and elocution (for strong lungs and clear diction); some colleges, though, hired specialists, often physicians, to teach hygiene and calisthenics. Although interest in preparing experts grew, only a handful of state normal schools and special programs, such as Dio Lewis's Normal Institute for Physical Education, offered training before the 1870s.

During the late nineteenth and early twentieth centuries, physical education emerged as a distinct vocation. The young field set out to secure an occupational niche, train practitioners, create a unique base of knowledge and expertise, and build an infrastructure for advancing and regulating itself.[2] In the 1880s and 1890s, viable jobs appeared as physical activities expanded in school and nonschool settings. By 1891–92, public schools in eighty-three cities employed a total of 137 specialists (including seventy-two women) to conduct required classes in physical education.[3] More colleges and universities established departments of physical education as well.[4]

Although many physical educators in the late 1800s had no formal preparation, opportunities for special training increased, especially for white men and women. At the end of the nineteenth century, several dozen institutions offered professional coursework in the field. These proprietary schools and summer programs awarded certificates, not college degrees; their curricula tended to be rudimentary and nonstandardized, and enrollees were predominantly, even exclusively, either male or female.[5] During the 1890s, some colleges, universities, and state normal schools opened teacher training programs in physical education, and several of the older, noncollegiate institutes evolved into degree-granting programs. These developments encouraged more rigorous requirements and curricula and, by the turn of the twentieth century, more gym teachers and recreation leaders had a modicum of good training.

These improvements were spearheaded by prominent physical educators, many of whom had medical backgrounds and held college positions. In 1885 white leaders founded the American Association for the Advancement of Physical Education (AAAPE) as a platform for discussion and reform; the organization is known today as the American Alliance for Health, Physical Education, Recreation and Dance. In 1889 more than two thousand people attended a historic conference on physical training in Boston, presided over by the U.S. Commissioner of Education.[6] In 1895 physical education became a recognized division within the National Education Association, the country's leading organization for white teachers.[7] Specialized books and journals also appeared. The AAAPE's *Proceedings* (1885–95) and its successor, the *American Physical Education Review* (1896–1929), were vehicles for professional reports, articles, and news.[8] In 1930 the organization founded the *Research Quarterly* to disseminate the field's scientific work. Numerous other groups supported the fledgling profession through meetings, literature, and public advocacy. The North American Gymnastic Union (the successor to the German-American *Turnverein*) lobbied for mandatory physical education in public schools and published the journal *Mind and Body* from 1894 to 1936.

The early decades of the twentieth century brought rapid gains in teacher training, employment, professional infrastructure, and social recognition.[9] World War I was critical to this progress, as physical educators' service in recreation, fitness, and rehabilitation brought favorable attention to their field.[10] The physical shortcomings of many military draftees raised concern about the country's lack of vitality, prompting large-scale conferences on health and fitness as well as the creation of the National Physical Education Service (NPES), the executive branch of a high-level committee to foster a vigorous citizenry. In the 1920s the NPES successfully promoted state and federal legislation for physical education in public schools. Scarce resources during the Great Depression, however, led many schools and colleges to curtail, even eliminate gym class and other non-academic activities.[11] With the revival of recreation and leisure activities in the late 1930s and early 1940s, physical education rebounded and, by many measures, qualified as an established profession. Leaders and rank-and-file teachers, though, still worried about the field's tenuous reputation of simply "'herding [youngsters] into a gymnasium, exercising them, and herding them out again.'"[12]

Men and women alike contributed to physical education's reforms in the early twentieth century and suffered from its precarious status. Gender and race, however, inflected women's experiences in unique ways. As women trained, sought employment, and built careers, they encountered firsthand the problems of difference and inequity in American physical education. This chapter profiles the country's early cohorts of female physical educators. The first generation included white women born during the 1850s and 1860s. The main figures represent the second generation—white and black women born between 1870 and 1900 whose work began between the 1890s and 1920s; information about white teachers, though, is more plentiful than details about black instructors.

Who Became a Gym Teacher?

Most of America's early female physical educators were white, native-born, and middle-class.[13] Their fathers worked in business, education, law, and other middle-tier professions. They hailed from small towns and cities in the Northeast. Gradually, young women from other regions as well as immigrant families also entered the field. Most gym teachers had at least a high school education; many pursued postsecondary education, ranging from normal school or college to advanced training in physical education or another health-related area. Most were young and single when their careers began. These attributes fit many white women who went into medicine, science, law, and other professions at the turn of the twentieth century.[14] What distinguished gym teachers was their enthusiasm for physical activity. As a new vocation, physical education offered women many avenues for converting this interest into a career.

The journey often began in childhood. Julia R. Grout (1898–1984), the daughter of a school superintendent in Massachusetts, was a "tomboy" who enjoyed "riding bicycle, throwing baseballs, and ice-skating." Julia's older brother taught her "how to wrestle and to throw and catch hard baseballs" and to hit tennis balls on a small court he marked out on the family's yard.[15] Dorothy Sears Ainsworth (1894–1976) learned German gymnastics in the public schools of Moline, Illinois. Inspired by her father, a draftsman with a passion for sports, Ainsworth excelled in basketball and tennis. "Our costumes," she recalled, "were longish skirts and shirtwaists for tennis and golf and for swimming black woolen suits with knee length skirts over bloomers and long black stockings. But we had a fine time."[16] While pursuing a history degree at Smith College, Ainsworth participated in intramural tennis and basketball, taking great pride in attaching a class-year numeral to her gymnastics blouse after team victories.[17]

Without help, however, young athletic women might not have realized that physical activity could be an occupation. Schoolteachers and other mentors often guided talented females toward the field. In the late 1880s, Ethel Perrin (1871–1962) attended a boarding school in West Bridgewater, Massachusetts, where a Sargent School graduate conducted physical training "twice a week in the attic of the schoolhouse." Unlike most of her classmates, Perrin relished the challenge of becoming "absolutely symmetrical" using the pulleys, adjustable weights, and other "exciting pieces of apparatus" in the makeshift gym. In 1890 Perrin enrolled in the Boston Normal School of Gymnastics (BNSG), because her principal's friend directed the program.[18] Similarly, Mabel Lee (1886–1985) had been "just wild about sports" as a youngster in Centerville, Iowa, during the 1890s.[19] She played games with neighborhood friends, learned to ride a bicycle, and enjoyed "swinging Indian clubs, jumping and running, [and] marching" at school, where she also led a girls military drill team.[20] While touting her athleticism, Lee also admitted being a "hollow chested and round shouldered and sadly underweight" child who "caught practically every illness that came to town."[21] Exercise's promise as both therapy and vocation dawned on her during high school and college. Lee's experiences as a gym class assistant at Coe College prompted her to enroll at the BNSG, where her teacher had trained.[22]

Many parents also encouraged their daughters to turn personal rehabilitation into a career. J. Anna Norris (1874–1958) suffered a foot injury during childhood when a piece of furniture fell on her; a high school gym teacher discovered that Norris also had a serious spinal curvature. Hoping to rescue his daughter from a life of disability, Norris's father enrolled her in a YWCA gymnastics program directed by a BNSG graduate. Following in her mentor's footsteps, Norris graduated from the BNSG (1895) and medical school (1900), and championed therapeutic exercise throughout her distinguished tenure at the University of Minnesota.[23] The daughter of a college professor and administrator, Gertrude Moulton (1880–1964) enjoyed the out-of-doors growing up in Colorado and Ohio.[24] Ill-health and frailty, though, led Gertrude to think of herself as an unskilled "dub." Her mother, a schoolteacher, steered Gertrude toward physical education, with the expectation that exercise would fix her daughter's deficiencies.[25] Some families, however, considered the field a questionable one for young women, whether sickly or robust. The mother of Anna Hiss (1893–1972) strongly objected when her daughter decided to satisfy her love of sports by becoming a physical educator. Anna mollified her mother by enrolling in the Sargent School, a reputable program in Boston, which her cousin attended.[26]

Although physical education troubled some Americans, others took advantage of its vague identity and diverse points of access. The new field's connection to health appealed particularly to men and women with medical and scientific interests. While teaching grade school in New York and Kansas, Delphine Hanna (1854–1941) became convinced that education should improve pupils' bodies as well as their minds. After studying physical training under Dio Lewis and Dudley Allen Sargent, Hanna augmented her scientific knowledge of exercise by earning a medical degree.[27] After studying with private tutors, Mary Channing Coleman (1883–1947) enrolled at the State Teachers College in Farmville, Virginia. More a scholar than athlete, Coleman then assisted a New York City orthopedic surgeon who taught her anatomy and kinesiology, and pointed her toward physical education.[28]

Medicine was even more pivotal for physical educators who were clinicians or researchers. Clelia Duel Mosher (1863–1940) taught hygiene and physical training at Stanford University during the mid-1890s and from 1910 to 1929. Mosher's undergraduate degree in zoology (Stanford, 1893), M.A. in physiology (Stanford, 1894), and subsequent medical training (Johns Hopkins, 1900) reflected her scientific inclinations. A practicing doctor and researcher, Mosher applied a biomedical approach to physical education, including hygiene instruction and medical exams.[29] Margaret Bell (1888–1969) was a distinguished teacher, administrator, and physician at the University of Michigan from 1923 to 1957. The daughter of a railroad official, Bell attended Chicago's John Dewey School, where she discovered her love of science and sports. A gifted athlete, Bell decided early on to pursue a joint career in medicine and physical education; she graduated from the Sargent School in 1910 and also earned a B.S. degree (University of Chicago, 1915) and an M.D. (Rush Medical School, 1921).[30]

Other routes to physical education were indirect or unplanned. Elizabeth Burchenal (1876–1959) had a cultured upbringing in Richmond, Indiana, as the daughter of a musician and a judge, who introduced their six children to literature, art, and dance. Burchenal did not envision a career in physical education and dance until the mid-1890s when she had gym class at Earlham College while earning her degree in English.[31] Raised in a small Texas town, Blanche M. Trilling (1876–1964) acquired the interests and education of a proper southern girl. She attended a boarding school in Virginia (where physical education comprised fancy marching drills), a private college in Tennessee, and a music conservatory in Cincinnati. After giving piano lessons in Texas for several years, Trilling changed course and entered the BNSG at the mature age of thirty-one.[32]

Black women's pathways were equally diverse. Some turned athletic talent directly into gainful employment. Inez Patterson (1911–?) was a multisport star in high school and Temple University during the 1920s. After college, she helped organize athletic clubs and worked for the YWCA in New Jersey and New York.[33] In other cases, opportunity knocked unexpectedly. Jessie H. (Scott) Abbott (1897–1981) was the daughter of a truck farmer in Des Moines, Iowa. She enjoyed walking, skating, and playing with her siblings and friends, white and black. Hoping to become a secretary, Jessie enrolled in business courses during high school and also took gym class. Shortly after graduation, she married Cleve Abbott, a college student-athlete, who soon took a coaching position at Tuskegee Institute. While working as a secretary for George Washington Carver and other prominent figures, Mrs. Abbott assisted her husband with the school's burgeoning program in physical education and sports. Besides coaching tennis and golf, she ran tournaments in these sports during Tuskegee's renowned Track and Field Relays.[34]

Although interest and circumstance sufficed for Abbott, the road to physical education increasingly traveled through formal mentors and special training. Anita J. Turner (ca. 1870–1941) attended Washington, D.C.'s premier high school for blacks and then the District's Miner Normal School. Observing Turner's exceptional performance in gym class, an instructor at Miner recommended additional training. After attending the Harvard Summer School for Physical Education under Dudley Allen Sargent, Turner taught and supervised physical education in the black elementary schools of Washington, D.C., for almost fifty years.[35] A New Orleans native, Azalie Thomas (1874–1935) graduated from Hampton Institute and then earned a diploma at the BNSG in 1899. She was the program's only black graduate during its first thirty-six years. Thomas taught physical education in the normal department of Tuskegee Institute from 1899 to 1904, and then moved to the Midwest to become a wife, mother, and nurse.[36] Maryrose Reeves Allen (1899–1992) became interested in health and physical education as a high school student in Indianapolis. After receiving a diploma from the Sargent School in 1923 and teaching in Trenton, New Jersey, Allen joined the faculty of Howard University. Within a decade, she also completed bachelor and master's degrees in physical education and undertook doctoral work.[37]

Physical education's multiple entryways were typical for any nascent profession. That said, admitting women presented unique issues in the late 1800s and early 1900s due to the field's questionable reputation. Few white Americans doubted that exercise benefited women or that teaching was an appropriate female job. Between 1870 and 1940, teaching never ranked lower than fifth on the list of women's occupations.[38] At the turn of the twentieth century, the majority of female schoolteachers were young, white, and middle class.[39] Yet some white Americans wondered, as Van Hagen's critic had, if respectable white ladies belonged in jobs identified with active bodies and sports.

Although some African Americans raised similar concerns in the early twentieth century, many sectors of the black community regarded femininity and athleticism as compatible. Of broader significance was black women's belief that work was normal and necessary, and that education represented the best avenue to meaningful jobs. From Emancipation on, African American women were far more likely than white women to be gainfully employed outside the home.[40] Both working- and middle-class black women viewed themselves as independent agents with multiple roles, paid and unpaid, in their families as well as communities.[41] At the turn of the twentieth century, black women were concentrated in menial labor and professional fields, with few options in between.[42] Despite many roadblocks, black women aspired to nursing, teaching, and other skilled positions that promised not only better incomes and more autonomy but also opportunities to promote racial progress.[43] Physical education met these criteria by enhancing the health and status of black Americans while improving a teacher's own social condition.

Preparing to Teach

Increasingly, the path to jobs went through education because employers expected, even required, gym teachers to have formal qualifications. During the early decades of the twentieth century, state certification laws for general classroom instructors became more common; a few regulations covered physical education and other special subjects. By the late 1920s some states required all teachers to have basic preparation in physical education; by 1930 thirty-eight states required specialists in physical education to be certified.[44] A similar, but less formal change occurred in higher education during the interwar period. As colleges and universities raised their standards for the academic professoriate, they also hired non-academic teachers with baccalaureate or higher degrees in their specialties.[45] These trends fueled the expansion of physical education training programs from two dozen in 1914 to eighty-one in 1921 to nearly three hundred in 1944.[46] Four-year professional curricula at predominantly white colleges, universities, and state teachers colleges supplanted older certificate programs in private normal schools. Some pioneering nondegree institutions evolved into collegiate programs; the YMCA International Training School became Springfield College, and in 1909 the BNSG affiliated with Wellesley College.

Second-generation white teachers (women born between 1870 and 1900) took advantage of these opportunities. Between 1900 and 1920 females constituted about three-quarters of trainees in programs admitting whites, either predominantly or exclusively.[47] White women enrolled in private programs such as the BNSG/Wellesley, the Sargent School (Cambridge, Massachusetts), the Anderson Normal School (Brooklyn, New York, then New Haven, Connecticut), the Savage School (New York City), the Posse Gymnasium (Boston), and comparable schools in Chicago, Battle Creek, Michigan, and other cities. Increasingly, young white women also attended degree-granting programs at Oberlin College, Temple University, the Teachers College of Columbia University, and various state universities, including Iowa, Nebraska, and Wisconsin.

Professional preparation for African Americans was far more limited. This shortage mirrored general patterns in teacher education for blacks in the late nineteenth and early twentieth centuries. Between the 1870s and 1910s, private schools trained most black teachers. Because these institutions did not offer specialized work in physical education, interested young blacks opted for predominantly white programs. The Sargent School trained many black women; the YMCA International Training School enrolled black men; Harvard University's summer school program admitted black students of both sexes.[48] Between the 1920s and 1940s, historically black colleges and universities assumed a larger share of teacher training in both general education and specialty fields. Howard University, Hampton Institute, and Tuskegee Institute began awarding diplomas, then professional degrees in physical education after World War I. By 1939 thirteen black institutions offered four-year degree programs in physical education.[49] When these programs proved too small to meet demand, land-grant institutions trained physical education teachers, upon achieving collegiate status in the 1930s.[50] Black women were well-represented in these programs. In the mid-1930s, they constituted about one-half of physical education majors at coed historically black institutions.[51] The schools' faculties also reflected the growth of professional training; in the 1930s the alma maters of female staff included private schools (particularly Sargent), predominantly white private and public schools (including Oberlin, Temple, and Columbia), and historically black institutions (especially Hampton, Howard, and Tuskegee).[52]

REQUIREMENTS

No training program, though, was egalitarian. In the early 1900s, prospective physical education majors at colleges and universities had to meet general requirements for undergraduate matriculation. By 1910 most predominantly white institutions specified that a physical education applicant be the graduate of an approved high school or pass a test in required subjects.[53] The Sargent School and other private programs also favored students with at least moderate resources and some prior education.[54] Initially, the BNSG required applicants to have the equivalent of a high school education. After the 1909 merger with Wellesley, an applicant to the Hygiene and Physical Education program had to

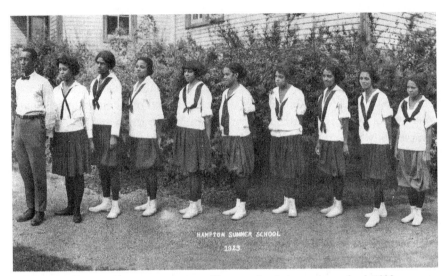

FIGURE 1.1 *Physical education trainees at Hampton Institute summer school, 1923 (Maryrose Reeves is third from left). Papers of Maryrose Reeves Allen, Moorland-Spingarn Research Center, Howard University.*

be a current Wellesley student, satisfy the college's entrance requirements, or hold a bachelor's degree from another institution. In the 1890s tuition at the BNSG averaged $150 per year; students also had to pay for room and board plus books, shoes, gym suits, and other miscellaneous items.[55]

These policies forced applicants and their families to weigh the value and price of specialized training. Because higher education stretched the resources of even middle-class families, many college and postbaccalaureate students got jobs to help cover costs.[56] Physical education majors were no exception. Alice Towne (Deweese) attended the University of Nebraska from 1901 to 1905. Although total costs were modest, "many students," she later recalled, "had to earn part or all of their expenses." During the school year, they "corrected papers for 15¢ an hour," did housework, or waited tables at restaurants; during the summer, boys worked on farms or joined "a steel gang, laying rails for the Union Pacific in Kansas."[57] As a master's candidate in physical education at the University of Iowa in the 1920s, M. Gladys Scott (1905–90) served as recreation director at the University Psychopathic Hospital; besides organizing activities, she was responsible for "chasing any of the patients who tried to run away during the walks around campus."[58]

Between the 1920s and 1940s, white leaders campaigned successfully to upgrade teacher education. After a coalition of white organizations issued national standards in the 1930s, entrance criteria rose, coursework became more rigorous, and requirements and expenses steadily increased.[59] Some black institutions adopted similar policies, but rarely had sufficient resources to implement them.[60] Many white and black schools also evaluated students' physical aptitude and personal qualities before admitting or graduating them. These academic, financial, and personal criteria favored middle-class men and women, while excluding young Americans who were poor or uneducated. The barriers were intentional; leaders believed that physical education would not become a respected profession if perceived quality was sacrificed for quantity.

LEARNING TO BE PROFESSIONAL

Formal and hidden curricula reinforced the field's aspirations. Training's official purpose was to prepare young adults for their everyday work as gym teachers, recreation leaders, or athletic coaches. In the early twentieth century, schools typically required general academic subjects as well as coursework in the theory and practice of physical education. Although content and quality varied widely, most programs taught human anatomy, movement, and psychology along with practical skills and pedagogy related to physical activity. During the interwar years, curricular and philosophical debates erupted; these often pitted male staff interested in preparing athletic coaches against female staff who defended physical education. Despite these battles, curricula still combined basic coursework in the biological and social sciences with essential ideas and methods pertaining to physical activity.[61] Competency, though, involved more than knowledge and skills. A physical educator, leaders observed, is not only an instructor, but also a member of an institution, a community, and a profession. To fulfill these roles, the argument ran, young teachers needed to personify virtue. Because schools were especially anxious about femininity and sexuality, they educated female students in "Phy Ed-iquette."[62]

At predominantly white institutions, codes of "Phy Ed-iquette" trained young women to be refined, intelligent, active ladies, free of masculine athleticism. Schools used both formal and informal means to instill this white, middle-class, heterosexual model of gender. The methods of Amy Morris Homans, the BNSG's early director, were legendary. No flaw, however small, went unnoticed or uncorrected. As one student approached "the end of her course, Miss Homans discovered that she bit her finger nails. Her diploma was withheld until some months after the class graduation, when she was able to present a perfect set of finger nails."[63] BNSG alumnae spread Homans's gospel of decorum across the country. Mary Channing Coleman (BNSG 1910) directed a mannish-looking major at the North Carolina College for Women to "'let her hair grow longer, get a blouse with lace and ruffles and take up knitting and crocheting,'" and the girl reportedly "did exactly as she was told."[64] At the University of Wisconsin, Blanche Trilling (BNSG 1909) and her staff advised trainees not to wear plaid shirts, "skimpy shorts," or brassieres that were "*too* pointed" and to avoid boyish haircuts, costume jewelry, and "vivid make-up."[65] Mabel Lee (BNSG 1910) expected majors at the University of Nebraska to adopt one cardinal rule: "To be a lady" and "to teach like a lady."

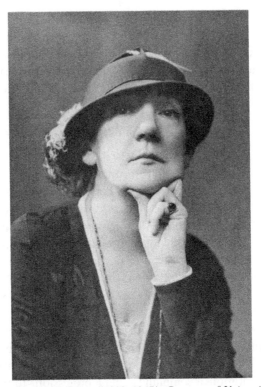

FIGURE 1.2 *Mary Channing Coleman (1883–1947). Courtesy of University Archives Photograph Collection, Martha Blakeney Hodges Special Collections and University Archives, University Libraries, The University of North Carolina at Greensboro.*

To polish students' rough edges, Lee modeled femininity for them by appearing at department teas (and everywhere else) in hat and gloves.[66]

Graduates of the Sargent School and other predominantly white institutions imposed similar norms. Gertrude Moulton, a protégé of Delphine Hanna at Oberlin College, recalled an incident at her mentor's house: "At one time she left a newspaper on the floor in an entryway. When the whole [senior] class had assembled and none had picked up the paper in the interest of good housekeeping, we had a little talk."[67] When Moulton herself joined Oberlin's faculty in 1923, she maintained Hanna's standards. On road trips with majors, Moulton never stopped at restaurants displaying beer signs and instructed students to leave public restrooms cleaner than they found them.[68] Staff members were expected to use students' proper names: "Not Pat, Pete, Brucie, Sloanie + Dutch but Gladys, Esther, Lucille, Edith and Ruth."[69] Despite holding mandatory etiquette classes for senior majors, the department had to issue reminders that students' off-campus apparel should emphasize "neatness and inconspicuousness."[70]

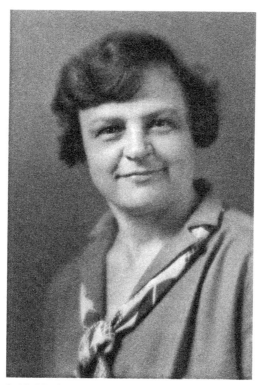

FIGURE 1.3 *Gertrude M. Moulton (1880–1964). Courtesy of Oberlin College Archives, Oberlin College.*

By quashing "phy ed" traits, programs intended to regulate personal relationships as well. White female leaders feared that improper friendships, whether casual or intimate, could ruin a young teacher's career and stain the profession. "Playing 'round with [a] questionable group—[especially] dating married men," declared Blanche Trilling, spelled professional disgrace and failure.[71] Faculty worried even more about lesbianism. Discussing "the 'crush' situation," Trilling's staff wondered how to impress upon students that "[a]ny attachment which excludes other people is not good."[72] Every physical educator at Wisconsin and other schools understood this oblique code for homosexuality.

To bolster heterosexual femininity, professional programs regularly evaluated their majors. Frank discussions of students' strengths and shortcomings occupied many departmental meetings during the interwar years. Staff naturally preferred healthy students who were proficient in their academic work, physical activities, and practice teaching. Their assessments of personal qualities were more telling. Trilling's colleagues at the University of Wisconsin were optimistic about girls who were "sweet, interested, industrious," and dedicated, despite modest talent. They gave low ratings to majors perceived to be untidy, stubborn, disagreeable,

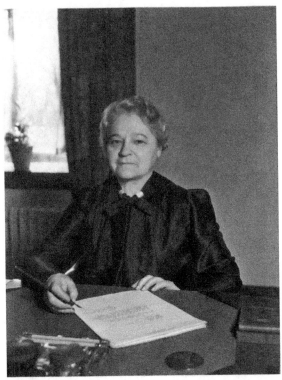

FIGURE 1.4 *Blanche M. Trilling (1876–1964). Courtesy of the University of Wisconsin–Madison Archives, Image #S05513.*

lazy, immature, ill-mannered, crude, conceited, or "uninterested and passive."[73] To make these ne'er-do-wells "'snap into it,'" the department sent them stern reports or called them to the office.[74] Pity the major of 1927 who "goes to all her classes on the hill in knickers. Affects masculine dress and hair cut. *Miss Trilling* to see her."[75] At the University of Michigan, Margaret Bell and her colleagues rated majors' cleanliness, sociability, tactfulness, vocabulary, hairstyle, clothing, posture, and weight.[76] Physical educators at Stanford University questioned the future of a student with "limited" intelligence and "a giggly manner" who did a "plodding sort of work" and was tentative, even "in tears some of the time," when playing field hockey. The teachers were ambivalent about a female major who had intellectual ability and a "nice personality" but was "'like a man' in movement" and rather "clumsy and uncoordinated in folk dancing and lacrosse." By contrast, the staff expressed enthusiasm about a young woman who was charming, "attractive, reliable, [and] efficient" and who moved remarkably well "for her size."[77]

To reinforce staff members' evaluations, departmental handbooks directed trainees to reflect on their own performance and deficiencies. Senior majors at the University of Michigan were supposed to consider if they "accept[ed] criticism cheerfully" and did "more than is assigned," or if they tended to lose self-control, "belittle others," "waste time," and "ask for exceptions."[78] Wisconsin's majors scrutinized their teaching abilities as well as conduct and appearance. Was their carriage "ungainly" and "masculine"? Were their facial expressions sullen or animated? Did they wear suitable shoes and apply the right color and amount of lipstick or rouge? Were they "rude; impudent; boisterous" or courteous and refined? Did they have interests and friends beyond the world of physical education?[79]

Finally, departments issued reports about their students and alumnae. By design, these documents concluded that female physical educators were normal. Blanche Trilling's informal survey in 1939 represented Wisconsin's successful graduates as resourceful, sincere, dedicated, and charming. By contrast, alumnae who failed struck Trilling (and their employers) as narrow-minded, selfish, "snooty," or lazy; they wore too much makeup, chewed gum, used "cheap slang," and looked "'phy-ed.'"[80] Numerous masters theses, doctoral dissertations, and journal articles on "the physical education major" reached similar conclusions. Comparing female trainees to other students, including male majors, most analyses depicted them as intelligent, well-rounded, extroverted young adults, who just happened to enjoy physical activity.[81] The studies provided good public relations for a field seeking legitimacy. They reassured home institutions, the profession, and the interested public that departments of physical education admitted only wholesome women, enhanced their many fine qualities, dismissed mannish candidates, and graduated young ladies who knit their talent and personalities into successful careers.

Featuring white norms, this model of middle-class heterosexual femininity was highly racialized. Although predominantly white institutions expected all physical education trainees, regardless of race, to embody this standard, they also signaled that black students were different. Sometimes, the objective was fairness. Recognizing that black students at the BNSG might encounter prejudice, Director Homans reminded a white student to include a black classmate in games and instructed a local hotel to treat a black trainee "graciously" during her stay.[82] Circumstances at the Sargent School were more complex. Despite its unusual accessibility to blacks, the program enforced segregation; African American students were not permitted to live in the school's dormitories until 1946.[83] The program's emphasis on unity and school spirit worsened black students' isolation and probably inspired them to devote their careers to racial uplift.[84]

State universities also had a preponderance of white students and faculty in the early twentieth century. Although their racial practices often went unrecorded, some clues remain. Recommendation letters for a black alumna of the University of Illinois mixed paternalism and lukewarm support. The young woman, observed a staff member in 1936, suffered "from all the handicaps of her race—lack of cultural background, lack of opportunity, and from the prejudices of those about her." Although the program had "colored students of better scholarship," none had shown such "outstanding qualities of leadership. . . . She is understanding, definite and clear, and, given the right kind of situation, should do a good piece of work." The letter concluded that the job applicant was "a very light-skinned colored girl. This may be regarded either as a handicap or an advantage."[85] By identifying candidates' race only when they were African American, white personnel marked black trainees as different.

Overall, teacher education at white institutions imparted lessons in gender, race, and sexuality as well as science and pedagogy. The field's preoccupation with trainees' character reflected its anxieties about social image and professional identity during the critical decades when physical education matured. Worried particularly about the taint of masculinity and lesbianism, white female leaders monitored their protégés closely. As an Oberlin alumna reflected, the gym "was not a place where girls became 'muscle builders' but where characters were molded."[86] The effort to instill white, middle-class, heterosexual norms stifled the individuality of female physical education majors, while accentuating their racial identity.

Finding a Job

Armed with lesson plans, feminine outfits, and missionary zeal, graduates fanned out across the country to teach exercise and games to girls and women. They got jobs at public schools, private academies, normal schools, colleges and universities, social service agencies, and the Girl Scouts, YWCA, and other voluntary organizations. Some worked at playgrounds, camps, recreation centers, doctors' offices, and physiotherapy clinics; others conducted private classes in general exercise or corrective work.[87] Determining the number of women in each category is difficult. Archival records suggest that 15 to 20 percent of female physical education majors from the interwar period became college-level teachers; the highest proportion from any training program ranged between 40 and 60 percent.[88] At mid-century, just over 10 percent of recent female physical education graduates with full-time jobs were employed by colleges and universities, while more than three-quarters taught at elementary and secondary schools.[89]

The concentration of gym teachers in academic settings reflected broad social forces. Developments in American education and the country's preoccupation with fitness and sports triggered significant growth in school-based physical activity programs. Between Reconstruction and World War I, a national drive for mass education, along with compulsory attendance laws and demographic shifts, brought thousands of youngsters from diverse backgrounds into America's elementary and secondary schools. In 1895 total enrollment in the nation's public high schools was 350,000; the number doubled by 1905 and reached 1.3 million by 1915.[90] Whereas fewer than 100,000 southern blacks were enrolled in school after Emancipation, their number exceeded 1.5 million at the turn of the century.[91] The influx of pupils coincided with major structural changes in public education. Between the 1870s and 1920s, secondary schools replaced uniform curricula with differentiated tracks of study, such as academic, commercial, and industrial, and also expanded their menus of non-academic subjects and extracurricular activities, including physical education and sports.[92]

The introduction of compulsory physical education was dramatic. Between the 1850s and 1890s, only a handful of cities and states mandated physical training, and the number barely increased between 1895 and 1915.[93] During and after World War I, concern over national fitness stimulated new regulations in both lower and higher grades. By 1922 twenty-eight states had enacted some physical education requirement; in 1929, the number was forty-six.[94] Between 1922 and 1934, the proportion of secondary school students who attended physical education classes grew from roughly 35 percent to 51 percent.[95] Requirements varied widely by region, school size, and pupils' age and sex. In 1930, elementary schools typically required physical education three to five times per week, and secondary schools required two or three sessions per week.[96] A 1939 survey of forty-nine accredited black high schools found that two- to four-year requirements were common.[97]

As exercise programs grew, so did the demand for special instructors, especially in secondary schools.[98] The number of full-time physical education teachers in Florida's public schools jumped from three to seventy-three between 1924 and 1927; in Minnesota, the number nearly tripled between 1924 and 1930.[99] A survey of 420 towns and cities in 1929 uncovered more than 4,600 public school physical educators.[100] Many school districts, counties, and states also established administrative positions. In 1929 most urban school systems employed a supervisor to plan and manage physical education programs.[101] Similarly, the number of state directors of physical education rose from four in 1917 to twenty-four in 1939.[102]

The structure of gym class and the duties of instructors followed the general configuration of American public education. Dual school systems—one for whites, another for blacks—prevailed in the South and many northern cities. In white elementary schools, a white classroom teacher or female physical educator led exercise for girls and boys together. In upper grades, white female gym teachers supervised girls, and white men handled exercise, military drill, and athletics for boys. In black schools as well, young children learned and played together, while physical activities for older girls and boys were separate; their teachers were white or black, depending on locale and grade level.[103] The division of exercise by sex and race meant that male and female gym teachers, white and black, were in demand.

From the outset, many public school gym teachers were female. In 1891–92 women constituted almost 53 percent of physical education specialists in urban schools.[104] In 1905, 65 percent of physical training personnel in 128 public school systems were female.[105] Women also held various administrative posts; urban school districts and state departments of physical education often employed a woman to direct the girls' division, while a man typically oversaw the entire program. Personnel in black public schools between 1900 and 1940 varied widely in number and background. Lacking a full-time physical educator, many black schools assigned regular teachers to supervise exercise class; some larger schools, though, did hire full- or part-time specialists, many of whom held college degrees.[106]

Activity programs and teaching corps also expanded at the collegiate level between the late nineteenth and mid-twentieth centuries. In the early 1900s, compulsory physical education was common for white college women, fairly standard for black female students, and sometimes prescribed but poorly enforced for male students, white or black.[107] Women-only institutions usually employed female physical educators. Most coed colleges and universities created separate men's and women's departments of physical education, and hired women to direct and teach in the latter. In the early 1900s, departments of women's physical education at white colleges and universities typically had only one or two members. Leading programs with professional curricula averaged five or six teachers. By the 1930s, women's departments in predominantly white institutions included between several members and a dozen.[108] Departments at historically black colleges and universities tended to be smaller and less homogeneous.[109] In the early 1900s, black institutions often hired black men or white women to teach women's physical education, but by the 1920s and 1930s a majority of the instructors were black women with professional credentials. At fourteen accredited black institutions (mostly coed), more than 60 percent of the instructors in women's physical education in 1939 were female and one-half of the women's programs had a black female director.[110]

The means by which colleges found new personnel and young teachers got jobs varied. Correspondence flowed regularly between employers and the directors of training programs; when presidents, deans, and department heads inquired about suitable prospects or particular candidates, mentors replied with names and recommendation letters. The information moving through these channels was very detailed. Colleges and universities looked for applicants with specific teaching expertise as well as acceptable age, race, physique, and religious affiliation. Mentors described their protégés' personal qualities and physical aptitude. Candidates filled out application forms that seem intrusive, even illegal by present-day standards. Professional networks were especially important during the hiring process, as colleagues in the field contacted each other about positions and candidates. Sometimes, regular relationships developed; whenever a school had an opening, a specific training program sent an appropriate graduate to fill it.

Two historically black institutions—Hampton and Spelman—illustrate how the college job market operated in the early decades of the twentieth century.

Founded in 1868, Hampton Institute, a coeducational school in Virginia, provided industrial and normal training along with "moral development" for blacks
and Native Americans. During Hampton's early decades, most administrators
and faculty, including female physical educators, were white. From the mid-1890s
to 1909, the Boston Normal School of Gymnastics sent one or two white female
graduates to Hampton each year; the Institute typically provided room and
board, while the BNSG covered teachers' salaries.[111] Director Homans micro-
managed the appointments: Was general exercise or athletics a young woman's
forte? Was she refined or "vulgar"? Was her hair too light or her skin too dark?[112]

After the BNSG/Wellesley merger, Hampton continued hiring the program's
graduates for another twenty years, while also appointing women from other
predominantly white training schools.[113] Regardless of alma mater, candidates'
personal qualities were decisive. In 1929, staff at the Central School of Hygiene
and Physical Education in New York City recommended a recent alumna as
a "girl of strong character and high ideals" who was a "good leader and an
excellent disciplinarian" with "robust physique."[114] The appointment lasted
eight years. Although Hampton's leaders found much to like, they could not
abide the teacher's emphasis on strenuous athletics and her supposedly "limited
cooperation" and "lack of refinement," including her smoking habit. For her
part, the young woman believed that Hampton's laissez-faire attitude about
extracurricular activities allowed students to waste valuable time on dancing
and casual socializing.[115] During the 1930s, Hampton's physical education staff
became interracial with the appointment of female graduates from historically black institutions, especially the Institute's own alumnae.[116] Applicants
leveraged professional experience and personal connections to their
advantage. Hampton officials certainly understood when hiring Charlotte
Moton as a physical educator and dance instructor in the mid-1930s that her
father was Robert R. Moton, an alumnus and former Hampton teacher who
succeeded Booker T. Washington as head of Tuskegee Institute.[117]

The hiring process at Spelman College, a private women's school in Atlanta,
also illustrates the formal and informal means by which employers and
candidates found each other. Opened in 1881, Spelman offered a liberal arts
education and some practical training to young black girls and women from
the rural South in a highly disciplined and religious environment. In its early
decades, Spelman's faculty was predominantly white, as were many senior
administrators; beginning in the 1920s, the staff became more interracial. The
school explicitly sought white women to teach physical education, and the
department did not include black instructors until the mid-1930s.[118]

During the 1920s and 1930s, many physical education staff members were
graduates of the Sargent and Posse schools. Spelman paid particular attention
to candidates' religious values, personal character, and racial sensitivity. As the
dean informed one prospect in 1925, "We need earnest Christian women who do
more than just teach their special subject in the class room."[119] Application forms

emphasized the same criteria. In addition to a photograph, the college requested information about education, professional background, age, marital status, race, and height and weight, along with various questions about the candidate's priorities, with every expectation that she would answer favorably: "What experience have you had in Christian work or practical missionary service? Would you enter heartily into the religious life of the school? Are you in full sympathy with the work that is being done for the elevation and education of the Negro?"[120] Candidates carefully matched their self-descriptions and Spelman's standards. A white applicant in 1924 stated that her "highest aim is to do some work for [the Lord] along with my other work," and that her conversion at a black mission had made her "especially fond of colored people."[121] Personal networks also helped; current staff alerted friends to job openings at Spelman, while other candidates relied on inside connections. The niece of a senior administrator at Spelman suggested that she contact a recent graduate of the Posse School who was "a Baptist and a peach."[122]

Spelman's inspection of physical educators did not end with their appointment. The very day one candidate accepted a position in 1924, she received a telegram with further instructions. "Of course," the dean wrote, "you will not bob your hair between now and the opening of school."[123] Throughout their stay, Spelman's physical educators—along with other personnel—were expected to set a good example in their professional work and personal conduct. Even small habits were crucial. In the late 1930s, the college chastised a black physical educator for frequently arriving late for breakfast and, to make matters worse, being "difficult" about it. The teacher's relationship with Spelman continued to sour and, within a few years, she resigned.[124]

During the first half of the twentieth century, physical education jobs in the United States were both plentiful and restricted. As activity programs grew, a complicated dance ensued between employers, training schools, and prospective teachers. Getting a job depended as much on gender, race, character, and connections as one's teaching potential. Moreover, as instructors at Hampton and Spelman quickly learned, employment was probationary and expertise was never the sole basis of evaluation. Departments weighed personal factors—from smoking and hairstyle to tardiness at meals—in decisions about hiring, retaining, or dismissing female physical educators.

Settling In

Besides adapting to campus culture, physical educators faced other tasks common to all incoming staff: finalize a contract, figure out daily schedules, locate housing, and get acquainted with new colleagues and surroundings. College administrators eased the transition by giving newcomers helpful tips. Spelman's dean told a novice teacher exactly what to expect. "You will live here

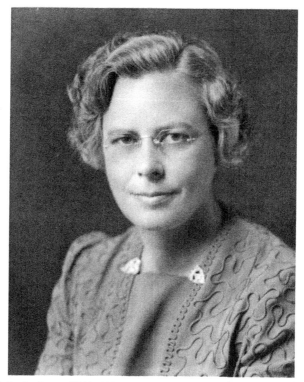

FIGURE 1.5 *Julia R. Grout (1898–1984). Courtesy of Duke University Archives.*

on campus. Our buildings are brick, with [steam] heat and electric lights. Our faculty has its own dining room." Given Atlanta's unpredictable climate, the dean advised the young woman to bring "warm clothing and high shoes for the winter weather. Teachers furnish their own towels, table napkins, bureau covers, and any little accessories they wish to use in making their rooms more attractive."[125]

Though delighted to have a job, new employees often wondered how far their salaries would go. Blanche Trilling and other department heads argued that the "splendid opportunity for experience and growth" at their institution would offset a teacher's seemingly modest income. Southern schools assured newcomers that the cost of living in that region was more reasonable than elsewhere in the country.[126] When Julia R. Grout arrived in Durham, North Carolina, in 1924 to direct physical education at the Woman's College of Duke University, she knew her salary would be $2,000 and that on-campus room, board, and laundry would be less expensive than up north. A native New Englander and recent graduate of Wellesley's training program, Grout was excited about her first job but uneasy as she traveled by train through the South's "fields of corn and cotton" and listened to the regional drawl. Greeted by the college dean, Grout toured the campus and settled into her spacious suite with a southern roommate, the college's new dietician. "Goodness," she wrote to her family, "I don't dare to think of what's ahead."[127]

Weekdays, Evenings, and Weekends

What lay ahead were many responsibilities. Between the 1920s and 1940s, college-based female physical educators averaged more than twenty hours of general instruction per week.[128] Service courses, though, comprised only one of their duties. Laura J. Huelster, who taught at the University of Illinois from 1929 to 1972, recalled academic life before mid-century as "rather relaxed," but her account of a typical semester belies this memory:

> Class and extra-curricular loads were heavy, but we were not required to publish or to conduct research. . . . We played on faculty teams in sports in matches with student teams, produced or helped colleagues produce swim shows or Orchesis [dance] performances, drove students to sports days, refereed games (not articles for journals), attended Major Club meetings, advised at least one student extra-curricular activity and even performed English sword dances at the Women's Faculty Club. And we were busy attending professional meetings.[129]

Similarly, Maryrose Allen and her colleagues at Howard University advised students from early morning to late afternoon, organized May Festivals and sports weeks, held public dance exhibitions, officiated at intramural games, served on all-campus committees, and even pitched in with janitorial chores.[130] College physical educators also performed physical exams, supervised the gym and pool, learned new games and sports, taught courses outside their specialty, and held office hours. Gertrude Moulton estimated that Oberlin's staff conducted more than one thousand individual conferences each year, with her share being nearly one-half.[131] Moulton and other department heads devoted much of their time to administration. Running seven days long, Margaret Bell's typical week at the University of Michigan included staff meetings for Women's Physical Education, the School of Education, and the Department of Public Health and Hygiene; individual appointments, committee meetings, and sessions of the University Council; various luncheons and parties for staff and students; sports events and special programs; and professional activities related to physical education and medicine.[132]

Splinters and Skunks in the Women's Gym

Female physical educators juggled these duties without the benefit of adequate resources. Most institutions—small and large, single-sex and coed—hampered women's programs. Because Milwaukee-Downer, a small women's college in

Wisconsin, lacked a swimming pool, it rented facilities at men's private clubs, an arrangement that director Althea Heimbach considered "very unsatisfactory." "If only one [Elks Club] member wished to swim, [our] classes were detained until he left." Circumstances improved when the local YWCA opened a new activities building and pool.[133] At Spelman College, the basement of Giles Hall, a classroom and residential building, served as a gymnasium for seventy years, despite its annoying center posts.[134]

Colleagues at coed institutions faced similar problems. When Delphine Hanna arrived at Oberlin in 1885, she made do with a 29′ x 44′ space from which she removed "a pile of oats, several unused camping outfits, discarded pictures and miscellaneous debris." Although Hanna's budget allowed some equipment purchases, the department made its own gym suits.[135] Her successor reported little improvement. If the women's program had a pool, Gertrude Moulton observed in the late 1920s, we would not have to drive "in rain and snow and sleet, in weather below zero, . . . twice a week to a [facility] nine miles away." Moreover, Moulton asked, how can the department thrive in a building with broken water pipes, falling plaster, and skunks in its frame? When the gym's wooden floor deteriorated, Moulton sent a collection of splinters to Oberlin's president; a new floor was promptly installed.[136] Prior to 1923, the women's pool at the University of Wisconsin had to be hand-scrubbed every Saturday night because it had no filtering system.[137] When rats chewed through women's lacrosse equipment at Ohio State University, staff and students stitched the nets back together and played on.[138] Good initiative, though, could not overcome tiny spaces. At the University of Michigan, the women's 19′ x 28′ swimming pool could not handle more than eight girls at a time and was condemned, "except under strict regulations," by the state's Department of Health in 1945.[139]

These hardships might simply reflect physical education's low status in academic institutions. At coed schools, though, an extra factor operated. When Oberlin finally constructed a new women's building, "the first thing the men did," Gertrude Moulton groaned, "was to ask if they could have it for their varsity [basketball] games."[140] Conflicts over facilities and resources were common at coeducational colleges and universities, and men's activity programs, especially athletics, often won. When Blanche Trilling arrived at the University of Wisconsin in 1912, women's playing fields were "only temporarily ours, and that by courtesy." The tennis courts were "scattered awkwardly over a wide area," and the location of the "bumpy, undersized hockey field" was equally "impossible."[141] Over time, these inadequate spaces were damaged, encroached upon, or taken over to accommodate men. On football weekends, heavy trucks often ruined women's archery and field hockey grounds. Wisconsin's fraternity men commandeered women's baseball diamonds for their intramural games without consulting the department.[142] New sites considered for women's sports were assigned instead to agricultural research, men's dormitories, and a football stadium addition. Sadly, Trilling concluded in 1938, "it is inevitable that the men will soon deem it essential to take over our entire field as they expand their athletic program."[143]

Even institutions committed to women's sports privileged men. In the 1910s, Tuskegee Institute authorized equipment purchases for girls' tennis, croquet, and other outdoor games; the program, though, received only hand-me-downs, when "equipment the young men had been using" was transferred "to the girls' play-ground."[144] Inequities continued through the 1930s and 1940s, despite the international fame of Tuskegee's female athletes. As late as the 1950s, recalled Nell Jackson, the famous runner and coach who taught at Tuskegee, "equipment ordered by coaches of men's sports [was] maintained by them for their sport. Equipment order[ed] by me for women's teams became property of the entire department."[145]

Financial practices amplified the disparities. In the late 1930s, the Women's Athletic Association at the University of Minnesota raised funds by selling balloons at carnivals and Homecoming—a practice that even male administrators viewed as unfair and almost "pathetic."[146] While women relied on small budgets and ad hoc revenue, money flowed to men's programs, especially intercollegiate sports. During Julia R. Grout's tenure at Duke, every male and female student paid an athletic fee that financed men's varsity teams; women students were charged an additional fee to support the activities of the Women's Recreation Association. "At one time," Grout recalled, "I urgently requested that a percentage of the athletic fee paid by all students be used for the sports program for women. The response was completely negative."[147]

In cataloguing their problems and demanding change, women physical educators positioned themselves as both victims and advocates. On the one hand, they pulled no punches about gender inequity, objecting to every policy that favored men and slighted women. Female teachers strategically connected fairness to institutional mission; since "present-day education emphasizes meeting the needs of the individual," they reasoned, the distribution of resources should serve every student's personal development.[148] This argument cast women physical educators as dedicated professionals who, as Julia R. Grout reminded her president, carry "on cheerfully in spite of [the] many inadequacies in facilities and maintenance."[149] The historical record certainly documents the grit and resourcefulness of women's programs amid adversity.

Looking for Respect

For many physical educators, meager resources were the most tangible sign of their campuses' broad disrespect for the field. Backed by their doctors, parents, and professors, undergraduates often claimed they were too frail, too healthy, too busy, or too uninterested to take physical education, especially if the class was required and graded. An English professor at the Woman's College in Greensboro, North Carolina, argued that one young lady should be exempt because "she had a horse and intended to ride every day." By that logic, Mary Channing Coleman replied, should the student also be excused from English Literature class because she brought a book to college and promised "to read a little every day"?[150]

Though shrewd, Coleman's question invited comparisons between active bodies and active minds. The consensus in early twentieth-century America that exercise was valuable did not guarantee physical education a place in undergraduate curricula analogous to that of academic subjects. Practical questions abounded: Should gym class be mandatory? Would students receive letter grades or pass/fail marks? Should evaluations reflect attendance or achievement? Would students who flunked gym class be denied their degrees? Simply put, should a college refuse to graduate a young woman "because she could not climb a rope"?[151] These matters were neither frivolous nor rare; between the 1910s and 1940s, many women's departments and their institutions used common benchmarks of higher education to judge physical education's standing.

Requirements were the core issue. During the late 1800s and early 1900s, widespread concern about women's health prompted colleges and universities to mandate physical education for female students. Nevertheless, campus politics made such policies hard to implement. Originating as the "Harvard Annex," Radcliffe College evolved during the late 1800s into a degree-granting institution with official ties to Harvard but with separate diplomas. Radcliffe was unable to require physical education until 1916.[152] Students resisted gym class because supervised exercise and an arduous swim test seemed far less attractive than independent sports. Harvard's governing board declared that Radcliffe could not make gym class compulsory unless the men's college also did, because the two institutions' equivalent degrees implied identical requirements. These objections struck Radcliffe's gym director as tangential. Higher education, Elizabeth Wright argued in 1908, should "hold students as strictly accountable for avoidable illness, faulty development, and crooked spines, as for failure in academic branches."[153] At other institutions, senior administrators opposed mandates because physical training seemed irrelevant to academic growth or students considered it onerous. Budget cutbacks during the Great Depression hit physical education and other non-academic subjects particularly hard. Finally, disputes over men's intercollegiate athletics often rendered women's activities guilty by association.[154] Undeterred, female teachers worked tirelessly between the 1910s and 1940s to protect physical education requirements, by writing memos, attending meetings, lobbying administrators, and building the case for "education through the physical."

Debates over gym class prompted questions about gym instructors. Could institutions of higher learning take teachers of "fun and games" seriously? In the early 1930s, the University of Minnesota rescinded its gym class requirement due not only to the subject's "physical rather than intellectual" content but also because "the staff, generally speaking, has not had training equivalent to that possessed by members of the regular college faculty."[155] Valid or not, doubts about credentials suggested that physical educators were not entitled to professional rank, promotions, and other rights and respect accorded academic faculty.

Some female physical educators were stars by virtue of their qualifications, intelligence, and power. Legendary examples include Dorothy Ainsworth at Smith College and Margaret Bell at the University of Michigan. Even national leaders, however, faced uphill battles on their own campuses. In Gertrude Moulton's view, colleagues and administrators at Oberlin simply did not understand the "meaning and scope of Physical Education," and gym teachers, being isolated and overworked, had few opportunities to enlighten them. Consequently, Moulton argued, her staff did not receive appropriate recognition or raises, despite their "loyal, forward-looking, efficient service."[156] Julia R. Grout's experience was illustrative. During her first sixteen years at the Woman's College of Duke, Grout remained an assistant professor, with a total salary increase of $1,100. Adding insult to injury, the school catalogue did not list Physical Education with the academic departments nor her teachers among the instructional staff.[157] "We are all teachers and leaders of students," Grout chided Duke's president in 1942.[158]

Sex discrimination was common at institutions of higher education in the early twentieth century, regardless of a faculty woman's field.[159] Physical educators, though, suffered unique burdens because their interests seemed suspiciously masculine. At Oberlin, Gertrude Moulton fought off numerous "remarks and insinuations" about department majors; even colleagues whom she respected were convinced that "the 'P.E. type'" was non-intellectual and became "less womanly, coarser, more conspicuous" through physical activity.[160] In the South, Julia R. Grout had an equally "hard row to hoe." For too long, she observed, physical education probably did attract "the extreme masculine type of woman," in a culture that considered it "unladylike for a girl to indulge in games."[161]

Campus disputes over gym class and gym instructors were intertwined. When institutions debated the purpose and efficacy of physical education, they called "women's work" into question. When colleges and universities puzzled over gym teachers' status, questions of femininity and sexuality loomed large. To be sure, debates also erupted over men's varsity athletics and the credentials and character of male coaches.[162] Women, however, represented the softer target in academic institutions and a broader culture that favored sports over exercise with hopes of bolstering masculinity through athleticism.

Administrative Structure and Power

Campus politics put women in an awkward position with respect to their male colleagues. At coed institutions, both men's and women's programs handled service courses, teacher training, and recreation and sports, and their curricula, facilities, and personnel were linked. When competing for resources, however, they often split over educational philosophy and priorities. As a female teacher at the University of Nebraska scoffed, "Men simply toss a basketball on to the court in the fall and pick it up sometime the next spring, and call that teaching."[163] Given these perceived differences, female physical educators wondered if men were their allies or rivals, while male teachers and coaches pondered whether to ignore, cooperate with, or control women's programs.

These dilemmas converged on the issue of departmental organization: Should women's and men's programs be separate or combined? During the interwar years, separation became more common but far from universal. A 1927 survey found combined departments at eleven of fifteen institutions in the West, Midwest, and East, although most experts regarded the system "as the least effective form of organization."[164] In 1941 nearly 50 percent of diverse institutions assigned the "responsibility for budget, requisitions, policies, and personnel of the departments of physical education for women" to a female department head; she also ran women's service and recreational programs about "two-thirds to four-fifths of the time."[165] Separate departments were especially common at large state universities.[166]

Structure, however, did not determine relationships. In a joint department, the senior director invariably was a man. Depending on his proclivities, women might enjoy equal treatment or be forced to defend their interests, especially against men's sports. A separate department promised women direct authority over policy and operations, with oversight by a college dean or president, and limited consultation with male colleagues. This arrangement, however, did not guarantee autonomy; the women's and men's units usually were connected administratively in such areas as budget, facilities, and curricula. Male teachers and coaches had no consistent opinion about separation versus merger; white and black female teachers, though, overwhelmingly favored independent departments.[167] These positions clashed when institutions prepared to divide or consolidate men's and women's programs. The state universities of Wisconsin and Minnesota illustrate what proved a familiar experience for female physical educators at coeducational institutions between the 1910s and 1940s.

When Blanche Trilling arrived at the University of Wisconsin in 1912, the men's and women's programs were housed in a single department under a male director.[168] Nevertheless, the women's division had "as much freedom as if it were absolutely separate."[169] Through the years, Trilling gained a relatively free hand over the curriculum, personnel, and business affairs of the women's division. She also ran the women's professional program and could consult the university's comptroller, president, or board of regents directly about any matter. Trilling attributed this unusual freedom to her long tenure and, during some periods, a fairly cooperative male director. For practical and philosophical reasons, though, Trilling was determined to have a truly independent department.[170] First, joint administration seemed inefficient.

Requiring the male director's approval for every purchase order created unnecessary delays, confusion, and aggravation for the women's program.[171] More importantly, Trilling regarded separation "a matter of principle."[172] Invoking the logic of sex differences, Trilling reasoned that women's unique bodies and character necessitated a special scheme of physical education with "a separate corps of instructors and a separate plant and equipment" supervised by a woman leader. At best, the male director of a combined department would focus on men's activities; his neglect or misunderstanding of women's concerns would render them "lost by default."[173] At worst, a man's "inability to recognize the needs of the [women's] department" might encourage him to interfere with their activities. "I think I shall never rest satisfied," Trilling therefore declared, "until the division is effected."[174] In 1930 Trilling's long campaign finally succeeded, and her newly independent department set about revamping its program.[175]

While Trilling pursued autonomy, her counterparts at the University of Minnesota fended off consolidation. Between 1939 and 1942 the school considered and ultimately rejected a plan to unite the men's and women's departments. The apparent instigator was the school's president, who viewed J. Anna Norris's retirement, after thirty years of service, as an opportunity to review women's physical education. From an educational standpoint, the president asserted, the women's program seemed outmoded and ineffectual; financially, it drained the university's maintenance budget, whereas a combined department could share the ample funds generated by men's athletics; administratively, the women's unit was "one of numerous floating kidneys around here" that needed a proper home.[176] A newly appointed Committee on Administrative Reorganization investigated the advantages and disadvantages of various schemes.[177] The committee discovered that male personnel were "more or less indifferent" to the proposed merger, whereas women definitely opposed it. The logic of sex differences persuaded the group to endorse the status quo; separation kept competitive athletics connected to men's physical education, where it properly belonged, while consolidation might undermine the unique strengths and philosophy of the women's program. The decision relieved Gertrude M. Baker, Norris's successor, who pledged to continue serving the "personal needs and interests of college women."[178]

Although colleagues at single-sex schools were free of men's programs, they too struggled to be self-governing. Many women's colleges combined the department of physical education with hygiene, health education, or student medical services; in some cases, a school's resident doctor headed physical training. Although such arrangements could be fruitful, friction often developed over priorities and administration as faculty members with strong personalities and professional allegiances tried working together. Between 1912 and the early 1940s Smith College had a joint department of physical education and hygiene, usually chaired by a physician. Although each unit enjoyed considerable independence, disagreements arose over appropriations and staff; more importantly, Smith's physical educators believed their profession deserved a status consistent with its growth and unique contributions.[179]

Whether a woman was subordinate to the male director of a combined department, headed her own program, or collaborated with medical services, the core issue was authority: Who controlled women's physical education? Political battles over structure and power were time-consuming but critical. By virtue of specialty and gender, female physical educators were marginalized figures at academic institutions. They worked unstintingly to legitimize their field and secure professional autonomy; they engaged every campus debate over department structure, physical education requirements, and policies on academic credit and grades for gym class. Department heads and rank-and-file instructors accepted these commitments on top of their regular duties. One has to wonder if they found time for professional or personal activities outside the office and gym. The answer is yes.

Professional Networks

Many white and black teachers participated in physical education organizations, served on professional committees, and developed informal networks with their counterparts at other schools. These activities, however, were divided by race and oftentimes by sex. At the turn of the twentieth century, the leading professional society for white teachers was the American Association for the Advancement of Physical Education (AAAPE). The AAAPE's organizational meeting in 1885 attracted sixty people, including six women.[180] Although relatively few women joined the group during its first decade, several did serve as officers. Between 1895 and 1905 women continued to hold important positions, and female membership in the renamed American Physical Education Association (APEA) mushroomed to 50 percent.[181] Somewhat reluctantly, the APEA became a platform from which female leaders influenced women's physical education around the country. In 1899 some white female teachers organized an independent group to devise rules for a women's version of the newly invented game of basketball. The committee became an affiliate of the APEA in 1917 and an official section in 1927. The National Section on Women's Athletics—the forerunner of the present-day National Association for Girls and Women in Sport—developed into a potent force in physical education and institutional sports.[182] Committed to female self-governance, the NSWA enunciated philosophies, issued athletic guidebooks, and built a national network of dedicated women teachers with "almost monopolistic hold over girls and women's sports in educational institutions" during the 1930s and 1940s. The NSWA also held sway in the APEA as male members "accepted or at least acknowledged" women's right to manage female sports.[183]

Several other organizations complemented NSWA's agenda, often guided by the same leaders. During the 1910s and 1920s regional associations for directors of women's physical education in white colleges and universities emerged. The groups banded together in 1924 to become the National Association of Physical Education for College Women (NAPECW) and soon opened membership to all white female collegiate teachers.[184] From 1923 to 1939, the Women's Division of the National Amateur Athletic Federation established standards and principles for female sports, especially in nonschool settings.[185]

Overall, the number of leadership positions available to white female physical educators during the first half of the twentieth century compared very favorably to opportunities in other professions.[186] At the same time, white women established autonomous groups precisely because male-dominated organizations did not represent their interests. Women's professional authority testifies not only to their political savvy but also the seeming paradox of their access to and marginalization in American physical education during its formative decades.

Black teachers' status was even more complex. Before mid-century, most white professional groups excluded them. The NAPECW did not welcome black members until 1947 when it adopted a policy of nondiscrimination based on race, creed, and color. The APEA barred African Americans from many activities, especially at the local and state levels; the organization finally addressed racial bias during the 1960s and 1970s, with mixed results.[187] Facing overt prejudice, black physical educators formed separate chapters of mainstream organizations as well as independent groups, such as the National Physical Education Association (NPEA), regional athletic conferences, and sports governance bodies. African American women also established separate organizations to promote interschool activities for black schoolgirls and undergraduates.[188] Racial discrimination was both an ingredient and outcome of professionalization. By relegating blacks to the periphery, white leaders believed that efforts to advance their young field would be more successful. As did many occupations in twentieth-century America, physical education emphasized the professional development of white members, casting blacks aside to train, work, and organize as "colonized professionals" who served other people of color.[189]

Personal Lives

White and black physical educators also created rich personal lives, enjoying an array of friendships, social activities, trips, hobbies, and volunteer projects. Known to family and friends as "Jerry," Julia R. Grout never seemed to rest during her forty years at the Woman's College of Duke University. Her correspondence and memoirs describe her many interests outside work during the period she called "The Happy Years."[190] Grout regularly attended campus lectures, concerts, and sports events, especially football games. She went to church, socialized with other female staff, organized a dining club with them, worked in her garden, listened to the radio, went on hikes, picnics, and weekend trips, and played tennis with ladies from town. Grout also completed a master's degree (Wellesley, 1928), developed a professional network, attended conferences, served as an officer in physical education organizations, and participated in the American Association of University Women as well as a local club for business and professional women.

Neither Grout nor most of her peers at Duke's coordinate college ever married. Reminiscing in 1947 about the school's original staff, Grout observed that "we ladies all still wear 'Miss' before our names."[191] Many collegiate teachers identified in this chapter also remained single. Before generalizing that most female physical educators made the same choice, various scenarios must be considered. Women may have trained as physical educators but married before being employed; others perhaps married after starting their careers and continued working or stopped either temporarily or permanently; some may have remained single throughout their careers. The common belief that gym teachers' low marriage rates signify lesbianism also requires examination.

Information maintained by physical education departments at three midwestern state universities provides clues about graduates' trajectories. Although the data do not specify race, the preponderance of alumnae from these institutions before mid-century probably were white. The University of Wisconsin training program graduated 950 women during its first thirty-five years (1911–46), of whom about one-half were married by 1946. Fewer than 20 percent of married alumnae worked outside the home. Employed graduates included doctors, physiotherapists, recreation directors, physical education teachers, and women involved in wartime service; about 10 percent of these women combined marriage and career, but their distribution by occupation is unclear.[192] Between 1922 and 1942 the University of Minnesota's physical education program graduated just over three hundred women, of whom nearly one-half were married by 1942.[193] Only about 18 percent of the married alumnae were employed outside the home. Almost one-half of graduates worked in physical education or a related area; about 15 percent of this cohort was married, with the majority being elementary and secondary schoolteachers. Similarly, about one-half of the women who majored in physical education at the University of Michigan between 1924 and 1941 got married during those seventeen years; more than two-thirds of this group did not work outside the home. Combining marriage and employment was even less common among alumnae who taught physical education or recreation; about one-fifth of this cohort, especially schoolteachers, continued to work after marriage.[194] Together, data from these schools suggest that about one-half of physical education alumnae remained single and one-half eventually married;

few combined marriage and employment in any field, but schoolteachers were the most likely to continue work after marrying.

These patterns are more informative when compared to other women's lives.[195] Marriage rates in early twentieth-century America were high; more than 90 percent of men and women born between 1895 and 1914 eventually got married. Despite warnings that higher education would turn women into childless spinsters, a majority of college alumnae—increasing from roughly 60 percent in 1910 to 90 percent in 1940—eventually married. Compared to this peer group, female physical education graduates were less likely to marry, and the disparity apparently grew as mid-century approached.

Whether they held a college degree or not, many American women faced decisions about marriage and employment. Overall, more women combined marriage and work as the twentieth century progressed. In 1900 about 16 percent of all females in the workforce were married; in 1950 the figure exceeded 50 percent. Circumstances varied considerably, though, by education and occupation. A 1930 study of women who earned a Ph.D. from 1877 to 1924 found that only one-quarter were married. Many women with doctorates eventually taught at a college or university, alongside male colleagues who were far more likely to be married. The average marriage rate among female scientists, irrespective of education, field, or workplace, also stayed relatively low, rising from about one-fifth in 1921 to just over one-quarter in 1938. By contrast, between one-third and one-half of female doctors and lawyers in the United States combined marriage and career during the first half of the twentieth century, while marriage rates among employed nurses and social workers more than doubled—from less than one-fifth to about two-fifths. Compared to many professional women between 1900 and 1950, white physical educators were distinctive; marriage rates among employed white teachers started low (10–20 percent) and remained so.

Although information about black female physical educators is limited, they apparently combined marriage and employment far more often than did their white counterparts. A 1958 analysis of 205 women physical educators at forty-eight historically black colleges and universities reported that 51 percent were married and 12 percent were divorced.[196] This pattern was common among African Americans of diverse social strata, from menial laborers to skilled professionals; in 1920, about one-half of married black women were in the workforce, compared to one-quarter of married white women.[197] Black academic women are a notable exception; in 1940, nearly three-quarters were not married.[198] These figures suggest that marriage rates among black collegiate physical educators fell between the low rates of black female professors and the higher national levels for all black female workers.

In sum, conventional wisdom about the marital status of female gym teachers can be misleading. No single generalization fits all white and black women in the profession, from recent graduates to in-service teachers. More physical education majors, especially white women, got married than previous scholarship has implied. Furthermore, their choices about employment and/ or marriage were far from uniform. One common belief, though, seems valid; marriage rates for white working teachers were lower than those of their black counterparts, many professional women, and the female population in general during the first half of the twentieth century.

Basing an analysis solely on marriage rates, though, obscures teachers' diverse identities and circumstances. Some female physical educators were heterosexuals who married or remained single. A significant number of unmarried teachers were lesbians; in all likelihood, some married physical educators also were homosexual. Careers in recreation, physical education, and sports not only nurtured lesbians' professional interests but also opened doors to nontraditional jobs and friendships. Many collegiate teachers had lasting relationships with other women. Their partners appear frequently in archival records as long-term housemates, daily confidantes, social friends, travel companions, and caregivers during old age.

These relationships were an open secret in physical education during the interwar years. Convinced that any hint of "deviance" would jeopardize the young field, national journals and organizations maintained an official silence. Male and female leaders carefully characterized physical educators as regular people—smart, well-adjusted, and heterosexual. Female professionals rarely mentioned lesbianism publicly, whether to protect colleagues or to mask personal prejudice. Lesbian teachers paid a considerable price for these biases. They were second-class members of a field that disadvantaged females, and worked in a society that marginalized their profession, women, and homosexuals. Given these pressures, the vibrancy and continuity of lesbian relationships among physical educators before mid-century is powerful testament to their courage and integrity.

Difference at Work

Between 1900 and 1940, opportunities to train and work in physical education were quite plentiful in the United States. The young field needed men and women, white and black, to fill positions in school and nonschool settings. Teachers' experiences, though, varied widely by gender and race. To boost the new profession, white leaders portrayed physical education as a vital instructional specialty that attracted competent, well-rounded individuals. Female trainees particularly had to seem wholesome—a code for middle-class, feminine, and heterosexual; insinuations about sexual orientation were especially injurious. Proper conduct was equally critical to hiring and retention, and employers scrutinized women's appearance and behavior as well as their professional expertise. Performing femininity on the job, however, did not guarantee respect or authority. As physical educators, women teachers held second-class status, especially in academic settings. As female employees, they usually had big workloads and tenuous autonomy. Because their institutions distributed power and privilege by gender, women physical educators typically had less clout and fewer resources than did men. Coeducational colleges and universities particularly slighted women's physical activities and female personnel, while advantaging men's sports and male staff members. Women thus incurred a double tax: discriminated against by virtue of gender, they also bore the brunt of physical education's precarious professional standing. These burdens fell especially hard on black women; they had fewer opportunities to train and advance in a white-dominated field and worked in segregated, underresourced institutions.

Female teachers were both complicit and defiant as inequities grew under the guise of professionalization and institutional priorities. To validate their femininity, many projected an acceptable image and expected the same of their students. To solidify the field's female sector, white leaders inculcated white heterosexual norms of "Phy Ed-iquette" and dutifully marginalized those who were lesbians or women of color. At the same time, many female teachers resisted second-class status by creating networks that enhanced their careers and professional power. On the job, white and black teachers protected curricular requirements, protested disparities in resources, and demanded equity and autonomy for their programs. In professional circles as well as on campus, women typically played the gender card—the very card that was played against them. Although deploying "difference" afforded many advantages, it also locked most female physical educators into conventions of gender, race, and sexuality deemed acceptable by their profession and mainstream society.

Active Womanhood and the Science of Sex Differences, 1890s–1940s

In their drive for professional authority, female physical educators argued that only independent programs could meet the unique physical and personal needs of girls and women. To make this claim stick, teachers had to develop their premise of sex differences into a cohesive philosophy of active woman-hood connecting female bodies, character, and exercise. This was no easy task between the 1890s and 1940s as American notions of fitness and femininity changed, and scientific debates over human differences intensified. This social and intellectual upheaval affected teachers' perspectives on sex, gender, and physical activity. The views of white female physical educators who taught at schools, YWCAs, recreation centers, and colleges and universities also reflected their status as white, middle-class Americans and their profession's search for legitimacy.

The Science of Difference

By concentrating on sex differences, physical educators joined a discussion that stretched back to antiquity. Distinctive Western perspectives on human nature had emerged during the sixteenth and seventeenth centuries as the Scientific Revolution's enthusiasm for applying empirical methods and mechanistic par-adigms in astronomy and physics spread to biology. Many anatomists, physiol-ogists, and doctors came to regard humans and other living things as physical systems governed by the same universal principles that regulated all natural phenomena. Reinforced during the Enlightenment, these trends accelerated between the mid-nineteenth and early twentieth centuries. Treating humans as ordinary creatures, Darwin and other evolutionists explored how specific physical, mental, and cultural traits emerged in individuals and *Homo sapiens* generally. Physiologists borrowed liberally from chemistry and physics to explain digestion, respiration, and energy production in material terms. By the turn of the twentieth century, neurologists speculated about the physical basis of mental aptitude and dysfunction, doctors proposed equally concrete ways to explain and manage disease, and geneticists sought the mechanisms of heredity. Overall, these developments produced a reductionist, determinist model of the human body as a physical system whose operations were either efficient or faulty—a mechanical metaphor reflecting industrial production, bureaucratic organization, and other symbols of modern society.[1]

The new paradigm of human nature transformed familiar conclusions about the origin and meaning of apparent variations among people.[2] During the Scientific Revolution and the Enlightenment, the established dualisms of male/female and white/black became more comprehensive as scientists asserted that sex and race penetrated every layer of human structure and character. By the mid-eighteenth century, anatomists, physiologists, and doctors maintained that the entire female body—from the brain to skeleton and skin—was sex-coded, just as reproductive organs were. As the logic of biodeterminism intensified during the nineteenth century, belief in the natural basis of difference hardened. If humans were physical systems, then variations and inequalities by sex and race must have biological roots. Physical anthropologists applied evolutionary theory to elucidate why women's development supposedly lagged behind that of men and why certain races seemed advanced or primitive. While psychologists and eugenicists helped solidify scientific racism, other experts sought the material essence of womanhood. The late-Victorian focus on women's skulls, ovaries, and energy usage gave way in the early twentieth century to genetics and endocrinology, which located femaleness in the sex chromosomes and hormones, respectively. Although their discoveries often refuted dualism, researchers nonetheless clung to a sexual binary and biological determinism.[3] Age-old debates about equality and the relative role of nature versus nurture in human development seemed to be over.

Between the 1890s and 1920s, however, a radically different perspective on gender, race, and culture emerged. A new cohort of American psychologists, sociologists, and anthropologists, including many women, contested dominant ideas about difference and the impact of heredity versus environment. Demonstrating that sex differences in personality and intelligence were minimal, they concluded that women and men were far more alike than dissimilar. They also argued that human character and behavior were not biologically determined and thus fixed, but responded to dynamic social and historical conditions. Whereas bioreductionists accentuated sex differences and located them in the body, maverick social scientists downplayed sexual dualism and attributed human development to cultural forces.

Although most researchers and intellectuals in the early 1900s emphasized either nature or nurture, few completely discounted the alternate explanation. Fervent environmentalists acknowledged that biology influenced, even governed certain individual traits, albeit not differences between groups. Although bio-reductionists were sure that nature determined physical attributes, most ceded some ground to social interpretations of behavior. In the early twentieth century, then, the nature/nurture debate presented American physical educators with a spectrum of ideas about human biology and behavior.

Active Womanhood, 1890s–1940s

Science, however, was not the only feature on the cultural landscape. Social conflicts over female recreation also affected teachers' ideas about sex differences. Between the late seventeenth and nineteenth centuries, more types of games, sports, and exercise became available to a wider range of girls and women in the United States, although many barriers persisted by region, race, and class.[4] From the 1890s to 1940s physical activities across all social strata became more regulated, institutional, and commercial. As industrial capitalism and mass consumerism steadily commodified daily life, health and athletics merged with national identity while diverse industries related to entertainment and sports sold the products and message of twentieth-century vigor.[5]

The commercialization of recreation and fitness was associated with new social values. Increasingly, material goods, physical appearance, and public behavior, rather than private character or moral bearing, became the hallmarks of bourgeois life. Although modern self-improvement entailed discipline, Americans were encouraged to view material acquisition and body management as enjoyable ways to find meaning and express identity.[6] Fitness entrepreneurs sold the promise of muscular, sensual bodies to a flabby, insecure public.[7] Health reformers coaxed Americans into regarding clean homes, personal hygiene, even high-bran diets and colonic irrigation as modes of self-enhancement and efficient living.[8] Movies, dancing, and other popular entertainments introduced less restrained styles of appearance and behavior. By the 1920s, new mores of sexual freedom spread from working-class culture to the middle ranks of society.[9]

BOURGEOIS WOMEN

The lives of middle- and upper-class females reflected these broad developments. To attain beauty, approval, and self-worth, girls and women embarked on body projects. White middle-class adolescents went on diets, worried about acne, selected the correct ready-made clothes, and learned to hide their menstrual periods.[10] Magazines popularized bourgeois standards of apparel, hairstyle, and behavior, while schools and clubs coached girls about deportment and athletic wholesomeness. Private secondary schools and elite white colleges cultivated healthy virtue through social regulations and extracurricular activities; physical education departments offered exercise classes, social recreation, and moderate intramural sports that encouraged healthy fitness without coarse competitiveness. Programs at many black colleges and universities promoted an equally wholesome version of athletic femininity. In large cities, middle-class white and black women played tennis on segregated courts, and learned social dance and good posture at local branches of the Young Women's Christian Association (YWCA). Girls and women from middle-class Jewish families found similar opportunities at community centers run by the Young Women's Hebrew Association (YWHA). Meanwhile, affluent Christian and Jewish women participated in tennis, golf, yachting, and other "enjoyable and carefree form[s] of elite sociability" at their country estates and exclusive athletic clubs.[11] Local and national tournaments in refined sports were open to wealthy women; wrapped in social respectability and unquestioned femininity, some well-to-do sportswomen, such as Eleonora Sears of Boston, became celebrities.

As new ideals of bourgeois womanhood proliferated, old models of the female body's shape and presentation faded.[12] For Americans in the late 1800s, true womanhood had meant either "voluptuous heaviness" (which, stripped of its working-class connotations, signified wealth and leisure) or delicate invalidism (which symbolized female weakness).[13] These images gave way in the mid-1890s to the iconic Gibson girl, who usually was portrayed as tall, proper, sophisticated, apolitical, and physically active. By the 1910s this ideal evolved into the athletic "American Girl" and the energetic "New Woman," who signified youth, freedom, health, self-confidence, and innocent sexuality. During the 1910s and 1920s the New Woman could be found hawking soap, cosmetics, and corn flakes in popular magazines, getting her hair bobbed at the beauty salon, and hitting tee shots with her husband at the golf course. Favoring individual games over team sports, the athletic New Woman sought fun and skill, not personal glory. During the 1920s, the flapper—with her boyish figure, unconventional habits, relentless vitality, and daring sexuality—introduced a more radical, yet tantalizing version of womanhood.

A new standard of physique and character also emerged for the middle-class white male at the turn of the century.[14] His build was athletic and muscular; his virtues included courage, decisiveness, discipline, and independence; his manner was energetic, forceful, and competitive. Every arena of life tested a man's strength and gumption; in business, politics, sports, and the military, a man encountered, even welcomed, new opportunities to lead and conquer. This masculine archetype contrasted sharply with feminine ones, as sex was mapped directly onto gender.

The interconnected binaries of sex and gender seemed to preclude any crossovers. Americans' disapproval of so-called feminine men and masculine women combined seamlessly in the early twentieth century with emerging prejudices about homosexuality.[15] For much of the nineteenth century, Americans did not use the labels "heterosexuality" and "homosexuality" to categorize sexual orientation nor did they automatically condemn same-sex friendships. During the late 1800s, however, doctors and sexologists in Europe and the United States began characterizing same-sex identities and relationships as signs of degeneration. By the 1920s the invention of homosexuality as social deviance and medical disease was complete. Although gays and lesbians continued to build loving relationships and viable subcultures during the early twentieth century, homosexuality was an identity best hidden and a label best avoided as suspicions about difference intensified.

The country's color line also hardened.[16] Enacted after Reconstruction, Jim Crow laws enforced racial segregation in southern schools, restrooms, restaurants, and other public facilities. In 1896 the Supreme Court's decision in *Plessy v. Ferguson* sanctioned "separate but equal" accommodations for white and black Americans as a legal doctrine and practice that endured for a half-century. Literature, music, cinema, and other forms of popular culture reinforced the heightened racial bifurcation of daily life. A corresponding change occurred in the conceptualization of race. Whereas older theories had recognized multiple races based on geography and other factors, evolutionists, comparative anatomists, and other scientists at the turn of the twentieth century asserted that innate physical properties established a sharp binary of white and black.[17]

The remaking of gender, sexuality, and race in the early twentieth century were interlocking processes.[18] Just as new representations of manhood connected male power to virile, civilized whiteness, the wholesome Athletic Girl and New Woman symbolized white, middle-class, heterosexual femininity. These female icons demarcated feminine and masculine character, respectable and uncultured behavior, white and black morals, and normal and aberrant sexuality. Unchecked, the New Woman's physical activities and pleasurable self-expression might drift into degraded forms of athleticism, sexuality, and independence. The flapper's androgynous physique and manner suggested—to bourgeois Americans, at least—a less disciplined, sexually liberated, lower-class style that could blur gender boundaries and undermine male supremacy. Respectable women might even assume the crude behavior that typified America's outcasts—the working class, blacks, and sexual deviates.

WORKING-CLASS WOMEN

While bourgeois Americans worried about degeneration, lower-class women considered assimilation. By imitating the American Girl and New Woman, disadvantaged groups could blend into mainstream society. On the other hand, by creating independent versions of womanhood, they could preserve cultural autonomy and challenge gender conventions. This dual process of integration and resistance was evident in working-class recreation.

At the turn of the twentieth century, social planners and municipal officials converted many city parks and neighborhood playgrounds into supervised sites;

organized by age and sex, these areas were designed to build character while inoculating the underclass against the hazards of urban, industrial life.[19] In Boston, the working poor lobbied successfully for more vigorous team sports; elsewhere, lower-class residents pushed park managers to introduce competitive events for girls.[20] In America's public schools, administrators, teachers, parents, and pupils negotiated over gym class and athletics. New requirements forced hard decisions about physical education resources and personnel just as the profession sought major curricular reforms. Devising appropriate activities for boys and girls, whites and blacks, and immigrant and native-born youngsters became increasingly difficult as student populations diversified. Physical activities at Native American boarding schools also engineered well-behaved citizens and sex-coded behavior.[21] Girls supposedly needed calisthenics and games to learn discipline, "passivity, sexual restraint, and domestic femininity."[22] Competitive baseball and football were designed to "civilize" Native American boys, but youngsters often subverted athletics to build a sense of dignity and solidarity.

Because educational institutions typically restricted sports to boys and men, lower-class girls and women turned elsewhere for athletic competition.[23] Blue-collar industries and ethnic communities sponsored leagues and tournaments in softball, basketball, and track and field. Between the 1920s and 1940s, talented females participated in elite events through the Amateur Athletic Union (AAU), the Olympic Games, and semiprofessional leagues. Although athletic success often earned black and ethnic women acclaim in their home communities, middle- and upper-class whites railed against such crass displays of masculine ambition and physicality.

Racial and class tensions over active womanhood escalated. In New York City, employers and social reformers organized recreation programs to acclimate working-class immigrants to urban, industrial life. What "do-gooders" envisioned as social adjustment, many young, single, wage-earning girls and women regarded as interference. They preferred commercial dance halls, amusement parks, movie theaters, and other heterosocial environments where personal and sexual freedom was possible.[24] In San Francisco, racial discrimination restricted Chinese immigrants to neighborhood playgrounds, recreation centers, and athletic leagues; meanwhile, Chinatown's inhabitants debated whether physical activities should promote Americanization or time-honored notions of gender.[25] In urban Jewish communities, established middle-class residents developed programs at settlement homes, aid societies, and the YWHA to help recent immigrants adjust. Women organizers and participants, though, chafed at the large gender gap in recreational opportunities.[26] Although racial segregation deprived black playgrounds, schools, and YWCAs of adequate resources, many African American churches and clubs sponsored physical activities for youngsters and adults. Skilled girls and women particularly benefited from an ideology of black femininity that affirmed athletic performance and racial pride.

Between the 1890s and 1940s Americans representing different social classes, political agendas, and racial and ethnic backgrounds battled over the meaning of womanhood. Meanwhile, scientists debated the biological and cultural basis of sex differences. Because the physical body seemed to reveal what a woman could do and should be, these arguments converged on female exercise and sports.

Female Body and Character

The controversies were unavoidable for women physical educators. They had staked their programs and authority on female-appropriate exercise. As one leader explained in 1928, women's physical education "should be based upon sound *educational psychology* as well as upon sound *physiological, anatomical and biological* principles. It should be based upon the *needs* of the girl and the woman. It should be governed by the fact that every girl is a potential mother, that every girl is a future citizen."[27] In elaborating these points, white teachers necessarily joined contemporary disputes over sex differences and female nature. They asked if the physical and psychosocial attributes of the two sexes were alike or dissimilar. They debated whether most sex differences were small or pronounced, trivial or important, changeable or fixed. They considered whether womanhood was the product of biological and/or social factors.

Women's physical form and functions seemed paramount. White teachers asked how the structure, movements, and skills of females compared to those of males and which abilities and limits distinguished women's bodies. Many structural features appeared to be handicaps: a female's oblique pelvis made running difficult; her small hands, narrow shoulders, and undersized muscles precluded certain basketball shots and baseball throws; inadequate strength and a low center of gravity rendered various track and field events impossible.[28] Physiological differences were equally important. Small hearts, low hemoglobin levels, and limited lung capacity, teachers believed, restricted women's stamina.[29] This lack of power, however, might be a blessing, one instructor reasoned, since it reduced the likelihood of injury.[30] Invariably, physical educators identified reproductive processes, especially menstruation, as the most critical sex difference. None doubted that strenuous exercise during menstruation was dangerous or, conversely, that menstruation limited a woman's vigor. Recognizing that current scientific knowledge was ambiguous, physical educators recommended prudence: girls could rest or exercise moderately during the early days of their periods, but should avoid vigorous activity and competition. The overall import of physical sex differences seemed clear. As Mabel Lee of the University of Nebraska concluded in 1933, "Physically women are not adapted by anatomical structure or physiological function to the intense forms of muscular activity and strain which are fundamental and normal in athletics as developed and carried on for boys and men."[31] Accepting male physicality as a benchmark, this generalization found female bodies and skill to be wanting.

To validate their conclusions, teachers could have cited extensive scientific data on physical sex differences. Between the 1890s and 1940s researchers studied variations in human metabolism, vital capacity, and strength as well as exercise's effect on blood pressure, heart rate, respiration, and gastric activity in one or both sexes. While some studies seemed to demonstrate women's physical liabilities, others minimized sex differences and the risks of exercise.[32] Published primarily in medical and physiological journals, such work appeared occasionally in physical education literature, and teachers including Gertrude Dudley, Alice Frymir, and Florence Somers conscientiously referenced the original studies. Others mentioned only like-minded sources or misrepresented scientific results.[33] Instead of citing evidence, though, most teachers simply portrayed women as physically distinctive, even disadvantaged.

Since this logic might undercut women's instructional programs, some teachers depicted physical disparities between males and females as complementary, rather than oppositional or hierarchical. As Helen McKinstry of the Pratt Institute suggested, "'Woman is not undevelopt man, but diverse.'"[34] Moreover, sex differences did not make fitness a man's special birthright, condemning women to inactivity and ill-health. The lethargic girls and fragile adults they encountered in the gym, teachers reminded each other, did not represent the upper limit of female vigor. Instructors warned against underestimating the physical capacity of young girls or coddling undergraduates with light exercise.[35]

Recasting women's athletics proved especially difficult. Having decided that females were physically ill-equipped for prototypic male sports, physical educators needed to measure women's aptitude by a yardstick other than men's performance. Although the female body is not built for "speed, strength and endurance," Agnes R. Wayman of Barnard College suggested, it is suited for activities requiring *neuromuscular skill, form* and *control.*"[36] By extension, women's sports were not pale copies of men's, as so many critics complained, but were interesting and challenging in their own right. Women's basketball is "not a modified, expurgated, imitation" of men's basketball, Helen McKinstry insisted, "but a different game," that "demands less endurance, but greater agility and speed, and puts a premium on strategy rather than on force."[37] Such arguments tempered teachers' sex-based hierarchy of physical structure and capacity, thereby valuing as well as stigmatizing women's bodies.

Turning to sex differences in personality and behavior, some white teachers regarded male and female psychology as polar opposites; others claimed that the two sexes had virtually identical dispositions.[38] Most physical educators took a middle position. Young girls struck them as unusually selfish, nervous, unrealistic, impulsive, and shallow. According to Blanche Trilling, girls are "habitually more excitable, more sensitive to opinion and more likely to give expression to emotional upsets than boys are. . . . [A girl] is overjoyed when praised and correspondingly cast down when blamed."[39] Unlike boys and men,

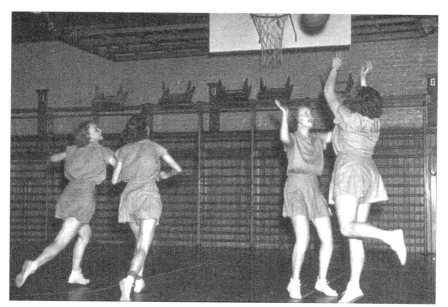

FIGURE 2.1 *Women's basketball at the University of Michigan, 1937. Courtesy of the Bentley Image Bank #BL001138, Bentley Historical Library, University of Michigan.*

females lacked a sense of cooperation, fairness, sound judgment, and focus. Frances A. Kellor, a sports advocate turned social reformer, lamented the inattentiveness of novices:

> They play "as though they had no heads on." . . . One day last summer, while working with a squad of green base-ball players . . . one of them made a splendid hit, good for at least three bases. She ran to first and when she was nearly to second came back to first. In desperation and amazement I rushed to first and asked the reason. "Oh," was the reply, "I noticed the first baseman was a friend of mine, and I came back to tell her something."[40]

Certain attributes, though, seemed common to both sexes. Humans "are endowed at birth with many instincts," observed Florence D. Alden, including "rivalry, desire to win the approval of others, love of being with others, pleasure in putting things through ('being a cause') and particularly in accomplishing this in co-operation with others, and joy in physical and mental activity in and of itself."[41] In modern times, women, not only men, should learn teamwork, honesty, loyalty, self-control, and decision-making—what one college instructor called "training in character and citizenship."[42]

Overall, white teachers envisioned the ideal female to be selfless, cooperative, and controlled as well as vibrant, wholesome, and confident. The athletic girl is not "loud and boisterous, with a tendency toward masculinity in dress as well as in speech and in general conduct," wrote Agnes Wayman, but a "strong, healthy,

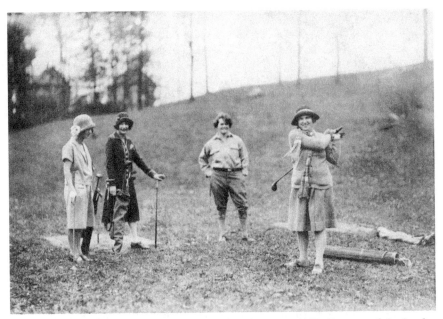

FIGURE 2.2 *Practicing golf at the University of Michigan, ca. 1922. Courtesy of the Bentley Image Bank #BL001141, Bentley Historical Library, University of Michigan.*

normal girl . . . a little saner, a little better balanced, and a little more capable of taking her place in life because of the training which she has received on the field or in the gymnasium."[43] Whether domestic or public, that "place in life" was, unquestionably, nurturing and heterosexual. Who would suggest, asked Helen McKinstry, "that the delicate, anaemic, hothouse plant type of girl, afraid of sun, wind and rain, timid, nervous and clinging, even though she have most womanly attributes, will make a better teacher, wife or mother than the strong, full-blooded, physically courageous woman, a companion for her husband on the golf links and a playmate with her children?"[44] Overall, teachers' portrait of white, middle-class, heterosexual femininity was both demeaning and uplifting. Notably, women's best qualities resembled those typically associated with white men, leaving masculinity as the paradigm of human behavior.

Navigating Difference

Teachers' complicated views on sex differences were not due to indecision but to multiple, interconnected factors—personal, social, and professional. Raised in white middle-class culture during the late nineteenth century, they absorbed traditional notions of women's nature and roles. As young adults and new professionals, they were equally comfortable with the re-imaging of bourgeois femininity in the 1910s and 1920s; in their view, the American Girl and New Woman symbolized perfect blends of fitness and femininity, health and virtue, service and self-improvement. By attaching heterosexuality to gender, teachers ruled out so-called masculine women and feminine men. Without explicitly naming class or race, they endorsed bourgeois whiteness; wholesome leisure contrasted sharply with the supposedly crude athleticism of lower-class women, especially immigrants and African Americans.

These prejudices reflected teachers' privileged status in American society as educated, white, and middle class. Conformity also bolstered mainstream physical education's pursuit of social legitimacy. In particular, women's endorsement of feminine heterosexuality deflected accusations of deviance and lesbianism in an era of rampant homophobia. Finally, conservatism buttressed their case for professional autonomy. The principle of sex differences, teachers declared, rendered female self-governance not just natural but essential; in the locker room and gym, only women could properly supervise girls, advise them about hygiene and menstruation, and understand their special needs.

Their orthodoxy, however, did not prevent physical educators from expanding the activities and qualities deemed appropriate for white middle-class women. Although white teachers often belittled women's physical abilities, their own lives refuted the dichotomy between male aptitude and female delicacy. As youngsters, many had enjoyed the freedom of spirited play. As professionals, they chose lives of exercise and vigor; some even participated in competitive sports during their teaching careers. Although few offered athletic opportunities to their students, they fully expected them to be physically active and fit. Teachers also presented female character as a gender composite. A modern girl or woman embodied morality, caring, and cooperation—redefined as human ideals, not uniquely female virtues. She displayed confidence, sound judgment, persistence, and other attributes usually associated with masculinity, while remaining free of men's shortcomings. Her less desirable qualities could be corrected through physical education.

Professional concerns also prompted women physical educators to downplay sex differences. Painfully aware of the superior resources that male colleagues enjoyed, white female teachers grew impatient with their subordinate status. At times, their demands for equity linked fairness to female distinctiveness; only special programs, they explained, could safeguard women's reproductive capacity. But they also justified equity by citing human similarities: Girls and women deserved fair treatment because their recreational needs and rights were comparable to those of boys and men. As presently constituted, Ethel Perrin complained in 1924, the "world of recreation is a boy's world."[45] "While the boys had the open school yard," Perrin observed, "the girls were forced to play baseball indoors in the gymnasium. And more often than not, after a short play period in the gymnasium, a whistle would blow signalling the girls to clear the floor so that the boys' basket ball team could get in their daily practice."[46] She called on schools to "REMEMBER THE GIRLS!" by providing them the "same opportunities for physical exercise as are afforded boys."[47] Girls and women, the logic ran, were entitled to comparable attention and resources because recreation was equally important for both sexes.

The mutual goals of developing active femininity through equitable programs led white female physical educators to put women's needs and interests on an equal footing with those of men. By identifying features common to both sexes, white teachers could promote physical activities and social traits that once had seemed inadvisable, if not impossible, for girls and women. Rather than settling for inferior facilities, secondhand equipment, and marginalized programs, they could demand fair opportunities for girls and women.

In sum, white female teachers were committed to both self-determination and equity. Neither exaggerating nor disregarding sex differences would satisfy this dual agenda; autonomy seemed predicated on the male/female dichotomy, while justice required gender convergence. This apparent contradiction was not unique to physical education. From the mid-1800s on, American suffragists had advocated women's enfranchisement on the grounds of both justice and expediency. On the one hand, they argued, women are entitled to vote as a matter of equal rights; on the other hand, women's special qualities would improve the democratic process. Likewise, female scientists, physicians, and civic reformers in the early 1900s contended that women's similarities to and differences from men justified female participation in the public sphere. For many women reformers and professionals, including physical educators, the "equal, but different" argument seemed a logical and viable position.[48]

Nature and Nurture in the Gym

Endorsing active womanhood, though, did not prove its feasibility. Could physical education enhance women's good qualities while correcting their deficiencies? Were female bodies and character subject to change? These questions thrust gym teachers into their era's heated debate over nature versus nurture. Beginning with the physical realm, white teachers decided that biology and custom contributed equally to sex differences in motor ability. Helen W. Hazelton analyzed a familiar example: What accounts for the "notorious fact that girls are poorer throwers and catchers [of a baseball] than boys"? "While there may be some slight structural handicaps," she concluded, "it is undoubtedly true that probably 75 per cent of the difference is due to lack of practice."[49] Similarly, Helen Smith argued that girls should not play basketball by boys' rules because female "organs are more delicately balanced and more easily displaced, the nervous system is more unstable, endurance and vitality is less." This was not, however, simply the biological legacy of "primitive woman and the labor and task of her period. Too many centuries of being held down by conventions and customs have intervened, too many centuries of physical inactivity."[50]

The average girl lacked stamina, Alice W. Frymir believed, because her lung capacity and hemoglobin count did not match a boy's. Male energy, however, had been "built up through generations of physical activity." With more opportunities, Frymir asserted, girls could develop sufficient endurance to run long, not merely short, distances.[51] Many colleagues agreed that experience would improve female skill, within the limits prescribed by nature. Although women would never be able to compete successfully with men, Hazel H. Pratt of the University of Kansas acknowledged in 1919, "during the past forty years, increased exercise and outdoor life to which women have been admitted have added to their weight, height, lung capacity and physical vigor."[52] By casting biology and custom as partners in women's physical development, most white female teachers avoided an extreme position in the nature/nurture controversy.

Their causal model of psychosocial traits was more one-sided. A few white physical educators were staunch biological determinists who attributed female character to evolutionary biology and endocrinology.[53] Others cited both nature and nurture. Beulah Kennard concluded that girls' artistic bent was innate, whereas their passivity and immaturity were acquired.[54] For most teachers, however, women's behavior owed little to biology; they considered female traits to be "largely the result of tradition and education." Whereas women's roles as "home makers and mothers" limited their "opportunities for social cooperation and team work," men had for centuries "experienced competitive and cooperative activities in the hunt, in tribal life, in war, and later in our industrial system."[55] This constant practice had fostered the very attitudes and behaviors that males utilized to be successful athletes. Expecting girls to be ready "emotionally and intellectually" for sports, observed Florence Alden, was like asking a child unfamiliar with fractions to do calculus.[56] By corollary, encouragement and practice would transform girls and women into team players, good sports, and responsible individuals. Kathryn E. Darnell, a high school basketball coach, enjoyed watching her "awkward girls grow into skillful players, lethargic minds become active and resourceful; explosive temperaments brought under self control; sulking girls learning to submit cheerfully, and all players learning the lesson of harmonious co-operation."[57] Convinced that women and men had similar interests and needs, most white female teachers asserted that environmental factors accounted for behavioral sex differences—a belief that America's new generation of social scientists also championed.

This complicated formulation of nature and nurture stemmed partly from teachers' professional identity. Biomechanical interpretations were attractive, even essential to them. By the turn of the twentieth century, empirical analysis of human form and function was replacing qualitative approaches.[58] Anthropometrists studied how physique related to athletic talent, personality, and other characteristics. Other researchers investigated the body in motion: What is physical efficiency and why does it vary? Does exercise affect respiration, metabolism, and other internal processes and, conversely, which vital functions enhance or limit motor performance? Borrowing this information helped physical education establish itself as an applied science. Armed with knowledge of the human machine, gym teachers were ready, one leader declared, to do the "work of biological engineering."[59] This outlook, though, carried risks. By implying that bodies and behavior were fixed, mechanical paradigms left physical educators little room for improving people's lives. Hoping to rectify cultural practices that seemed backward and unfair, female teachers were averse to blaming nature and excusing society for women's apparent shortcomings. In short, they aimed to be reformers as well as bioengineers.

When physical education reinvented itself as a social science in the early 1900s, teachers embraced the tenets of environmentalism and portrayed their work as constructive character building.[60] By contributing to psychological and moral development, they explained, "education through the physical" cultivated the values and traits that a democratic, industrial society required. Pure environmentalism, though, seemed unwise. If physicality was more cultural artifact than concrete reality, then physical education would lose its much-valued affiliation with science. The profession therefore retained biophysical interpretations of activity while emphasizing its psychosocial aspects. As bioengineers, gym teachers enjoyed the cachet of contemporary science by remaining body-centered. As environmentalists, they secured a place in educational reform and social improvement.

This unusual blend of roles distinguished physical educators from other exercise experts in the early 1900s. The expansion of leisure-time pursuits, the institutionalization of recreation, and the growth of technical information about fitness opened the door to many self-proclaimed authorities on exercise.[61] Doctors, nutritionists, athletic trainers, and fitness entrepreneurs volunteered to teach ordinary Americans about their bodies and guide them toward health. Government officials, private interests, and social reformers lined up to regulate popular recreation. As the crowd of experts grew, physical educators staked their claim on female bodies. Citing special knowledge of women's physical and psychosocial nature, female teachers identified themselves as educational engineers who built character as well as health. This represented a bold move. For decades, male doctors and scientists had defined womanhood, deploying the theory of sex differences as an especially powerful tool of subordination. Along with female physicians and academics, physical educators demarcated areas in which women's insights and expertise seemed crucial.

Political Valence

Although many biological and social scientists debated the issue of human differences in the early twentieth century, physical educators' interpretations were unusually complex. Both harsh and reassuring, white teachers' assessment of active womanhood neither minimized nor inflated sex differences. Discerning physical disparities between the sexes, white teachers regarded female form and function as both inferior and complementary to men's. Although teachers doubted women's physical aptitude, they qualified every liability. They viewed the female body as disadvantaged but trainable; women's skills as limited yet important; women's sports as tame compared to men's but challenging in their own right. Likewise, female physical educators found similarities and differences in human personality. Describing female traits as both commendable and flawed, they concluded that women's character was stable and malleable—a work in progress that should be neither valorized nor disparaged. While convinced that biological identity influenced behavior, they also exposed the stifling effects of society on female life and physical activity. Although physical educators respected natural dualities, they softened the sharp edges of binary difference and biodeterminism. Rejecting simple extremes, teachers' intricate logic usually returned them to middle ground in critical debates over sex differences.

Scholars often underestimate this complexity. Some have depicted early gym teachers as conformists who dutifully replicated middle-class standards of gender and sexuality. Others have characterized them as proto-feminist radicals who incisively critiqued masculinist values and sports. Still others have portrayed them as essentialists who glorified women's values and promoted an independent, woman-centered culture.

To some extent, each label fits white female physical educators between the 1890s and 1940s. Their endorsement of white, middle-class, heterosexual femininity was consistently orthodox. They accepted white male bodies and character as an appropriate standard by which to judge women. Though firm, this conservatism was nuanced. In cautious ways, white teachers redefined femininity and difference. They deserve credit for dispelling some Victorian myths and popularizing broader ideals of white female character and physicality. They also found fault with male-centered culture. As an alternative to win-at-all-costs elite competition, women physical educators typically favored "*democracy in recreation*," to allow everyone, regardless of sex or ability, to learn skills and play games.[62] An ideal program, female teachers maintained, should encourage "form and skill," rather than "great strength and speed," physical activity, not athletic expertise, and personal growth and lifelong habits, rather than short-term glory or other shallow goals.[63] Teachers' rhetoric resembled that of other women professionals and reformers who opposed the emergent ethos of masculinity, scientism, and technocracy in early twentieth-century America. At the same time, criticizing male values did not mean valorizing womanhood, nor was teachers' defense of separatism the equivalent of cultural feminism. Women physical educators did not accept, much less celebrate an intrinsic female character; their independent gyms were not enclaves of essentialism but rather political headquarters for developing physical education on their own terms. In sum, a rigid typology of conservative, progressive, or essentialist does not adequately capture the complexity of white teachers' views.

The history of women's physical education also demonstrates that people's interpretations of sex, gender, and body can be circuitous. Multiple, often conflicting forces pulled white female teachers in the early twentieth century away from simple perspectives on active womanhood toward highly nuanced ones. As women in American culture, they contended with prevailing notions of physicality and gender—norms that felt both comfortable and grating. As physical educators, they sought to uphold the social value and scientific authority of a new profession, while securing their exclusive claim on female health and fitness. As teachers of women, they were caught on the horns of the difference dilemma, pursuing both autonomy and equity in a society that favored men. Given these conditions, teachers could neither overlook nor belabor sex differences; they could not attribute differences solely to biology or culture; they had to both criticize and value women's character. To completely denigrate women would marginalize, even destroy their separate gym; if female skills and attributes were unimportant, then physical education for women had no rationale and little claim to resources. By devising a convoluted theory, white female gym teachers could affirm bourgeois whiteness and heterosexual femininity, sustain the importance of their profession, justify both sex segregation and equity in the gym, and still leave room for new ideas about womanhood and fitness.

Gym Periods and Monthly Periods, 1900–1940

For many Americans, the reproductive system represented the physical essence of womanhood and the principal sex difference. This belief pushed women's reproductive health to the center of many social conflicts in the early twentieth century. As more immigrants arrived from southeastern Europe, middle- and upper-class Americans warned that "race suicide" would ensue if birth rates among educated white women fell behind those of working-class ethnic families. Despite persistent claims that education diverted bourgeois women from motherhood, formal schooling seemed necessary for the American Girl and New Woman. The appearance of more female students and teachers at all levels of education, however, triggered further controversy; the prospect that America's schools were being feminized—a proxy for concerns over masculinity— revived old assertions that education damaged female health. The rise of academic and professional women coincided with the suffrage movement as well as debates over abortion, birth control, and occupational safety that engaged medical experts, public officials, and political activists. These wide-ranging controversies drew upon new research in physiology and endocrinology on the interactions between reproductive functions and other internal processes, emotions, work, and physical activity. Amid all this commotion, ordinary girls and women handled the immediate and personal implications of puberty, menstruation, pregnancy, and menopause while navigating adolescence, school, relationships, marriage, employment, and recreation.

Questions about exercise and reproductive health fell squarely in the domain of physical educators. Because most female teachers supervised schoolgirls, college students, and young, single workers, they focused on menstruation rather than pregnancy or menopause. Of particular interest was the impact of posture, clothing, diet, and mental outlook on the ease or difficulty with which girls and women negotiated their monthly cycles. Above all, physical educators wondered if exercise and menstruation were compatible: Did physical activity disturb the monthly cycle? Conversely, did menstruation influence motor skills and performance? Teachers addressed these questions frequently in public and private venues. Professional organizations conducted surveys of menstrual health and issued reports and recommendations. At schools around the country, physical education departments implemented policies regulating students' participation in gym class and sports during menses.

This chapter examines teachers' perspectives on the relationship between gym periods and monthly periods, and their guidelines about exercise and menstruation between 1900 and 1940. It draws upon professional textbooks, journals, reports, official sports manuals, teachers' writings for popular audiences, and unique materials from institutional archives. Since relevant documents by black physical educators are scarce, the chapter's primary figures are white teachers and administrators in secondary and postsecondary institutions.

Menstrual Health and Problems

Between 1900 and 1940, most white teachers described menstruation as a natural, not pathological, process. As Katharine Wells of Wellesley College declared in 1939, "The menstrual period is a normal physiological function in women. The term 'sick period' should be forever banished."[1] Such optimism was especially common among women who had trained in both physical education and medicine. According to Margaret Bell, Helen McKinstry, and Clelia Duel Mosher, healthy cycles should be relatively uneventful—as routine and inconspicuous as digestion or respiration. Even conservative teachers thought that menstruation might inconvenience, even handicap a girl, but should not incapacitate her.[2]

Though ordinary, monthly cycles were not uniform. Moderate variations in periods' frequency and the amount or duration of flow, teachers believed, were common during an individual's life and between women. In terms of frequency, Helen McKinstry declared, a girl

> may be perfectly normal . . . who menstruates regularly as often as every
> 21 days or as infrequently as every five weeks. Regularity of appearance
> is the important factor, but even this may be disturbed without any cause
> for alarm. Change of climate, a great mental or nervous strain, a radical
> change in habits of living may cause marked irregularities in the perfectly
> normal, healthy woman.[3]

Although a significant "deviation from [one's] customary condition at menstruation" might warrant medical attention, McKinstry advised, there was no standard length or amount of flow; patterns varied widely according to a person's general health, "individual and racial peculiarities," body size, and even hair color.[4]

Nevertheless, some abnormal and unhealthy conditions did exist. Physical educators expressed concern about delayed onset, excessive flow, irregular or absent periods, and vaginal discharge. Two problems—infertility and dysmenorrhea, that is, painful menstruation—seemed especially troubling. Because females are "responsible for the future of the race in the bearing of children," teachers repeatedly observed, the impact of physical activity on reproductive health demanded special attention; sensible exercise and sports, they pledged, would protect, even strengthen women's unique capacity.[5] Equating female health and reproductive fitness was axiomatic among middle-class professionals and reformers in early twentieth-century America. Whatever their view of women's rights, most white doctors, educators, and social activists accepted fertility as the ultimate sign of female health and promised to respect women's special role as mothers.

Gym teachers' preoccupation with dysmenorrhea was more distinctive. Between 1900 and 1940, they wrote extensively—and often compassionately— about the prevalence, causes, and management of painful periods. Professional leaders, graduate students, and college physicians also conducted research on the subject.[6] In all likelihood, teachers' accounts of dysmenorrhea among their students were accurate. Given cultural assumptions about menstruation at the turn of the twentieth century, painful periods were an expected and commonly reported occurrence among young, white, middle-class females—the very population that white physical educators usually encountered.[7] Teachers understood the link between anticipation and experience; as Agnes Wayman observed in 1925, an "extremely large percentage of girls and women . . . suffer from menstrual disorders" partly because of a "universal feeling among girls that pain and discomfort of some kind is to be expected and endured."[8]

Teachers attributed both reproductive problems and dysmenorrhea to the structural mechanics of women's pelvic system. Because only a few overworked ligaments held the uterus in place, they argued, the organ was inherently unstable and thus ill-equipped to carry heavy loads. The days before and during menstrual flow were especially risky. As Margaret Bell explained, "The small, pear-shaped, freely movable uterus—slung in bands of ligaments—is topheavy and engorged with blood during menstruation."[9] Bell's shift from lyrical images to more ominous ones dramatized the womb's vulnerability. Once menstrual blood was discharged, teachers reasoned, the uterus regained some stability.

Many habits seemed to aggravate women's precarious situation. Poor posture, restrictive clothing, insufficient or ill-advised exercise, and other faulty practices, teachers explained, weakened a woman's abdominal muscles and ligaments, making uterine cramps and spasms more likely. Similarly, excess pressure on the womb compromised its structural integrity; the ensuing displacement or collapse could endanger fertility and childbirth. Teachers singled out competitive sports as especially risky; collisions, falling, and other accidents, they argued, were particularly dangerous before and during menses. "Girls should not be allowed to compete" in track and field events "during the menstrual period," Alice W. Frymir warned, "nor to participate in the practice of any of the jumping events, or hurdling, as the uterus during this period is slightly heavier, and the jar may cause too great a pull on the ligaments sustaining this organ."[10]

Menstrual Paradigms and Authority

Teachers' mechanical model of female physiology harked back to ancient theories. Greek and Roman philosophers had described menstruation as periodic congestion and elimination. In the fourth century BCE, Aristotle's nutritive theory of menstruation contrasted male and female processes. Men had sufficient internal heat, he argued, to transform nutriment into blood and then blood into semen—purportedly the purest and most useful state of matter. In women, however, the conversion of nutriment was incomplete; limited by their cold, moist nature, females could produce only blood. Except for nourishing a fetus during pregnancy, Aristotle claimed, such matter was superfluous; it collected in women's blood vessels and, once a month, was expelled.[11] Building on these concepts during the second century CE, Galen's plethora theory of menstruation stated that the accumulation of extra matter in women's bodies (due to their supposed inactivity) created pressure and congestion that was relieved by periodic discharge.[12] Some eighteen centuries later, American physical educators also viewed menstruation as essentially a hydraulic process.

By contrast, most Western scientists and physicians had steadily abandoned ancient theories of menstruation between the classical and modern eras.[13] During the sixteenth through eighteenth centuries, anatomical and physiological discoveries led to new concepts of "normal" menarche and menstruation as well as diverse treatments of functional disorders.[14] By the late 1700s, investigation of the ovaries focused attention on the probable relationship between ovulation and menstruation. During the second half of the nineteenth century, many scientists endorsed a neurophysiological model positing that "ovarian influence on the uterus was . . . mediated through the central nervous system."[15] With the discovery of ovarian secretions in the late 1800s, scientists examined the role of hormones in regulating the monthly cycle. Deploying an economic metaphor, many doctors likened women's complex hormonal fluctuations to disruptions in information and control during industrial production.[16] However appealing, this metaphor did not identify an underlying mechanism—which internal organs, alone or together, governed women's periodic hormonal secretions? As scientists tested various hypotheses, the biochemical interpretation of menstruation became increasingly detailed and persuasive.[17]

Gym teachers' ideas owed little to this ascendant paradigm. Throughout the early decades of the twentieth century, stark differences separated medical science and physical education. Viewing physiology through a biochemical lens, endocrinologists sought menstruation's biological purpose and mechanisms by studying hormonal patterns in humans and other primates in experimental settings. By contrast, teachers were more interested in menstruation's implications for the daily lives of ordinary girls and women, and their sources of information included gymnasia, homes, and workplaces. Snubbing modern biomedicine, physical educators adopted a more classical model to describe how the mechanical process of menstruation affected and was affected by practical habits and individual circumstance.

Scientists and gym teachers were not the sole interpreters of menstruation, nor were their divergent perspectives simply intellectual disagreements. During the nineteenth and early twentieth centuries, control over menstrual ideas and practices in the United States shifted from mothers and other adult women to public authorities.[18] Increasingly, medical specialists and a burgeoning hygiene industry directed how American girls and women thought about, prepared for, and managed their periods. Guided by neurophysiological and biochemical paradigms, gynecologists and other clinicians often reduced patients' experiences to hormonal events and pathologized menstrual phenomena that physical educators regarded as natural variations.[19] Meanwhile, hygiene companies sold sanitary pads, belts, and eventually tampons via retail stores, direct mail, and vending machines in women's restrooms. Advertising their products in trade catalogues and professional journals, businesses cultivated profitable relationships with medical writers, school nurses, and physical educators.[20]

The process by which medical and commercial interests became dominant was contested. Ordinary girls and women, their families, and diverse health professionals also affected menstrual ideas and practices.[21] Pharmacists dispensed advice as well as products; obstetrical nurses taught their patients about personal hygiene; doctors wrote popular guidebooks and secured patents on innovative "catamenial appliances." The new science of menstruation also impelled school personnel to rethink how biological maturation affected the intellectual progress and physical well-being of their female students. School administrators often turned to medical staff, physical educators, and other in-house experts for guidance.

As they jostled for influence, each group adopted a theory of menstruation that conferred intellectual and practical advantages. Every menstrual paradigm, past and present, specifies how "regular" cycles can be maintained and "disordered" ones can be prevented or fixed. The biomedical model of the early 1900s legitimized biomedical intervention: analgesics to suppress pain, hormone injections to regulate cycles, and surgery to reposition the uterus.[22] Many male doctors were skeptical of nonmedical approaches; at a conference in 1930, for example, some physicians disputed a colleague's efforts to connect dysmenorrhea with poor posture, weak muscles, and other structural problems.[23] Biomedical discourse afforded doctors exclusive power over women's monthly cycles while discrediting intervention by other professions.

By contrast, the plethora model favored gym teachers. It suggested that girls and women could avoid problems by reducing mechanical strain in the womb through proper dress, hygiene, diet, and exercise. Conscientious females might wonder, however, which sort of physical activity and how much was safe or harmful and where they could find reliable answers. Available scientific research, teachers insisted, was too incomplete and inconclusive to be useful.[24] Between 1900 and 1940, investigators from around the world studied the empirical relationship between physical activity and menstruation. Every extravagant report of dysfunction, even sterility, due to exercise was countered by equally zealous arguments that activity during menstruation was safe, even therapeutic.[25]

Recognizing that scientific ambiguity might drive girls and women to seek advice from other experts, female physical educators explained the shortcomings of each potential source. Male physical educators were unqualified, the argument ran, because they could not understand the physical dynamics of womanhood, and girls felt uncomfortable discussing their periods with men. As one female teacher explained in 1935, "A man can never supervise the health of girls as a woman can. . . . [I]t is imperative to have a trained woman who understands the physiology of girls, their problems and troubles; a woman in whom the girls can confide."[26] Nor could American females rely on male sports promoters—the men who coached girls and women in interscholastic, municipal, and industrial athletic leagues; they were too willing to exploit players by sacrificing their health in pursuit of victories and trophies.[27]

Some teachers trusted students' decisions about gym periods and menstrual periods. Margaret Bell declared that the University of Michigan "never had any difficulty . . . with our women trading on painful menstruation as an alibi for absence from class."[28] Others shared Bell's optimism that students could abide by an "honor system."[29] Most teachers, though, were skeptical. On the one hand, they noted, students who enjoyed exercise or felt obligated to a team might conceal their periods and overexert. In the early 1930s, three-quarters of high school girls in Ohio acknowledged that they "always" or "sometimes" participated in athletic activities during the first two days of menstruation.[30] Such choices struck many teachers as uninformed, defiant, and risky.[31] On the other hand, girls who disliked exercise might use their menstrual periods (real or alleged) as a reason to be excused from physical activity. Teachers at Stanford University were suspicious about the unusual frequency of students' periods. According to staff members in 1939, the girls' custom of skipping gym class with claims of menstrual distress had become a "racket."[32]

Having dismissed other arbiters of exercise and menstruation, physical educators asserted their unique qualifications in helping women maintain or restore menstrual health. Teachers' preference for a classical model of female physiology proved strategic. By emphasizing mechanical problems and practical answers, rather than biological causes and cures, their perspective brought women's cycles, both normal and disordered, within the purview of physical education.

Statements and Regulations

Having seized the question, teachers needed to formulate an answer: Which physical activities were safe or risky during which stages of the monthly cycle? Physical educators announced their conclusions in articles, textbooks, and official statements from professional organizations. More directly, they tried influencing how American girls and women thought about and behaved during their monthly cycles at schools, colleges, YWCAs, and summer camps across the country. Some instruction was formal; by choice and occasionally by default, physical educators often handled classroom sessions on physiology and hygiene. Other lessons were more subtle; teachers characterized menstruation whenever they excused girls from gym class during their periods, admonished them about overexertion, or responded to complaints about cramps. Departments also developed rules and procedures for policing students' activities before and during menses. Together, published guidelines and departmental practices brought teachers' mechanical theory of menstruation into the everyday world of the classroom, locker room, and gymnasium.

Between 1900 and 1940 white physical educators and their professional organizations took a clear, consistent stance on physical activity and menstruation.[33] Female teachers advised girls and women to continue their usual routines, including moderate exercise, throughout the month. One need not—in fact, one should not—become inactive during menstrual flow; light exercise during menses, teachers insisted, was therapeutic. Both research and experience had demonstrated, they explained, that exercise and correct posture strengthened women's abdominal muscles; better muscle tone stabilized the uterus, thereby alleviating, even preventing menstrual cramps and congestion. By following "Nature's methods," teachers promised, girls would experience less pain, more energy, and a brighter outlook during their periods.[34]

At the same time, most instructors opposed vigorous activity before and during menstrual flow because it could damage an already overburdened uterus. They were especially adamant about athletic training and competition: sports that involved jumping, kicking, or hurdling and ones that exposed girls to collisions or falls endangered the womb during the accumulation and expulsion of menstrual blood. To reinforce this logic, teachers cited stories of women who "'sapped [their] vitality and strength'" and suffered "'internal derangement'" through "'violent physical exertions'" during their younger years.[35] A few physical educators suspected that the womb's vulnerability had been exaggerated. If pelvic organs were so delicate, remarked Ethel Perrin, how did most girls navigate adolescence without incident?[36] Similarly, female physiologists at the University of Wisconsin pointed out that women had endured the rigors of work and motherhood throughout history "without obvious deterioration."[37] Nevertheless, most women gym teachers strongly disapproved of strenuous exercise during menses.

This injunction applied regardless of condition or age. As Mabel Cummings of Wellesley College stated in 1927, "No girl, however well and husky, should take part in the most vigorous exercise during her menstrual period."[38] Physical educators were especially concerned about adolescence because the likelihood of overexertion and menstrual difficulties seemed greater and the long-term consequences more dire. "The danger of strain is greater than after maturity," remarked one teacher in 1917, "and exhaustion should be guarded against [so] that the development of the generative organs may not be retarded."[39] Mary Channing Coleman of the Woman's College in Greensboro, North Carolina, conveyed this point with a mechanical metaphor. Comparing adolescent bodies to newly constructed bridges, Coleman noted that people "do not allow heavy loads to pass until the structure has settled." Like engineers checking a new bridge, she continued, teachers, principals, and parents must judge carefully if and when a youngster's structure had stabilized enough to handle substantial pressure.[40] Once girls matured, teachers concluded, their reproductive systems could accept larger, though never extreme, burdens.[41]

In sum, published guidelines charted a middle course between what one prospective teacher called "excessive caution" and "reckless disregard."[42] Girls and women need not be immobilized during menstruation, nor should they invite trouble through willful misbehavior. Gym teachers apparently practiced what they preached; during their own periods, most continued their usual routines but eliminated intense activities.[43] This "sane middle position" on exercise and menstruation seemed particularly sensible because science had yet to render a clear verdict. As we await better data, one teacher advised in 1925, "we can best err on the side of safety."[44] Although the Amateur Athletic Union and other sports organizations disputed gym teachers' conclusion, many women doctors and physiologists agreed with it.[45]

To disseminate and enforce their position, physical education departments developed rules about which activities were approved or forbidden during different stages of the monthly cycle, and how students would be monitored and disciplined. Historical documentation of such regulations can be found primarily at colleges and universities where national leaders headed departments, including Wellesley, Smith, Stanford, and the state universities of Michigan, Minnesota, Nebraska, and Wisconsin.[46]

These institutions were more likely to codify menstrual policies for their instructional programs than for intramural or interschool competition. Although teachers regarded organized sports as uniquely hazardous, the logistics of regulating participation in such activities may have seemed too difficult. Departments therefore focused on gym class: Is attendance during menses excused, voluntary, or mandatory? Must absent students make up missed work? If attendance is required, which activities should a girl undertake or "sit out"? To some extent, answers depended on local circumstances. Nonetheless, most colleges and universities—private and public, coed and single-sex—followed the same general pattern. Between 1900 and 1940, lenient policies that allowed girls to skip class during some or all of their menstrual flow gave way to more stringent rules that mandated some participation throughout the month. In the process, most departments instituted disciplinary systems that enabled teachers to monitor students, encourage compliance, and impose penalties for violations.

Case Study: Smith College

The evolution of rules at Smith College is representative.[47] Founded in 1875, Smith College was a private, single-sex, predominantly white institution in western Massachusetts. Its policies in the early twentieth century reflected traditional concerns about exercise during menstruation.[48] From 1910 to 1915 the physical education department excused students from gym class during their periods; a girl could take as many menstrual days as she "conscientiously need[ed]" and was not required to make up the missed work.[49] Although menstrual absences were automatic and free, students could not disappear at will; they had to notify the department using the "excuse box" and, upon returning to class, had to explain their absence to the instructor.[50] Unexplained or excessive absences led to serious penalties. Smith required physical education of all first- and second-year students; because exercise classes were "regarded as academic requirements," the department warned, the college's usual reprimands for attendance violations applied and penalties for unwarranted absences had to be removed promptly through appropriate makeup work.[51] In egregious cases, delinquent girls could be banned from playing on intramural teams or holding office in the students' athletic club; this was tough punishment given the school's spirited culture of sports in the early twentieth century.[52]

Between 1915 and 1920 Smith continued its two-year physical education requirement, and penalties for poor attendance or unsatisfactory performance also remained in effect. In two respects, though, regulations stiffened. First, menstrual excuses could not exceed three a month. Students who went beyond this limit had to see their instructor, whose disciplinary discretion had increased.[53] Second, the price for menstrual absences and other missed sessions was now identical; as the department stated unambiguously in 1918, absences due to menstruation were considered "regular excused absences and must be made up."[54] The department warned students that unexcused absences (and even excused absences when too numerous, regardless of cause) would adversely affect their grades and might constitute grounds for an "Incomplete" or "Failure"—a nontrivial burden given the two-year requirement. From 1910 to 1920, then, Smith College treated menstruation as a physical liability, but not an ethical free ride. Only the most pain-ridden or determined girls likely sought menstrual excuses, and only a brave or foolish student would have tempted fate through poor attendance.

Between 1920 and 1940 the department's regulations changed considerably. In 1921 it began requiring attendance throughout the month. At first, menstruating girls took "special supervised work," probably light exercise. By 1927 they participated in regular gym class; as the department manual tersely stated, "work will be continued as usual" during menstruation.[55] Unexcused absences entailed makeup work, and extreme delinquency triggered penalties. Many undergraduate institutions joined Smith in switching to mandatory attendance during the interwar years, although the transition was rarely fast or smooth.[56] In some cases, physical education departments favored the new requirement but lacked sufficient staff or facilities to handle the growth in student participation and administrative oversight that such a policy entailed. At the University of Minnesota, J. Anna Norris preferred a no-absence rule over her department's system of one-day menstrual excuses; limited resources, however, plus the likelihood that many girls would disappear for a day anyway, dissuaded Norris from changing the policy in the mid-1920s.[57] At the University of Chicago, Gertrude Dudley reluctantly permitted girls to miss class on the first two days of their periods because the school was nonresidential.[58] Elsewhere, administrators, staff physicians, and parents objected when departments moved to require class attendance during menstruation, questioning whether physical exertion during menses was safe and appropriate for undergraduates.[59]

Expressing similar concerns, physical educators at Smith College allowed several exceptions to mandatory physical activity. The school's physician could exempt girls suffering serious menstrual disorders from participation and makeup work. More broadly, certain activities were off-limits to *all* undergraduates during menses. Between 1931 and 1936 menstruating girls were not permitted to ride horses but simply observed equitation class in their street clothes.[60] From 1932 to the early 1970s students were not allowed to swim during their periods.[61] This ban persisted at Smith and other schools long after tampons became commercially available following World War II. Overall, Smith's rules between 1920 and 1940 sent mixed messages. Although mandatory attendance normalized the monthly cycle, exceptions to the new policy continued to stigmatize female physiology.

Menstrual Politics

This ambiguity typified physical educators' general assessment of sex differences in the early twentieth century. On the one hand, they regarded the monthly cycle as problematic. Echoing Galen, teachers' mechanical paradigm depicted the womb as a fragile organ that might collapse under duress. When Smith College excused menstruating students from gym class in the early 1900s and prohibited horse riding during the 1930s, it construed women's bodies as encumbered and menstruation as uniquely perilous. Teachers also perpetuated the old belief that menstruation was unhygienic. Some encouraged frequent bathing to control the extra perspiration and odors that supposedly accompanied menses.[62] Fears about sanitation drove Smith's long-standing ban on swimming—despite a growing conviction among health professionals, including some physical educators, that menstrual blood was not impure.[63]

Above all, teachers prioritized reproductive health over physical activity. They rarely asked how the menstrual cycle affected women's motor skills or learning, despite current scientific investigation of the topic. Between 1900 and 1940 researchers disagreed vigorously over the cause and extent of periodic variations in women's muscle efficiency, blood pressure, metabolism, respiratory rate, even tight-wire walking, as well as their mental abilities and temperament.[64] Menstruation's minute effects, however, did not interest most physical educators; instead, they focused on the opposite question, namely, the impact of daily life and exercise on menstrual health. When Smith College prescribed light exercise during menses and banned strenuous activity, it signaled that the fact of menstruation and the promise of pregnancy were more important than athletic talent. Simply put, no woman should trade her reproductive health for an hour of basketball.

This conservatism derived partly from physical educators' ambition to govern female exercise. Unlike obscure biomedical theories, teachers' old-fashioned description of monthly periods and practical rules about gym periods surely made sense to average students and parents. Instructors' social locus also shaped their ideas. Following the conventions of their race, sex, and class, white female instructors frowned on competitiveness and other masculine values, equated health with reproduction, considered women's bodies to be somewhat flawed, and worried about exercise during menses.

Even so, gym teachers challenged menstrual mythology. By depicting the monthly cycle as a normal occurrence, physical educators encouraged women to worry less and exercise more. "Most happily," one teacher cheered in 1916, "actual facts and statistics are absolutely disproving previous theories of women's physical and mental inferiority and particularly this antiquated temporary shelving of woman for the menstrual period and permanent retirement to caps and knitting at 50."[65] Having disputed female frailty, physical educators translated their optimism into new regulations. The mandatory attendance policies of the 1920s and 1930s normalized menstruation as a routine process during which moderate physical activity was possible, safe, and beneficial.

Several factors enabled teachers to question old notions of the monthly "handicap." Experience alone refuted tradition; gym teachers themselves proved that women could be (even had to be) physically active and competent throughout the month. The American Girl and New Woman—as symbols of white femininity—projected the same theme. Physical educators both benefited from and contributed to these important (albeit limited) reconceptualizations of women's bodies as active and wholesome, cleansed of sickness, menses, and other physical disturbances. Finally, a broadminded view of menstruation enlarged the profession's scope. If physical educators merely comforted girls during dysmenorrhea and taught therapeutic exercise, they would have accepted purely custodial and corrective roles. By naturalizing the monthly cycle, however, their field could assume the more educative function of incorporating menstruation into students' general program of physical activity and personal development.

As did other Americans in the early twentieth century, physical educators regarded reproductive functions as the primary sex difference. Their perspective on menstruation at once perpetuated and questioned long-standing prejudices. Similarly, their policies both stigmatized and demythologized the monthly cycle. Although physical educators moderated their views between 1900 and 1940, social, intellectual, and professional forces prevented them from completely overturning the menstrual politics of active womanhood.

Managing Students

Menstrual rules necessitated administrative procedures. At Smith College and other institutions, staff members tracked students' attendance, checked their excuses, verified makeup work, and enforced penalties.[66] Although gym teachers had rarely allowed undergraduates much latitude, supervision became increasingly elaborate and intrusive during the interwar years. Since this trend coincided with teachers' relative optimism about exercise and menstruation, its timing might seem odd.

The explanation lies in concurrent developments within higher education. In the early 1900s, many American colleges and universities applied their general policies about academic work and student behavior to physical education. During the interwar years, these codes of conduct became more stringent. As undergraduate populations grew more heterogeneous and campus culture seemed rowdier, many administrators and faculty members regarded student deportment and discipline as urgent problems. Institutions ranging from private female colleges to coeducational state universities decided to regulate student behavior more closely.[67] Physical education departments joined this march toward micromanagement. Strict rules about attendance, absences, notification, and makeup work imposed standards of discipline and accountability on female undergraduates. Menstrual policies gave physical educators considerable knowledge of and control over students. Although this authority entailed extensive paperwork and was limited to a few hours each week, gym teachers gained some power to manage young women by policing their bodies.

Physical educators kept an eye on their colleagues as well. Menstrual policies helped women physical educators clarify their relationships with other institutional units, especially student health services and hygiene instruction.

Some colleges and universities combined these entities and physical education into a single department and appointed the college physician as adjunct faculty, regular staff, or program director. Bringing disparate professions together could be productive or corrosive. Smith College merged its medical service, hygiene department, and physical education program into a single administrative unit around 1911. The college physician headed the department, and the senior physical educator directed the activity program, its budget, and staff. Over time, friction arose within the department's three units as well as between them; questions about staff members' work often masked deeper conflicts over professional philosophies and expertise.[68] In the early 1940s, the physical education division requested and was granted a formal separation.[69]

Whether a school's health service, hygiene department, and activity program were combined or independent, the groups interacted frequently.[70] They conferred on health instruction, posture studies, physical exams, and students' participation in gym class and sports. Inevitably, these deliberations provoked jurisdictional disputes. Did decisions about a student's physical activities, which depended partly on her menstrual history, belong to medicine or physical education? Most institutions made gym teachers responsible for devising and enforcing menstrual regulations, while health service doctors certified which girls needed special dispensation for medical reasons. This arrangement suited physical educators; other than deferring to doctors' clinical judgment about the severity of students' problems, gym teachers determined which activities were appropriate at various stages of the monthly cycle. Using menstrual policies to demarcate their authority with respect to other campus personnel, female physical educators institutionalized their claim on undergraduate bodies and professional authority over women's health.

"The Modern Period"

Teachers' influence was neither unique nor automatic. General physicians, gynecologists, research physiologists, hygiene companies as well as ordinary Americans also affected how girls and women thought about and managed their periods in the early twentieth century. These groups sometimes intruded on the gym. Family doctors and school medical staffs determined which girls could or could not participate in gym class due to menstrual problems. Hygiene companies supplied gym teachers with pamphlets and films about menstruation for in-class instruction. By the 1940s young girls fidgeted during "the film," grabbed Kotex samples and brochures, and decided what to do when "their aunt came to visit," regardless of gym teachers' policies.

Negotiations over menstruation were part of a larger conversation about sex differences and active womanhood between 1900 and 1940. Who would describe normal menstruation, separating regularity from irregularity? Who would mark the boundary between "health" and "abnormality"? What was the relative importance of reproduction, work, education, and leisure in women's lives? In the early 1900s as today, how female biology was constructed and by whom had concrete social impact. Whoever controlled paradigms and customs of menstruation exerted considerable power, in both public and private settings, through medical care, employment policies, and the ways in which women understood and experienced their bodies.

Women physical educators chose ideas and policies that enhanced their authority. By asserting that the exercise-and-menstruation question was up for grabs and then grabbing it, gym teachers positioned themselves as arbiters of active womanhood. By adopting a mechanical model of physiology, physical educators strengthened their involvement in women's lives while neutralizing the power of other experts. For the average woman, they claimed, sensible living, not medical intervention, was the best path to reproductive health. In effect, physical educators became menstrual police—marking and patrolling the border between female fitness and dysfunction. By regulating when, how much, and in what way girls and women exercised during the monthly cycle, female gym teachers advanced their general campaign for professional authority during the early development of their male-dominated field.

{4}

Gender, Race, and Equity

HOWARD UNIVERSITY AND THE UNIVERSITY OF NEBRASKA

Men's authority over physical education and sports was not an abstract or distant problem. Female teachers experienced it, in large and small ways, every day at their home institutions. As case studies of the University of Nebraska and Howard University illustrate, even well-known women professionals grappled with questions of equity and autonomy.

The University of Nebraska was founded in 1869 to educate and serve the state's citizens through liberal arts curricula. A half-century later, vocational and professional training had displaced general education as the school's central mission. The university also had grown from less than two hundred students to seven thousand sons and daughters of predominantly white families from Nebraska's farms, small towns, and expanding cities. Physical activity was a fixture of student culture and required coursework during the 1920s; men's and women's programs, though, differed sharply. In 1924 the university hired Mabel Lee, an experienced white teacher, to head its department of women's physical education. Lee promptly overhauled the program by introducing Danish calisthenics, interpretive dance, elective sports, and more stylish gym suits. She also revitalized intramural recreation along with various pageants and demonstrations. By contrast, intercollegiate sports, especially "king football," overshadowed basic instruction for male students. The school dedicated a new stadium in 1923, followed in 1925 by the Coliseum for men's basketball and other large events. Despite awkward changes in staff, the football team opened the 1925 season by beating the University of Illinois and Red Grange, the legendary Galloping Ghost, in what has been called "one of the most brilliant moments in Cornhusker history."[1] In the year's final game, the Cornhuskers shut out Notre Dame and its famed coach, Knute Rockne, amid allegations that Nebraska's spectators had abused the Irish's players and fans.

Halfway across the country, men's athletics also preoccupied Howard University during the 1920s. In 1924–25, questions about a football player's eligibility prompted the athletic conference for black institutions in the upper South to ban competition between Howard and other members for one year. The scandal tainted Howard's increasingly successful sports program and, more generally, intensified an internal debate over education, athletics, and racial progress. Chartered in 1867, Howard began as a small institution "for the education of youth." Steadily raising its entrance requirements and faculty credentials, the university leveraged federal and private funds to develop a comprehensive curriculum ranging from classical studies to programs in education, law, and medicine. During the 1920s it became a recognized center of higher learning for middle-class blacks under the tutelage of black teachers. The football incident led many to wonder if men's athletics advanced or detracted from Howard's academic objectives. Meanwhile, women's physical education evolved quietly under the leadership of Maryrose Reeves Allen. Hired in 1925, Allen, a young black woman, spent the next forty-two years promoting feminine health and body awareness through recreation and dance.

Physical activities at Nebraska and Howard were distinctly gendered: elite competition for men versus mass participation for women, athletic prowess and specialized training versus diverse skills and lifelong recreation, and the public display of masculinity versus the inconspicuous cultivation of femininity. A *separate world* was exactly what female teachers wanted. Deploying the principle of sex differences, Mabel Lee and Maryrose Reeves Allen advocated and to some extent achieved programs for, of, and by women. Autonomy, however, came at a price. While men's athletics garnered massive resources and attention, Lee and Allen ran women's physical education with modest budgets and second-rate facilities. Chafing at the disparities, both teachers struggled to reconcile sex differences and gender equity; they hoped to be separate *and* equal at institutions that privileged men. To analyze how Lee and Allen handled the difference dilemma, this chapter compares their concepts of active womanhood, instructional programs, and efforts to attain fair treatment.

Disparate Paths to a Shared Philosophy

Mabel Lee (1886–1985) is a well-known figure in the annals of American physical education.[2] Several events marked Lee's rise to national prominence: her oft-cited, but inaccurate surveys of women's athletics, her contributions to the Women's Division of the National Amateur Athletic Federation from 1933 to 1940, and her rapid ascent in the American Physical Education Association, serving as its first female president in 1931–32. Lee held office in many professional organizations at the state, regional, and national levels and also represented her field in federal programs, especially during World War II. An officer of the American Academy of Physical Education, Lee received many honors for distinguished service, including AAHPER's prestigious Gulick Award in 1948. She was a prolific writer and tireless speaker for professional and public audiences.

Born in 1886, Mabel Lee grew up in small-town Iowa.[3] Her father owned a lumber company in Clearfield and later ran a coal business in Centerville with his brothers. The second of four daughters, Lee had ready companions for games, play-acting, and other pastimes. Her close-knit family also welcomed neighborhood children into its home for spirited get-togethers. After attending local schools, she enrolled in Coe College, graduating in 1908 with a degree in psychology and philosophy and a minor in biology. Lee combined her academic studies with a busy schedule of physical education and sports.[4] Inspired by several semesters as a gym class assistant, Lee decided to pursue physical education at the Boston Normal School of Gymnastics, where her college teacher had trained.[5] She earned a two-year certificate in 1910, shortly after the BNSG merged with Wellesley College. In 1910 Lee returned to her alma mater for an eight-year stint as Coe's director of women's physical education. She then accepted a similar position at the Oregon Agricultural College, but a severe bout of influenza cut short her stay. After convalescing, Lee directed women's physical education at Beloit College for four years. In 1924 she went to the University of Nebraska, where she oversaw female majors and non-majors for nearly thirty years. Between her retirement in 1952 and her death in 1985, Lee remained professionally active with conferences, speeches, and writing as well as documenting her field's history through various publications and the establishment of AAHPERD's official archives.

Maryrose Reeves Allen (1899–1992) was a pioneer among black physical educators in the United States who inspired and mentored many female teachers between the 1940s and 1980s.[6] Her protégés taught at public schools and historically black colleges and universities or worked as recreation directors, physical therapists, and social workers. In 1953 Howard alumnae constituted 80 percent of the female gym teachers in the black public schools of Washington, D.C.[7] Allen influenced many other black instructors during summer workshops at Hampton Institute (1923–45).

Born in Louisville, Kentucky, Maryrose Reeves was raised in Indianapolis. By age twenty, her dual interests in the performing arts and physical education were apparent. She studied at the Cosmopolitan School of Music and, in 1923, earned a diploma at the Sargent School for Physical Education. After teaching in Trenton, New Jersey, for two years, Reeves joined Howard's staff and soon headed the women's program. She married in about 1927 but later divorced. In 1933 Allen received a B.S. degree in Hygiene and Physical Education at the Sargent School, which affiliated with Boston University in 1929. She earned a master's degree in Education at Boston University in 1938 and also undertook doctoral work. An influential teacher, administrator, and

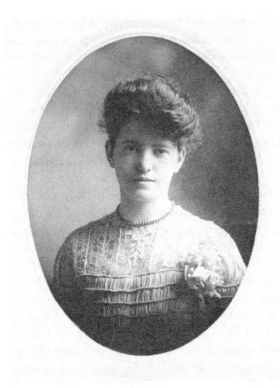

FIGURE 4.1 *Mabel Lee as a high school junior, 1902–03. Courtesy of Springfield College, Babson Library, Archives and Special Collections.*

mentor at Howard, Allen organized public demonstrations and outreach activities in Washington, D.C., especially during World War II. She joined several predominantly white organizations, including AAHPER and the eastern and national associations of Physical Education for College Women. Allen's primary network, however, comprised black female physical educators in mid-Atlantic and southern states. In 1938 this cohort established the Women's Sports Day Association (WSDA), which organized nonvarsity athletic events for female students at black colleges and universities in Virginia, North Carolina, and Washington, D.C.

Lee and Allen agreed that physical education should focus on girls, each girl, every girl, and only girls. A good program must respect the physical and psychosocial characteristics that distinguished girls and women from boys and men. Because females were not uniform, however, physical education should attend to individual needs and interests. Regardless of ability, though, every girl could and must be physically active. Finally, female physical education ought to be just that—by and for women. Self-governance, Lee and Allen believed, allowed qualified female teachers to insulate their programs from the transgressions of men's sports. With her usual flair, Lee explained the logic:

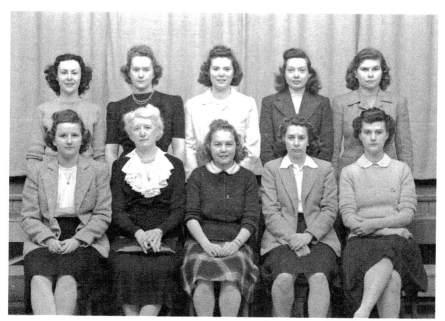

FIGURE 4.2 *Mabel Lee with student members of the Women's Athletic Association, University of Nebraska at Lincoln, 1943. Courtesy of Publications and Photography Collection: Athletic Series, Archives & Special Collections, University of Nebraska–Lincoln Libraries.*

Because of the particular physical conformation and emotional makeup of girls let us promote for them an athletic program free from emotionalism, free from intense competition, free from heart and pelvic strain, free from all attempts to imitate the boys. . . . Let us keep the girls out of spectator athletics, keep them out of the boy's realm of sports. Let us build for them a sports realm of their own, a realm of Play Days, founded on physical safeguards and moderation.[8]

Amid their profession's many debates over active womanhood, Lee and Allen adopted a conservative doctrine early in their careers and never wavered.

Mabel Lee and "Girl Nature"

To describe "'girl nature,'" Lee said, we must understand "those scientific facts" relating to a female's "physical, mental, social and racial welfare."[9] Science left no doubt that the two sexes differed "physiologically, psychically and socially."[10] Compared to male anatomy, Lee explained, the typical female has narrow shoulders, a wide pelvis, and a small leg-to-trunk ratio.[11] Along with complicated reproductive systems, girls and women tended to have hyperthyroidism and low red blood cell

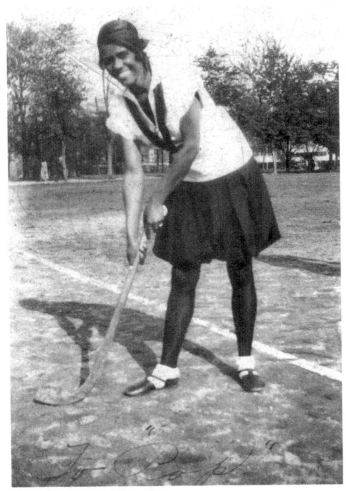

FIGURE 4.3 *Maryrose Reeves in her youth. Papers of Maryrose Reeves Allen, Moorland-Spingarn Research Center, Howard University.*

counts. Besides limiting women's strength and endurance, these features made running, jumping, and other basic movements awkward and inefficient. Physical sex differences were so extensive and "deep seated," Lee concluded, that girls should be treated "as separate entities and not as slightly modified patterns of the boy type."[12] Accordingly, sports gear must be sex-specific; light bowling balls, for example, would prevent the "severe wrist and finger strain and arm muscle soreness" that girls suffered using boys' equipment.[13] Lee reinforced these generalizations by depicting herself as weak and inept. As a child, she recalled, "I caught practically every illness that came to town. . . . I was hollow chested and round shouldered and sadly underweight, a veritable beanpole with two scrawny pigtails."[14] Feeling like a "sorry dub at performance" in field hockey, Lee longed as a young adult to find a sport in which she excelled or just felt comfortable.[15] These negative views

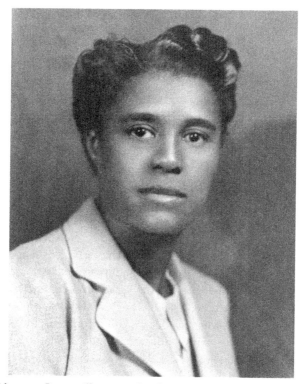

FIGURE 4.4 *Maryrose Reeves Allen, around mid-career. Papers of Maryrose Reeves Allen, Moorland-Spingarn Research Center, Howard University.*

hardened when her BNSG instructors discussed activities that were unsafe, even impossible for girls and women.[16]

Lee's distrust of female bodies led her to objectify them as unruly systems that had to be tamed. Her curiously disembodied view of physicality was evident in Lee's remarks on three subjects: exercise, sexuality, and menstruation. Throughout her life, Lee stressed the regulatory role of exercise. Physical education, she declared in 1933, should enable a child to discover that "she can command her body, can make it submissive to her thoughts, an instrument to obey her will!"[17] Creativity was by no means irrelevant; attributing her love of sports to its "life-restoring, life-refreshing, life-enriching values," Lee wanted other girls and women to experience the "Religion of Health through Physical Activity and the Religion of Happiness through Play."[18] Nevertheless, her true religion was self-control. From her teens through her thirties, Lee's diary reported her physical accomplishments: how far and fast she walked, how well she skated or played golf, which stunts she executed in the gym.[19] Performance, not self-discovery, attracted her, and confidence, not freedom, was its chief reward. The same conviction suffused her teaching. A lifelong advocate of formal gymnastics, Lee was skeptical of her field's enthusiasm for progressive education in the 1930s; natural, interest-based exercise, she objected, only "succeeded in deleting discipline and effort from education."[20]

Lee was equally vigilant about sexuality. As an adolescent and young adult, Lee was interested in heterosexual friendships and dated quite regularly, and the pain of lost loves lingered for years. Her family's silence about intimate matters, however, left Lee unprepared for romance.[21] Rather than exploring her sexual feelings, Lee's memoirs and diaries recorded only cryptic remarks and petty irritation. In college, ardent and "sentimental" suitors made Lee uneasy; she particularly disliked the "dinky fellows" who pursued her "with the tenacity of bull-dogs."[22] When asked why she remained single, Lee often declared that combining career and marriage seemed impossible or at least undesirable.[23] This answer masked her anxiety about the internal chaos that sexual passion implied.

Her uneasiness about female bodies extended to menstruation. Lee's diary depicted monthly visits by her "grandmother" more as a challenge than natural process. At Coe, Lee prided herself on attending gym class during menses no matter how bad she felt; she despised the "gold-bricking" students who used their periods as an excuse to skip class.[24] Lee's body, however, sometimes triumphed over her stoicism; when headaches and cramps became too severe, she reluctantly crawled into bed with a hot-water bottle.[25] Although instructors at the BNSG required trainees to attend class during their periods, Lee endorsed menstrual excuses when she returned to Coe College as a staff member in 1910.[26] Similarly, during Lee's early years at the University of Nebraska, the physical education department exempted girls from regular gym class during the first three days of their periods but required "very light and relaxing exercises" at the "Restricted Gymnastics Room."[27] In the late 1920s and 1930s, Lee followed colleagues at other schools by mandating attendance throughout the monthly cycle.[28] This new policy, however, hid lingering qualms; for example, in the 1940s, Lee expressed strong reservations about the hygienic viability of commercial tampons.[29]

Lee's misgivings about physicality inspired her career choice as much as her love of activity did. Accepting old myths, she never doubted that women's unique anatomy and physiology disadvantaged them or that volatile female bodies, including her own, needed management. Physical training promised to overcome frailty and ineptitude; silence helped conceal sexual feelings; menstrual periods usually were no match for perseverance. This gloomy outlook makes Lee's endorsement of the iconic American Girl and New Woman seem inconsistent. Not only can girls and women handle vigorous activity, Lee insisted, but most want "'roast beef'" in the gym, not "'milk toast.'" Instead of "mollycoddling" young girls, teachers and parents should promote fitness and self-confidence through "some good honest sweat."[30] Lee had learned this very lesson. As a youngster in the 1890s she was "just wild about sports."[31] She played games and went skating with friends, learned to ride a bicycle, and enjoyed "swinging Indian clubs, jumping and running, [and] marching" at school, where she also led a girls' military drill team.[32] As a teenager and college student, she loved basketball and also played croquet, ping pong, and tennis.[33] For all her professed weakness, Lee enjoyed exertion and eagerly mastered new activities, even risking pain. During college, she did not mind that hard work-outs on the gymnasium ladders left her hands "raw and beastly sore" or that she "could hardly wiggle" after field hockey practice.[34] Seeing female bodies as both a troublesome instrument and source of empowerment was not unusual. Many of Lee's professional peers also clung to traditional views of physical sex differences while welcoming a wider vision of active womanhood. More broadly, new forms of leisure and self-management in the early twentieth century left many Americans both more relaxed and more anxious about their bodies. As did other middle-class white women, Lee struggled to make sense of the country's shifting mores of the physical self.

The psychosocial self seemed less confusing. The two sexes, Lee believed, shared certain needs and interests. In gym class, both girls and boys should learn discipline, responsibility, "worthy citizenship," and "constructive living"; likewise, both sexes enjoyed self-testing activities and informal coed recreation.[35] In most respects, however, Lee regarded personality and behavior as sex-specific. Girls and women naturally focused on posture, weight, cosmetics, and clothes; they understood that fitness was essential for life's demands, from marriage and motherhood to outside employment or wartime service.[36] Recreation and sports, Lee continued, expressed each sex's innate character. Being instinctively combative, boys and men liked athletics, which conferred external rewards for success. By contrast, females' modesty and cooperativeness inclined them toward activities featuring social interaction and long-term enjoyment.[37] For an undergraduate woman, "the joy of participation is its own reward," whereas "her college brother . . . must have his gift of a sweater, or a blanket, or a watch fob every so often to bolster up his pride and to prove to the world that he is a real 'he-man.'"[38]

Lee performed femininity expertly. A gracious, well-groomed lady, she scoffed at less disciplined individuals and often described herself as timid, submissive, and insecure.[39] Nevertheless, she also had a rebellious streak. Resenting the rules that Coe College's "old peanuts" imposed, Lee and a "little clique of pranksters" found many ways to have fun, such as "midnight spreads in each other's rooms by candlelight" and an annual "progressive bunk party."[40] Her appetite for success and recognition was equally strong. Relishing athletic victories, particularly against overconfident opponents, Lee had a ready explanation whenever she did not win a game or capture an honor.[41] The BNSG tested her willful independence even more. Chafing at Director Homans's rigid standards, Lee exclaimed, "Land! What can we do that would please that woman!"[42] Each scolding from Homans tormented her, just as every compliment thrilled her.[43] In Boston, Lee learned to temper ambition with ladylike decorum. Claiming disingenuously to never having been "a fighter in my own behalf," she "decided from the very start that submissiveness was the path of wisdom to achieve the ultimate goal."[44] As her colleagues and acquaintances later speculated, Lee's public propriety probably hid a calculating shrewdness and tenacity.[45] More than any other trait, this fusion of decorum and ambition characterized Mabel Lee, emerging early in life and never waning during her ninety-nine years. Wrapping her iron will in a velvet glove, Lee both defied and fulfilled her own model of sex differences and became the *grande dame* of white physical education.

Lee did not, however, represent every female teacher or athlete, nor was her paradigm of "girl nature" all-inclusive. Her interlocking criteria were white, middle-class, and heterosexual. She slid easily from white codes of bourgeois femininity to condemnations of homosexuality. Conscious of her field's precarious reputation, Lee worried particularly about the sexual orientation of women gym teachers. She railed against "abnormal attachments" among colleagues and "exclusionary" friendships between physical education majors. Claiming naiveté about such matters, Lee considered relationships between females of different ages to be repugnant and called students' and colleagues' "crushes" on her a "great annoyance."[46] The "great rank and file" of physical educators, Lee insisted, are "women of culture and refinement," despite being more athletic than the typical female.[47]

She did not mean, however, that exceptional sportswomen necessarily surrendered their femininity. Despite opposing high-level competition, Lee praised star athletes who embodied white heterosexual femininity. Her favorite examples were Helen Wills and Alice Marble, the white tennis champions of the 1920s and 1930s, two "charming and attractive" women who played for pleasure, not fame, and wore their talent with modesty.[48] By contrast, Lee denounced the ambition and vulgarity of "that other type."[49] Her usual target was Babe Didrikson, the blunt, gifted "tomboy" from Texas who became an Olympic medalist in track and field, and a successful professional golfer. Didrikson's "bad manners, social ineptness, and poor sportsmanship," Lee declared, set an appalling example for the "thousands of normal average girls" in America who enjoyed sports.[50] Whereas middle- and upper-class white women exemplified heterosexual charm, working-class women seemed deviant by virtue of social standing and ambiguous sexuality.

Although Lee talked freely about white athletes, she was silent on the many black females who starred at the Olympic Games and other venues between the 1920s and 1950s. Having little contact with African Americans as a child and young adult, Lee had casually adopted racist conventions. Her diary recorded the memorable day as a teenager when she met a "nigger boy," and at Coe College, she and several girl friends "looked just killing" in black face and "darkey dress" for a gymnastics exhibition that brought the house down.[51] In later years Lee finally acknowledged America's long history of discrimination. In 1950, for example, she threatened to stop sending university classes to a local bowling alley because it refused admission to a black student.[52] Lee's delay in writing about racial inequity, much less contesting it publicly, spoke emphatically. By featuring only white females, her gender construct left no room for black girls and women—whether ordinary or talented, unrefined or cultured.[53]

Lee regarded her standard of femininity as absolute.[54] The distinctive attributes of men and women, she declared in 1937, are located "in the very depths of their inner natures."[55] She nodded occasionally toward the other side of the nature/nurture debate. Since males acquired positive qualities through sports, she reasoned, comparable experiences might teach girls and women the "game of 'Give and Take'" and other social skills.[56] Generally, though, Lee depicted female character, along with norms of sexuality, class, and race, as biological facts. In her view, other versions of womanhood not only contradicted nature but offended society as well.

The task of bringing American girls and women into the fold of white, middle-class, heterosexual femininity sometimes looked formidable. At the University of Nebraska, Lee was "struck by the overweight and lack of sophistication of most of these corn-fed girls."[57] The Jazz Age was in full swing when Lee arrived in 1924; much to her chagrin, Nebraska coeds joined their eastern sisters in exploring new freedoms, such as smoking, sex, and *nouveau* fashion.[58] Nevertheless, Lee recalled, most of Nebraska's "students were eager, earnest, sincere, grateful, fun-loving, and cordial."[59] They just needed help with body mechanics, personal grooming, impulse control, and constructive values. Lee had every expectation that her students would fit into American society. However unpolished, midwestern girls were entitled to a place in the world and were capable of learning womanhood. After all, Mabel Lee—a headstrong white girl from middle-class Iowa—had done just that.

"She Walks in Such Beauty"

Although Lee considered her students unexceptional, they were members of an exclusive club. In 1917 fewer than 5 percent of Americans between eighteen and twenty years old attended college; two decades later, the figure was 15 percent.[60] Among African Americans, higher education was even more unusual; in the early 1940s, whites were four times more likely than blacks to enroll in college.[61] Despite belonging to this very select group, undergraduates at Howard University still faced discrimination and uncertain futures. Offering them a more positive vision, Maryrose Reeves Allen pledged "to mould every one of my girls so that wherever they go the world will whisper, 'I can always tell a Howard woman when I see one because she walks in such beauty.'"[62]

Allen's signature philosophy of "Beauty-Health" centered on the distinctive "biological, physiological, sociological and psychological phenomena" of women's lives.[63] She regarded female beauty in all these dimensions as the fundamental sex difference. The female body sets the "norm of beauty for the world," by virtue of "its tenderness, grace, curves, loveliness, plus the sacredness of motherhood."[64] Womanly health entailed correct "form, proportion, symmetry, posture, grace, rhythm, and poise in the body."[65] Nevertheless, science had documented that women's unique anatomy and physiology rendered them "physically inferior to men." Their "smaller muscles, waists, sloping shoulders, broad hips, and shorter legs" hindered agility and strength, while menstruation disallowed any exercise associated with "pelvic disturbances."[66] The risks were as much psychosocial as physical. "If practised to excess after the twenties," Allen stated, vigorous sports "tend to develop lumpy muscles and an almost masculine abandon of movement. There is nothing charming in a striding, weather beaten hockey player."[67] A woman's true nature entailed "feminine characteristics and wholesome group associations, such as loyalty [and] unselfishness."[68] Another hallmark was wholesome heterosexuality. Allen regarded sex between a man and a woman as a sacred relationship and motherhood to be a woman's primary responsibility.[69] By linking body, femininity, and heterosexuality, Allen—much like Mabel Lee—proscribed identities outside the man/woman binary that nature supposedly created.

Beauty-Health also articulated, however, a keen racial consciousness. Observing the varied looks, clothing, and physiques among Howard women, Allen declared that every black female was entitled to an individual style, so long as it reflected African American norms. White prescriptions—such as "only straight hair is good hair"—led black females to experience their bodies as a "source of shame and discouragement and a cause of social maladjustment."[70] By seeing "beauty in their dark skins, their wooly hair, white teeth, sparkling eyes, [and] full mouth," Allen stated, black women could attain health and pride.[71] Beautiful thoughts and actions were equally, if not more, important. A "proper attitude and outlook" along with "a clean wholesome life," one colleague agreed, fostered "beauty and poise . . . regardless of looks."[72] Combining outward and inner beauty, a black woman exuded confidence and dignity by standing tall. Good posture derived not simply from "exercise and body mechanics," Allen explained, but expressed "an inner spirit and self-respect which makes all people feel upright and grand."[73]

Racial uplift seemed critical. Black Americans, Allen argued, suffer both physical and psychological degradation—a legacy of slavery, oppression, and prejudice. Compared to whites, she elaborated, blacks have poor health, high death rates, and short life spans. Poverty and substandard education restricted blacks' access to medical services, their knowledge of hygiene, and their appreciation of the "finer conceptions of healthy living."[74] Although all African Americans feel demoralized, Allen observed, self-hatred is especially debilitating among black women. "Taught from childhood to be ashamed of their kinky hair and dark skins, many [females] go on through life with an inferiority complex."[75]

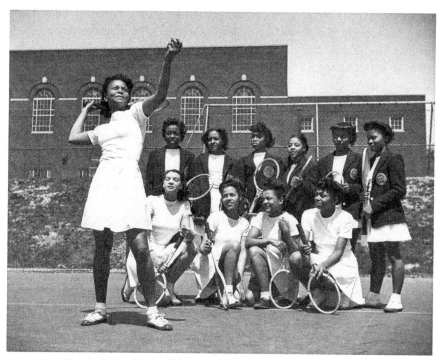

FIGURE 4.5 *Tennis class at Howard University, ca. 1940s. Courtesy of Scurlock Studio Records, Archives Center, National Museum of American History, Behring Center, Smithsonian Institution.*

Allen's analysis of black womanhood responded to long-standing racism. Since antiquity, Western culture had depicted "black" as inherently depraved and loathsome, whereas "white" denoted dignity and civilization. From the eighteenth through the twentieth centuries, this duality focused increasingly on black physicality as the signifier of inferiority and described black female bodies as brutish and depraved.[76] To counteract this hostility, African American women created three distinct self-representations.[77] *Decorporealization* concealed black women's maligned physicality while accentuating their intellect and "potential for civilization." *Normalization* portrayed women of color as the embodiment of virtue and domesticity, in effect, "as culturally white," thereby signifying their ability to enter American society "as full citizens." Finally, *affirmation* enabled some African Americans to celebrate black women's holistic beauty and sexuality on their own terms, a stance that validated the physical and social realities of their lives without comparisons to dominant ideals.

Decorporealization was impractical for Maryrose Allen and other black physical educators. Recognizing that white Americans typically judged blacks by their appearance, Allen could not purify the black female body through secrecy.[78] Instead, she directly resisted racist stereotypes of the black female as licentious and repugnant. Coaching her students about the "duty of restraining and governing the appetite of sex," Allen warned that vulgarity, prostitution, and unwed motherhood were degrading. Whereas "obscene conversation, sexy conduct [and] dress" disrespect the female body and spirit, chastity "includes purity of thought, speech, and action."[79] By schooling Howard undergraduates in white, middle-class morality, Allen opted for the common path of normalization. In the same way, contemporary black intellectuals and activists portrayed African American women as feminine and virtuous, historically black schools instructed female students about grooming and decorum, black nurses and teachers adopted the rules of respectability, and black beauty pageants and commercial cosmetics sometimes absorbed white norms of attractiveness and charm.[80] Normalization implied that because white and black women shared the same qualities, they must be equal.

Equal but not identical. Rather than simply reproduce white ideologies, black women's self-representations drew explicitly on their own values and experiences. Allen stressed the relationship between Beauty-Health and religion, a critical foundation for many middle- and working-class blacks. By finding her true self, Allen argued, a young woman moved closer to God and her spiritual center. Although Mabel Lee and other white teachers appreciated the interdependence of body and identity, Allen's direct references to Christianity probably mystified them. Personal harmony, Allen continued, also served a broader social mission; self-improvement enabled a Howard alumna "to radiate moral and spiritual beauty as she moves with physical beauty, rendering constructive service to herself, her family, and her community."[81] To model this responsibility, Allen's department sponsored outreach programs in Washington, D.C., and prepared majors for "race work," such as teaching in poor black communities.[82] The department also provided officials for segregated sports events. As of the late 1940s, the white-dominated organization responsible for certification had "never granted a Negro woman a national rating," but several staff members and students at Howard broke the race barrier in the early 1950s.[83] Sharing Allen's belief in womanhood as a civic condition, many African American reformers also highlighted black women's obligation to community service, racial uplift, and social justice.[84] This validation of racial difference often evolved into celebration. Declaring that "Black is Beautiful," Maryrose Allen extolled the dignity and diversity of her race, as African American magazines and beauty contests had done since the early 1900s.[85] Similarly, Howard's renowned dance program displayed blacks' international cultural heritage along with confronting race relations and religious prejudice.[86] Such affirmations of blackness were uniquely powerful because they challenged, even inverted, racial hierarchies so dramatically.[87]

In sum, Allen simultaneously espoused white standards, deflected prejudice, and asserted self-worth. Her normalizing images undercut racist stereotypes and afforded black women respectability in a white-dominated society. Rejecting biodeterminist views of difference, Allen exposed whites' historical denigration of people of color and encouraged black females to discover their all-encompassing beauty as both a possibility and a right. At the same time, she dignified racial difference. When a Howard woman learned to "walk in such beauty," she would attain not only white approval but also black pride and authenticity. By addressing the interplay of race and gender in black women's lives and their double consciousness as Americans of color, Allen engaged questions about active womanhood that Mabel Lee never contemplated.

A Gym of Their Own

Having differentiated the two sexes in theory, both Lee and Allen advocated independent programs of female-appropriate activities under female supervision. "How or why should [men] be expected to know what girls need or should have?" Lee exclaimed in 1928. "Women, on the other hand, are apt to know girls, to understand their physical limitations, their needs, [and] their conditions."[88] She was especially adamant that sports be "controlled by women, coached by women, officiated by women, trained by women, protected by women physicians and we say to those men of America who are not concerned with ideals, men who would like to commercialize the growing force, men who seek notoriety through women's athletics—we say [to those men] 'Hands Off'— and we mean just what we say."[89]

Self-governance, though, seemed insufficient. Few women's departments enjoyed real autonomy for their staff or adequate resources for their students. "Who is it," Lee asked rhetorically, "that gets the choicest hours of the day for the use of the gymnasiums and the play fields? And the choicest equipment? The girls?"[90] Paraphrasing Virginia Woolf's *A Room of One's Own*, Lee complained that "while men are served caviar and wine, women are subsisting on corn beef and cabbage."[91] Identical meals, however, were not the solution. Fairness, Lee explained, did not require "that the girls should have exactly what the boys have," but rather that "each should have their needs provided for with equal consideration according to their proportionate needs."[92] In short, fairness did not mean equality through sameness, but equity through difference. Although the logic of difference and parity justified independent departments, Lee and Allen both discovered that autonomy was fragile and equity virtually impossible.

LEE: FOUR JOBS, COUNTLESS PROBLEMS

Mabel Lee headed women's physical education at four coeducational institutions. Although she personalized every difficulty and rarely admitted fault, Lee justifiably complained of being a second-class citizen in a man's world. At Coe College she resented having multiple responsibilities without commensurate authority.

Despite handling everything from teaching classes to cleaning lockers, Lee had no separate departmental budget, little protection from administrative interference, and (to her mind) an inadequate salary.[93] Lee's brief job at the Oregon Agricultural College proved even more difficult. "It [was] nothing but quarrel, quarrel, quarrel about something or [with] someone from morning till night and I loathe it."[94] Many OAC students and professors favored women's varsity athletics, but Lee abhorred them. Due to wartime restrictions, the laundry room in the Home Economics building served as the women's gym. Apparently everyone from her secretary to the dean told Lee how to run her program. "Guess being Head of Dep't. allows me no privileges to decide matters for myself as I think best. Some queer world," she muttered in 1919.[95] At that point, a case of influenza offered her a welcome excuse to leave.

After recovering, Lee became director of women's physical education at Beloit College. Conditions were all too familiar; her department had

> no equipment of its own, with the rights to go into the men's gymnasium on occasional hours during the week for exercise, with the use of one open room in the basement for a dressing room, no lockers or bathing privileges, a cubby-hole off a hall way in a distant building for the director's office and the impression that . . . the director's influence upon the young women start[ed] only with roll call for any particular class and end[ed] with the dismissal of that class.[96]

Four years of effort yielded adequate facilities, a diverse program, and a system of medical exams and conferences that helped "the weaker girl and her development."[97]

From the outset, Lee's challenges at the University of Nebraska in Lincoln looked daunting.[98] Because the men's and women's divisions were structurally and financially linked, Lee's boss was the men's department director, whom she regarded as an obstinate troublemaker.[99] She could not even trust him to purchase decent field hockey balls; she tossed the "worthless" balls in the wastepaper basket, as "samples of the type of equipment the men ordered for the women when they had charge of things."[100] Initially, men also controlled the teacher training program although, as Lee bitterly noted, "almost all of the actual work of that division is performed by the women, there being 68 women to 2 men who major" in physical education.[101] Facilities were woefully inadequate. The women's playing field was "an old dump pile" that coughed up dust, stones, and even "broken crockery."[102] Freshman girls got from the gym to their dressing room by means of a trap door that released an odd "contraption that was a cross between a stairway and a ladder."[103] The women's "crowded, disagreeable" locker room handled more than twelve hundred students in "only one-half the space assigned the mere hand-full of men who [took] gymnasium work."[104] The women's staff was a collection of overworked, underpaid professionals, including some "lazy and indifferent" teachers who just wanted easy schedules and regular paychecks.[105] Finally, Lee had to contend with professors, doctors, and "doting parents" who, in her view, failed to understand physical education.[106]

Attributing these problems to her lack of autonomy, Lee parlayed an argument about difference, efficiency, and fairness into a demand for self-rule. The activities of male and female students, both majors and non-majors, she observed, differ fundamentally; a separate department would meet the needs of female students and staff more effectively. Lee negotiated departmental separation in 1925, followed by professional programs and the budget. Within a few years, she had upgraded women's facilities, resources, personnel, and curricula, and continued on that path for two more decades.[107] With this record, Lee defiantly asked in 1933, why should women "be content to play so conspicuously 'a second fiddle,' when they might so easily be 'first fiddle in their own orchestra'"?[108] In many respects, however, Lee did not manage her own orchestra even after separation. Throughout the 1930s and 1940s, male administrators and colleagues challenged her power at Nebraska. Every transfer of women's physical education from one university division to another jeopardized her authority. Even at mid-century, when approaching retirement, Lee still protested gender inequities in salaries, workloads, and resources.[109]

The separation of men's and women's programs in 1925 did not create gender disparities at Nebraska, nor was Lee's argument about sex differences responsible for persistent discrimination. Instead, university officials appropriated the logic of difference and fairness to cement long-standing practices and further marginalize women's activities. Treating men and women differently seemed imperative during the interwar years.[110] While men's athletics at Nebraska enjoyed a "Golden Age" in the 1920s, concern grew over female students' experiments with cigarettes, alcohol, sex, and risqué clothes. Despite the sobering effect of the Great Depression and the New Deal on undergraduates, Nebraska cracked down even harder, especially on women, in the 1930s. Following World War II, the university welcomed the male veterans who revitalized campus life. Throughout these changes, Nebraska's leaders were determined to strengthen gender boundaries and preserve male privilege through sex-differentiated regulations and extracurricular activities; drawing a sharp line between men's sports and women's recreation was particularly effective. Shielded by the logic of sex differences, Nebraska's neglect of Mabel Lee's program symbolized women's lesser worth at the university.

GENDER AND RACE AT HOWARD

Maryrose Allen's appointment in 1925 coincided with a major overhaul of athletics and physical education at Howard University. Before the turn of the twentieth century, physical activities consisted primarily of military training and competitive sports for men, organized by the students themselves. In the early 1900s, faculty control of athletics increased and formal, but voluntary physical education for both sexes also appeared. By 1915 the school required physical education of most undergraduates. A military officer or athletic coach directed the overall program, while a female instructor handled women's classes. Following World War I, several disputes erupted over men's sports, including the football team's violation of eligibility rules in 1924–25 and Howard's subsequent one-year banishment from the Colored Intercollegiate Athletic Association. During the late 1920s and 1930s, budget cuts, losing records, ongoing scrutiny, and temporary suspensions of various teams continued to disrupt men's athletics.

Howard's problems were not unique. Allegations of corruption and commercialization forced many institutions to examine the relationship between sports and higher education in the early twentieth century. Debates were especially heated at historically black colleges and universities. Did athletics serve racial pride and equality? Or might sports fuel white prejudice and detract from assimilation through intellectual and social channels?[111] At many schools, questions about the purpose and management of sports "began to play into larger controversies concerning student autonomy, presidential authority, and the aims of black education."[112] At Howard, these widely discussed issues contributed to President J. Stanley Durkee's resignation in 1926. Durkee's successor, Mordecai Wyatt Johnson, was the university's first black president. Early in his thirty-four-year tenure, Johnson reined in men's sports by abolishing athletic scholarships and training tables. His controversial decisions were part of general deliberations over Howard's identity as an academic institution of and for blacks.[113]

The school's sharper educational mission had far-reaching consequences for physical activities. Undergraduate requirements in physical education gradually increased. Each successive professionally trained male director brought a stronger commitment to physical education than to athletics and coaching.[114] The university eventually transferred physical education to the College of Liberal Arts, separated the department from military science, and introduced a curriculum for majors. Against this backdrop, Howard's senior administration welcomed Maryrose Allen's Beauty-Health philosophy of feminine recreation as an educational counterpoint to men's competitive athletics.[115] In 1930 the university institutionalized this distinction by splitting men's and women's physical education.[116]

Despite these auspicious beginnings, Allen's department faced many challenges. Her staff was small and overworked, secretarial and janitorial support was hard to come by, and resources and facilities inadequate.[117] After World War II, the women's program inherited the men's old gym but still shared a pool with them; in the 1950s, a lack of playing fields forced women to use Howard's football stadium and other spaces if and when they were available.[118] In the late 1930s, a significant threat to Allen's authority arose when Howard debated whether to consolidate men's sports and women's intramural recreation under a single (male) director of athletics. Emphatically opposed, Allen spelled out her philosophy of self-governance and gender equity. A merger was unfair and ill-advised, she argued, because "women's interests in all directions [would] become submerged in the interests of men's athletics."[119] Male leaders probably would convert women's recreation into a "modified man's program," because "men naturally set their own standards and fail to appreciate the anatomical, physiological, emotional and functional limitations of women."[120] Allen's warning was prescient; during the 1940s Howard's football coach and soon-to-be men's department head pressured her unsuccessfully to institute varsity athletics for women.[121] Female students, Allen continued, deserved to learn in "an atmosphere of dignity and refinement," free of the "unfavorable publicity, exploitation and rowdyism" that plagued men's sports.[122] Because women's training and experience enabled them to understand female nature, only they could design an appropriately educational program.[123] Finally, Allen asserted, a merger would exacerbate current inequities. Unlike men's sports, women's intramural recreation received no supplementary funds through student fees or the school's Athletic Board. Consolidation might further short-change women; a male director would concentrate available resources on athletics, Allen reasoned, whereas under female leadership, "women's salaries . . . are likely to be more just and more money is likely to be spent for women students."[124] Allen and her allies prevailed. Howard's Board of Trustees left women's intramural activities under the purview of the Department of Physical Education for Women.[125]

Though effective, Allen's stance on gender equity was more cautious than her critique of race relations. People's ignorance, she surmised, converted natural sex differences into gender disparities; by contrast, she concluded that American society had created racial difference to justify discrimination. Although Allen clearly understood that segregation enabled whites to disadvantage blacks, she believed a separate women's gym could be equal to men's programs. Allen's seemingly contradictory views served Howard well in its quest for more prestige. Women's recreation demonstrated the school's commitment to academic integrity, wholesome femininity, and social assimilation through physical activity. Meanwhile, the men's department, senior administrators, and outsiders were free to debate black masculinity.

The structural and philosophical divide between men's and women's programs concealed the privileges that Howard conferred on many athletic teams and the benefits it reaped from their success. Few constituencies at Howard probably recognized women's hardships, much less men's favored status, as gender discrimination; only proposed mergers and similar initiatives exposed the inequities in resources, facilities, and salaries. Regardless of Allen's interpretation of parity and self-governance, women's programs were disadvantaged before and after 1930, when her separate department was founded, and also suffered before and after 1939, when the partial merger was considered. Institutional politics, not Allen's philosophy, doomed fairness. Portraying its program for women as a model of educational uplift and black femininity, Howard could devote substantial resources, even divisive attention to men's intercollegiate athletics.

Individuality and Inclusiveness

Although parity *between* men's and women's programs proved elusive, Lee and Allen had another option: they could pursue justice *within* their own gyms by meeting each person's needs and interests. Attention to each girl guaranteed attention to all girls. While proclaiming equity within diversity as their guiding principle, neither Lee nor Allen fulfilled her twofold promise of individuality and inclusiveness.

LEE: PREACHING AND BETRAYING DEMOCRACY

Every girl in gym class, every member of an intramural team, every woman at leisure, Mabel Lee declared, needs and deserves recreation. This tenet covered individuals with "weak hearts, goiters, crippling defects, flat chests, round shoulders, flabby abdominal muscles, weak feet, over-weight, under-weight, laziness, over stimulation towards activity, anemia, ingrowing temperaments, outgrowing temperaments, sulky dispositions, those who think they hate to exercise, and the so-called 'dub.'"[126] Personal development went hand in hand with democratic participation. Shrewdly invoking American values, Lee noted that a true democracy serves the many rather than catering to the few. Inclusive recreation "recognizes not only those who are highly skilled but also the motorly retarded who need athletic training and, too, that great middle class of athletic performers who will never excel but who will find life greatly enriched by training for wise leisure."[127] Her principle seemed absolute: if ping pong was the only activity that appealed to just two girls, then their school should offer it, even if the game seemed "worthless" compared to other sports.[128] Risking mediocrity was the necessary, but small cost of inclusiveness; a "*good* program," Lee asserted, "is one that gets *many* girls out to play even though they play a poor game rather than one that gets a *few* girls out even though they play a technically super fine game."[129]

The contrast with men's approach was stark. "While we women are most interested in THE GIRL herself," Lee chided a male sports promoter in 1933, "you men are most interested in the SPORT and champions for the sport."[130] Lee deplored men's "fruitless worship of the great God 'Superior Skill' and his inevitable companions 'Intense Competition' and 'Desire to Win.'" This obsession with victory diverted resources from ordinary participants to elite stars. The "novice is neglected [while] the man already an adept is over trained, too severely exercised, over disciplined, [and] robbed of all initiative." By stressing "hard grinding work," Lee lamented, men's abusive, aristocratic system all but crushed the "play spirit" and educational content of physical activity.[131] Reaching similar conclusions, some male physical educators and administrators also called for extensive reforms in boys' and men's athletics during the early 1900s.[132]

Lee declared that all right-minded girls and women instinctively agreed with her innate values—an essentialist claim that concealed how the experience of unfairness and exclusion had shaped her philosophy.[133] As a college athlete, she was bitter when competitors gained an advantage by cheating or other devious means; if a contest was clean and her opponents were superior, she lost more graciously. Perhaps, Lee gradually realized, fairness and skill mattered as much as victory did.[134] During her studies in Boston, Lee felt the sting of being mocked at the swimming pool and excluded from field hockey because she herself was a "dub."[135] The BNSG code of "sacrific[ing] the winning of a game rather than one girl's health" hit home when Lee returned to Iowa in 1910. Refereeing basketball games for high school and college girls, Lee found the players' fatigue and the boorish behavior of coaches and spectators appalling; their hunger for victory, she decided, had superseded the rules of health and femininity.[136] By the time Lee arrived at Oregon, her philosophy was set. Facing a campus that supported the "Varsity idea," she was determined to "nip [it] in the bud."[137] At Beloit and Nebraska, she steadfastly rejected "that type of physical education which stands for the over training of the strong and the neglect of the weak."[138] She resolved that "our sporting sisters" must be saved "from their madness."[139]

Nebraska's core program remained much the same during Lee's tenure.[140] To prepare non-majors for "constructive living" through democratic recreation, instruction included individual medical and physical exams, a mix of required and elective work, and classes in body mechanics, swimming, dance, games, and sports.[141] Dance classes and pageants emphasized basic movements and prohibited vulgar expression, especially in coed settings.[142] Sports focused on individual and dual recreation with "carry-over" value, such as archery, golf, and tennis. Team sports and highly specialized activities were available, but de-emphasized. Embedded in the formal work was a hidden curriculum of good behavior: wear a proper gym suit, do not use facial rouge, do not leave class early or skip your shower, and boost your grade by showing "spirit of work."[143] Supplementary programs included intramural sports, a dance club, annual pageants and demonstrations, and Play Days with neighboring schools.[144] Two student groups— the Women's Athletic Association (WAA) and the Physical Education Club for majors—organized most of these events under Lee's watchful eye.

Lee's staff taught thousands of young women, whether gifted or inept, about their bodies and physical activity. As a democratic counterpoint to men's

intercollegiate sports at Nebraska, the importance of her alternate approach
and trenchant critique should not be underestimated. That said, Lee's own gym
was discriminatory. Her prescription for active womanhood was rigid and uniform, irrespective of a student's background, interests, ability, race, or sexuality. Many undergraduates adhered to her formula. Shortly after Lee's arrival,
the WAA agreed

> to make a program of sports attractive to every girl in school; to get the
> girls out, and into the game just for the fun of the game; to if possible
> grow away from this old idea of playing to win, of getting out to practices
> to pile up points toward a big letter to wear on a sweater; to reduce the
> desire for individual awards, and to increase participation.[145]

Between the mid-1920s and late 1940s WAA tournaments encouraged fair
play, while penalizing teams for lateness, defaults, illegal players, and arguing with referees. In distributing certificates, pins, and other awards of
symbolic value, the organization favored good sportsmanship over skill.[146]
When talented athletes resisted Lee's dogma, she acknowledged that "the
skilled few may never attain their dream of a place in an interscholastic
sun."[147] Rather than pursuing personal glory, she opined, these atypical students should be satisfied with organizing activities for the majority. Rejecting this advice, Nebraska's female athletes pushed the WAA to sponsor
more high-level competition and to reward individual skill and superior
achievement.[148]

Lee's philosophy enabled many female students to learn and play, while con-
ferring professional authority and social acceptability on women's physical education. Her gym, though, had no room for supposed deviance. Gifted athletes
had few outlets, lesbians were not welcome, and working-class girls learned
middle-class manners. By constructing femininity so narrowly, Lee thwarted
genuine equity in her gym. By equating masculinity, skill, and competition, she
allowed athletics to stand as the exclusive and supposedly natural domain of
men.

ALLEN: TEACHING AND DILUTING DEMOCRACY

For majors and non-majors alike, Maryrose Allen believed, physical education
should develop a "sound body and mind, good moral character, amiable personality, poise and good body-grooming" and a deeper understanding of daily
life as an artistic expression with spiritual and social value. Because students
varied, Allen promised to help each and every one discover her unique "road
to a finer, more noble life."[149] The process began with an individual evaluation.
Does a student lack "grace of movement"? Is she "clumsy in the feet"? Is "Miss
Co-ed" introverted or gregarious? Customized plans might involve remedial
work for students with serious handicaps, swimming and dancing for those

lacking balance and poise, social activities to relieve shyness, and individual exercise to complement an extrovert's personality.[150] Howard's core program for first-year non-majors included "Body Aesthetics" and "Body Sculpture through Movement."[151] The former ranged from elementary physiology and sex education to practical workshops in first aid, grooming, cosmetics, and clothing.[152] While new students practiced posture, gymnastics, and dance, sophomores sampled a menu of individual and team sports, from archery to field hockey.

To supplement required classes, Howard offered voluntary activities that suited each girl's "health status, physical capacity and skill," whether average or exceptional.[153] Non-majors could participate in intramural sports and coed recreation, take part in the Women's Athletic Association (WAA), earn awards for their accomplishments, perform in exhibitions, the annual May Festival, and other pageants, or join one of Howard's renowned dance groups.[154] The main criteria for WAA points and honors were sportsmanship, participation, service, and character rather than athletic talent or achievements.[155] To avoid the taint of masculine athletics, women's tournaments were intramural. When interschool activities developed, they too emphasized social interaction and friendly competition. In 1938 female physical educators at historically black institutions in the upper South established the Women's Sports Day Association. For several decades the WSDA was a key sponsor and philosophical compass for women's athletics at Virginia State College, Howard University, Hampton Institute, and North Carolina's Bennett College. The organization proposed to "develop in women the qualities of beauty of movement, poise, [and] femininity by affording each individual who participates an opportunity to play in an atmosphere of dignity, courtesy, and refinement."[156] The typical format was a Play Day, that is, competition between teams comprising girls from different schools rather than between intact groups from each institution. Although Howard's participation in the WSDA waxed and waned, Allen held true to its principle of sports as a social experience.[157] Howard's professional program instilled the same values. Weaving Allen's Beauty-Health philosophy into every course, from theory and pedagogy to physical activity, the staff trained model teachers who disseminated her ideals to black schools and communities.[158]

Overall, Allen's work both honored and belied her commitment to individuality and inclusion. She enabled young black women, general students and majors alike, to explore their physicality and racial identity and, as Allen intended, "to recreate in a manner befitting a Negro woman."[159] Her Beauty-Health vision suited Howard's image as an institution for respectable, middle-class African Americans destined to join what W. E. B. Du Bois called "the talented tenth" of educated black leaders. Nevertheless, Allen's model of refined, heterosexual black femininity precluded a truly democratic gym that encouraged diverse identities and abilities.

The Difference Dilemma

Both Mabel Lee and Maryrose Reeves Allen set out to build a gym of, by, and for women. Their separate space was intended to respect femininity and individuality, enabling each and every student to become a wholesome, active woman, free of masculine coarseness and competitiveness. The principles of difference and autonomy reaped considerable benefits. Managing their own departments, Allen and Lee taught exercise and recreation to thousands of majors and non-majors during their long careers. Literally and symbolically, the women's gym was a sphere of professional authority that served female students while critiquing masculine values.

Women's departments, however, were not isolated boxes on an organizational chart. Enmeshed in systems of power and politics, Allen and Lee had to contend with senior administrators, faculty committees, and male coaches and physical educators. Howard University and the University of Nebraska marginalized women's activities while privileging men's varsity sports, and Lee and Allen chafed at the inequities. Being different and separate, they objected, did not justify being treated unfairly. Teaching every female student about health and fitness while attending to individual needs, both declared, complemented a university's educational mission and America's democratic values. Yet, by discouraging identities outside a narrow standard of womanhood, Lee and Allen's gyms precluded individuality, inclusion, and parity.

Lee and Allen focused on difference—its salience between the sexes and its absence among women. Although they probably viewed the two sexes as complementary, they spoke of female bodies and character as both superior and inferior to men's. This essentialist logic was compelling but risky; in a nonegalitarian society, "difference" too easily implied inferiority and excused discrimination. Their expectation that separate meant equal was, at best, naïve. The advantages enjoyed by men's programs put Allen and Lee constantly on the defensive—monitoring inequities, demanding resources, and fighting encroachments on their turf. Finally, by universalizing "womanhood" as middle-class, feminine, and heterosexual, their sexual binary discriminated against female students whose identities fell outside this norm.

Lee and Allen's work illustrates an enduring paradox in American physical education: Can a field organized around "difference" advance fairness? Can separate be equal? Other women professionals in the United States during the first half of the twentieth century faced a similar conundrum. Seeking access to male-dominated fields, some female doctors, scientists, and academics deployed "difference" to carve out unique areas of expertise, while insisting that nontraditional did not mean less meritorious. Fusing difference and justice in women's physical education was especially tricky. Lee and Allen pursued fairness while training the bodies they represented as innately different from, even lesser than, men's. Although difference and equality are not inherently incompatible, Lee and Allen's argument facilitated gender discrimination in the gym.

To fully understand their predicament, however, one must look beyond Lee and Allen's personal philosophies and examine institutional dynamics: How did their schools interpret "difference" and who benefited from inequity? Gender disparities existed at Nebraska and Howard whether budgets were flush or lean, whether the universities indulged men's athletics or questioned them. By supporting an independent women's gym, both schools obscured gender inequities in the name of difference and fairness. Separation was, by design, an asymmetric relationship that disadvantaged female staff and students while equating athleticism and masculinity, and ensuring men's privileges. Howard University, the University of Nebraska, and other coeducational schools exploited the logic of difference and independence to institutionalize and mask discrimination. This practice rendered gender equity elusive, even impossible.

"The joy of hard play"

COMPETITIVE ACTIVITIES FOR COLLEGE WOMEN,
1920s–1950s

In 1927 J. Anna Norris, the director of women's physical education at the University of Minnesota, decided to organize the school's first Play Day. Because the event involved participants from other schools, it deviated from her department's usual program of general instruction, noncompetitive exhibitions, and intramural tournaments. When Norris approached her president about using university facilities, she felt obliged to clarify that the novel activity "will be a step in the direction of interest in play for all, for purely recreational purposes, and will demonstrate to the participants the joy of hard play without bitter rivalry."[1] Low-key, inclusive, healthy, and fun, the event was designed to avoid the mistakes of men's intercollegiate athletics.

Norris's professional peers who shared her philosophy assumed their ideals were a common reality. Surveys in the 1920s and 1930s reassured them that extracurricular sports for most college women featured intramural and benign extramural activities, but rarely included varsity-style competition. Reports often attributed this pattern to young women's natural interest in social recreation and distaste for "bitter rivalry." Such claims strengthened the agenda of the "Great White Mothers" in American physical education and usually relied on studies that they or their protégés conducted.[2]

Through the 1970s, most historians also believed that Norris, Mabel Lee, Blanche Trilling, Agnes Wayman, and other white leaders had successfully popularized inclusive recreation and quashed elite competition in secondary schools and colleges. During the 1980s and 1990s, however, more extensive research revealed that extracurricular competition before mid-century was hardly tame or uniform. At some colleges and universities, physical education classes became a platform for intramural contests that, unwittingly, entailed "bitter rivalry." Elsewhere, undergraduate organizations ran high-powered tournaments involving dormitory groups or class years. During the 1920s and 1930s, many institutions participated in Play Days, telegraphic meets, and other mild intercollegiate events. By the 1940s, Sports Days—which kept teams from individual schools intact—became common. Endorsing even more vigorous competition, some institutions played against local high schools, amateur clubs, and YWCAs during the interwar years. Others routinely sponsored intercollegiate athletics for elite varsity teams. Some schools offered multiple forms of extracurricular competition, thereby accommodating skill levels from average to exceptional.

To explain this variety, sports scholars in the 1990s and early 2000s considered several factors. Perhaps teachers' ideas about gender and sexuality, the presence of male versus female leadership, or an institution's location and racial composition affected its decisions about competitive activities. Although such studies greatly enhanced the historical investigation of college women's sports, few conclusions seemed generalizable. Instead, contradictions abounded: like-minded teachers did not establish identical programs, comparable institutions had divergent policies, and individual schools often changed their positions. Despite a wealth of case studies and analytical insights, historical work has not yet produced a comprehensive interpretation that integrates diverse factors across time and disparate settings, and incorporates both national developments and local conditions.

Deliberations over women's sports occurred amid major changes in American higher education. In the 1920s the United States was home to more than one thousand four-year colleges and universities, including public and private, large and small, coed and single-sex, religious and secular, academic and vocational, and predominantly white or black. Between the world wars, these diverse institutions faced demographic shifts, financial challenges, and debates over academic and extracurricular priorities.[3] As high school graduation rates increased, a steady march to college began across the country. During the interwar years, America's undergraduate population expanded more than fivefold, with public institutions absorbing most of the growth.[4] In 1918 more than one-half of postsecondary institutions had fewer than three hundred students, with only 5 percent of the schools enrolling over two thousand.[5] By the late 1930s combined enrollments in undergraduate, graduate, and professional programs at most state schools ranged between twenty-five hundred and seventy-five hundred, with some campuses exceeding twenty thousand.[6] College students also became more diverse.[7] By 1920 females constituted about 47 percent of undergraduates, and by 1940 women's total enrollment had more than doubled, reaching about six hundred thousand.[8] This influx included not only young women from affluent and middle-class families but the daughters of farmers and immigrants as well. Meanwhile, total enrollment at historically black colleges and universities grew from about two thousand in 1920 to fourteen thousand in 1930.[9]

Regardless of composition, most campuses were embroiled in curricular debates.[10] Tired of vague elective programs, educational reformers pushed for prescribed courses of study with utilitarian objectives. Around the country, John Thelin notes, "teams of termites" worked "industriously beneath the surface of campus life" to transform university curricula.[11] They found many allies among philanthropists and foundation heads who endorsed a corporate model of higher education, epitomized by multipurpose research-based institutions.[12] For most students and average citizens, though, academic reform was hardly the real story in higher education. Mass media portrayed college life as endless parties, athletic events, and frivolity—an extension of the youth culture that swept the country during the 1920s. For the archetypal College Man, undergraduate life was a "social opportunity rather than an intellectual experience"; his fraternity, clubs, and sports teams became an incubator for "the pursuit of pleasure" and future success.[13] Some educators welcomed the publicity and donations that intercollegiate football and other spectacles generated; most administrators and faculty members, however, regarded young men's exploits as "trouble in paradise."[14]

Women's conduct seemed no less disturbing. The heterosexual tone of postwar campus life at coeducational and women's schools alike apparently signaled an end to the same-sex "smashes" and "crushes" so common in earlier decades.[15] Yet parents and administrators worried that decent undergraduates might go too far with their brash heterosexuality. Would books and self-control, adults wondered, give way to petting and other forms of independence, from the gin flask to trendy clothes? These forays onto once forbidden ground seemed to reflect college women's general outlook.[16] Pulled simultaneously toward conformity and rebellion, matriculants in the 1920s focused more on men and campus life than on world politics. Though more somber than her predecessors, the female collegian of the 1930s also concentrated on her prospects for work and marriage rather than on larger social dislocations; above all, she insisted on self-determination, "with the rights of access to the opposite sex, to privacy, and to pleasure."[17] Fiercely independent, female students did not stand by while social scientists and cultural pundits analyzed them or parents, teachers, and administrators told them what to do.

As concern over undergraduate behavior escalated, colleges and universities revisited their services and regulations.[18] Many expanded their offices of student affairs, a cadre of administrators who counseled and disciplined undergraduates. Another strategy for nurturing well-rounded young men and women focused on clubs, student government, and other extracurricular programs. Schools relied particularly on intramural and extramural sports to foster appropriate pastimes and values. When colleges and universities decided which female students would play which sports against whom and for what purpose, they embodied specific ideologies of active womanhood along various axes of difference. Competitive activities could not only accentuate or minimize supposed differences between men and women; they could also homogenize women or affirm variations among them by race, class, sexuality, religion, and physical ability and interests.

Institutional decisions depended on local factors. Each school's mission and identity, demographic makeup, donor base, governance structure, and campus culture affected its deliberations and policies about women's extracurricular sports. The process was rarely smooth and the outcome never permanent. Every significant change in personnel, finances, or power arrangements reopened the negotiations. The result was by no means predictable; even schools with seemingly identical characteristics reached divergent conclusions.

This chapter examines how postsecondary institutions thought about and practiced "difference" in women's extracurricular sports between the 1920s and the 1950s. It comprises a series of case studies of diverse colleges and universities in different regions: first, predominantly white institutions—public and private, coed and single-sex—where competitive activities were either banned, emergent, or prevalent; second, historically black colleges and universities (HBCUs)—vocational and academic, coed and female-only—where women's athletics were either common or nonexistent. Emphasizing each school's unique features, the examples trace negotiations between female physical educators, senior administrators, academic faculty, trustees, donors, and students across several decades. Together, the analyses of individual campuses permit some conclusions about which systems of "difference" either facilitated or thwarted competitive activities for white and black undergraduate women in the United States before mid-century.

The Old Guard at Work

The Great White Mothers of American physical education and their protégés taught at institutions representing the full gamut of higher education. They worked at private white female colleges, from Mills College in California, Agnes Scott in Georgia, and Milwaukee-Downer in Wisconsin to Wellesley, Smith, and other Seven Sister schools in the Northeast. Their conservative philosophy also took hold at private coeducational schools, large state universities, and public and coordinate women's colleges. Although such institutions differed in size and purpose, they all clung to mainstream social values as American higher education adapted to the "prosperous twenties, [the] struggling thirties" and the turbulent forties and fifties.[19] Institutional leaders promoted curricula, student organizations, codes of conduct, and physical activities that delineated white, middle-class, heterosexual norms of educated manhood and womanhood. The iconic New Woman epitomized this standard. Distinctly white and bourgeois, she stood above America's degraded black and ethnic underclass. She exuded feminine health and confidence, without the rough edges of masculine egotism or athleticism. Focusing her heart and pastimes on men, she avoided the flapper's sexual excesses and the lesbian's perverted tendencies. To embody this ideal, many predominantly white institutions turned the women's gym over to a Great White Mother or her surrogate.

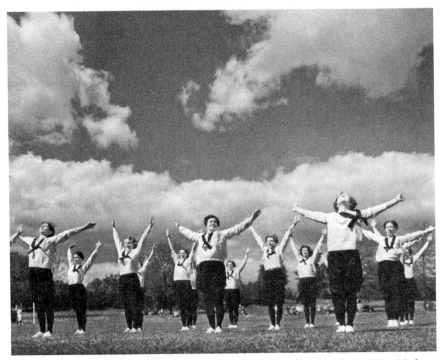

FIGURE 5.1 *Outdoor calisthenics for the "New Woman" at the University of Wisconsin, Madison, ca. 1920–29. Courtesy of the University of Wisconsin–Madison Archives, Image #S05514.*

Blanche Trilling cheerfully accepted this assignment at the University of Wisconsin. "The wasp waisted, pale-cheeked, clinging vine type of Victorian woman, easily moved to tears and fainting over the least provocation has become history," Trilling announced in about 1940. Modern society required women to be "vigorous, wholesome, well-balanced, physically and mentally competent to carry their share of the world's work"—the very qualities that gym class imparted.[20] Instructional games and sports, Trilling and other Great White Mothers explained, built teamwork, perseverance, and self-control, encouraged leisure-time interests, and steered an undergraduate's "misdirected feelings into a natural channel."[21] This allusion to sexuality warned against the release of inhibitions bordering on masculine hypersexuality and, even more so, abnormal same-sex attraction.[22] To replace "'crushes' or morbid girl friendships" with restrained heterosexual relationships,[23] the Old Guard prescribed co-recreation or at least activities that drew male attention, including archery and other individual sports along with dual games such as badminton. With proper guidance, one teacher elaborated, an undergraduate might realize that participating in team sports after college was unlikely, but she could learn to "play a smashing game of tennis or to execute diving and swimming in such good form that the boy friends at a swimming party will sit up and take notice."[24]

The principle of feminine heterosexuality also permeated schools' extra-curricular programs of intramural and extramural activities, whether compet-itive or noncompetitive. Typical intramural offerings for white undergraduates between the 1920s and 1950s included activity clubs, field days, and demonstra-tions as well as campus tournaments in individual and team sports. During the 1920s, Wellesley College sponsored field days each fall and spring; organized by class year, several hundred students competed in ten or so sports. To keep the occasion low-key, the admission fee was ten cents and spectators were limited to faculty, other students, and girls from local preparatory schools. Staff mem-bers were "on constant guard" to ensure that participants, especially Wellesley's enthusiastic rowers, did not overexert.[25] To distinguish such events from men's athletics, physical educators portrayed them as a natural extension of depart-mental curricula. All activities at Milwaukee-Downer's annual competitive gymnastic exhibition, the staff proclaimed, "represent[ed] regular work done in class without special preparation for this drill."[26]

Interschool events also were available. At the turn of the twentieth century, some white colleges and universities sponsored varsity-style extramural com-petition for women; by 1915 though, most schools banned such contests and replaced them with events that avoided head-to-head rivalry. Telegraphic meets, for example, enabled students to participate in archery, riflery, or track and field on their own campuses; each school then transmitted its scores telegraph-ically to other institutions or a central office. Even more common was the Play Day, involving games between teams comprising players from different institu-tions. Because composite membership usually weakened team play, many white colleges and universities switched by the mid-1930s to Sports Days, in which teams representing individual schools remained intact. To avoid snobbery and preserve decorum, selection criteria emphasized personal qualities as much as skill.[27] Participants in a Play Day at the North Carolina College for Women in 1928 were chosen "because of health, sportsmanship and leadership." The event, Mary Channing Coleman explained, was "a simple invitation" to other schools "to 'come play with us,' with no winning teams or awards; the objectives are limited to good fellowship and the joy of playing together."[28] To enhance social interaction, organizers held post-match mixers. After "an afternoon of fun and recreation" at the Woman's College of Duke University in 1938, mem-bers of the school's athletic association "served as hostesses to the visitors at a tea."[29]

Conceding that most participants wanted recognition, not simply refresh-ments, physical educators devised systems whereby students accumulated points and received awards for intramural and extramural activities. As the fall or spring season ended, a department might name varsity teams in various sports and present modest awards such as pins, school letters, badges with spe-cial insignia, or sweaters. To ensure that honors delivered the right message, departments assigned points for effort and sportsmanship as well as victories;

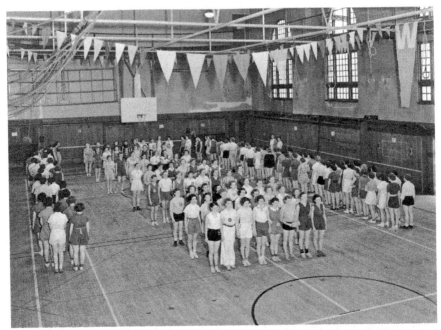

FIGURE 5.2 *Interschool Play Day at the University of Wisconsin, Madison, 1936. Courtesy of the University of Wisconsin–Madison Archives, Image #S05512.*

all-star teams existed in name only and rarely competed; tangible awards carried mostly symbolic, not material, value. During the 1920s, for example, Wellesley College named honorary varsity teams and awarded "a large old English letter" for achievement "in several sports together with health, posture, sportsmanship, and other considerations."[30]

This arrangement appealed to the Great White Mothers because it promoted health and exercise for the majority of students, while distributing a department's scarce resources economically. Above all, teachers said, democratic recreation was a matter of principle. We are committed, Blanche Trilling declared, to "relaxation and fun for all, instead of over-exertion for a few. Maximum activity for maximum numbers."[31] While male athletes sacrificed their health and education for fleeting moments of personal fame and school pride, their female classmates learned the value of fitness, community, and heterosexual appeal through recreation. After all, Margaret Bell of the University of Michigan observed, a "girl should be a girl."[32]

Physical educators expected students not only to participate willingly in feminine recreation but to promulgate it as well. Departments asked majors and non-majors to administer extracurricular sports through their women's athletic association (WAA). Under the faculty's watchful eye, WAAs ran athletic events, recorded results, determined point values, and conferred awards on classmates.[33] The Great White Mothers were also instrumental in forming regional and national organizations for collegiate WAAs. In 1917 Blanche Trilling and other professional leaders established the Athletic Conference of American College Women. The ACACW and its successor, the Athletic Federation of College Women (AFCW), helped white undergraduates interpret and apply the central dogma of feminine competition.[34]

Many WAAs dutifully complied by organizing stunt nights and May Festivals, holding mass participation tournaments, downplaying competition, and tabulating points for symbolic awards.[35] Some students toed the line even more closely than their mentors did. In March 1926, the Ohio State University WAA penalized several classmates who competed extramurally. The offenders were "disqualified from all W.A.A. activities for the remainder of the year," their intramural team forfeited its points and rank from a recent tournament, and the team captain and manager lost their individual athletic points. In 1927, to encourage students to "'play for play's sake' rather than 'play for point's sake,'" the organization switched to awards based on participation in sports or any WAA activity. One year later, it abolished awards altogether. OSU's physical educators fully supported the students' decisions, despite the notoriety the department gained in previous and later decades for sponsoring high-level intercollegiate competition.[36] The University of Minnesota's WAA took a similar path. In 1931 the group stopped giving points for "athletic accomplishment" because the scheme favored girls with "native ability or special training" and promoted the "adolescent-minded stage wherein every act had to be rewarded with so many points." Under its new system, the WAA explained, awards would recognize loyalty and "personal participation," qualities that any and all girls might possess.[37] These signs of obedience encouraged one college instructor to predict that the story of women's sports, written by teachers and faithfully read by students, would conclude with the words, "They all played happily ever after."[38]

Case Studies in Resistance

Some undergraduates, however, defied the Old Guard. Tension was especially acute at private nonsectarian women's colleges. Established in the late nineteenth century, these institutions were noted for their exclusive student bodies, elite social ethos, and rigorous codes of behavior. The absence of male classmates allowed female undergraduates to exercise unusual privileges and autonomy.[39] During the 1920s and 1930s, their cliquish subcultures gave way to more secular, heterosexual, free-spirited activities.[40] Fearing a lapse in discipline, private women's colleges intensified their enforcement of white bourgeois femininity, with the enthusiastic support of the Great White Mothers. Athletes at Agnes Scott, Smith, and Milwaukee-Downer, though, pushed back by creating forms of competition and ambition within the bounds of mass recreation.

On paper, extracurricular activities at Agnes Scott College, a small residential school for white women near Atlanta, look conventional.[41] Students helped plan the annual May Day Festival and joined clubs devoted to bicycling, roller skating, hiking, and tennis. Each year, dozens signed up for intramural tournaments in basketball and field hockey. In 1931 the school's athletic association stopped awarding a silver cup for outstanding achievement and endorsed Play Days. Our objective, the yearbook declared, should be "Sports for Fun for Everyone" and "Personal Progress in Pep and Play."[42] These mottos befit the school's ideal of wholesome educated femininity. Founded in 1889, Agnes Scott College prepared elite young white women for Christian motherhood. Although its vision gradually broadened, the institution remained quite insular and conservative through the mid-twentieth century.[43]

Despite these constraints, students at Agnes Scott discovered the camaraderie and freedom of sports competition. Interclass rivalries and rowdy spectators energized the college's intramural tournaments. The yearbook hailed athletic classmates, especially those who earned the coveted ASC letters—which stood for "agility, strength and courage" as well as the school's name. Sensing students' enthusiasm, physical educators slowly approved higher-level competition; by 1940 the college's best golfers participated in a national tournament, and its quasi-varsity tennis team played against several nearby schools.[44]

Undergraduates at Smith College were just as restless. Founded in 1875, Smith attracted young, predominantly white women from well-to-do families and prepared them for lives of intelligence and virtue in the private and public spheres.[45] A tight-knit residential institution in Northampton, Massachusetts, Smith emphasized academics, community, discipline, and decorum. These values, administrators and faculty members believed, should also guide extracurricular activities. After publicly rejecting intercollegiate sports at the turn of the twentieth century, the college emphasized general recreation and intramural competition for decades thereafter.[46] Director Dorothy Ainsworth herself had embraced this system as a Smith undergraduate in 1912–16. She had "loved the whole sports program," whether canoeing with friends or practicing with her basketball team.[47] Upon returning as an instructor in the 1920s, Ainsworth strengthened the school's intramural tradition, believing that every undergraduate—from the "genius in sports" to the "average good sportswoman" to the "'motor moron'"—should "learn to perform as well as she possibly can."[48] Campus tournaments took two forms: the "class competition for the more ardent and skillful athletes, and the house competition for all who wish and are able to enter."[49] Extramural activities were closely regulated as well. Until the 1960s Smith rarely participated in telegraphic meets, play days, or sports days, unless the competition promised to be relaxed or declining another school's invitation seemed impolite.[50] Learning to justify the staff's "seemingly 'isolationist' policy," the students' Athletic Association rewarded classmates not only for ability but also "proper attitude," "poise and self-control," and "appearance, including posture, good health, and neatness and appropriateness of dress."[51] By accommodating diverse abilities and avoiding the drama of intercollegiate sports, Smith College brought elite, white femininity into the gym.

Field days and intramural games, however, were not as genteel nor the participants as demure as the school hoped. Interclass tournaments, especially basketball, were major events, and students vied eagerly to be selected as team members.[52] Players often ignored Smith's training rules, teachers conceded, by deciding for themselves "how far and how much" to train.[53] When big contests arrived—such as Rally Day for the junior and senior basketball teams—tickets were scarce, crowds were raucous, and the fierce competition exercised students' emotions as well as bodies. Without appearing to defy their mentors' ideology, undergraduates at Smith used intramural sports to re-create white femininity and physicality in ways that Ainsworth herself had relished as a student.

Athletic points and awards proved equally subversive. The original system at Milwaukee-Downer, a small, private women's college in Wisconsin, seemed consistent with the Old Guard's conservative philosophy.[54] Adhering to the tenets of the ACACW and Althea Heimbach, a staff member who trained at Oberlin, Milwaukee-Downer's athletic association made activities and awards readily accessible, thereby minimizing competition and stardom. To be sure, athletic ability was not irrelevant when the group organized field days and intramural teams. During the 1910s, basketball players who performed poorly were dropped from squads; similarly, the WAA initially issued no awards after introducing baseball because the participants "have not been skillful enough."[55] Generally, however, the organization's criteria downplayed raw athleticism. Members of rowing crews were "chosen essentially for their ability to maintain correct form" as well as for "speed and endurance." To earn top honors in the spring regatta, a crew had to accumulate the "greatest number of points, both in form and speed."[56] Character mattered even more than aptitude. To join a team or receive points, students needed sportsmanship, regular attendance in gym class, and solid academic standing.[57] Lest some participants feel unappreciated when Milwaukee-Downer celebrated its most proficient swimmers, the school also named an honorary class team of girls who were competent, but "had not quite come up to a perfect standard."[58]

Because some students objected that distributing points and honors so generously cheapened them, the WAA set out to make the scheme more meaningful—a process occupying several decades. Many reforms dealt with eligibility: Who deserves points and for which activities? For example, are injured players, cheerleaders, referees, and other nonparticipants entitled to points? What about relatively inactive team members? Surely, students did not deserve points simply for "filling up space on a team." Some loyal substitutes, though, probably did play enough to qualify for points and a numeral.[59] The WAA's emphasis on performance was tied to its passion for success. Since winning seemed even better than participation, perhaps the revised system should favor talented athletes, despite

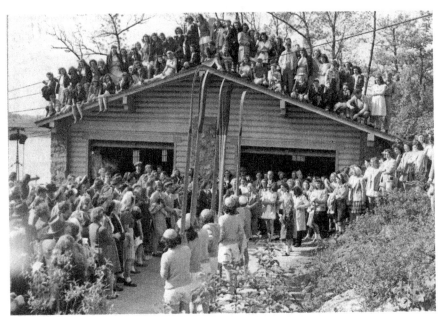

FIGURE 5.3 *Students and staff at Milwaukee-Downer College gather after a rowing regatta for presentation of the winner's trophy and naming of the honorary "all college" crew team. Courtesy of Lawrence University Archives, Appleton, Wisconsin.*

their shortcomings. In 1919, as the annual basketball game between the college and its preparatory academy neared, the WAA wondered if a particular undergraduate should be disqualified simply because she had failed one course; maybe the board could relax its academic regulations for the sake of fielding the best team and securing a victory. The WAA decided to assemble its squad from the best players on the college's class teams based on "only three of our four usual requirements, namely: Sportsmanship, Faithfulness and Skill, disregarding scholarship."[60] In this case, victory on the court mattered more than penalizing poor schoolwork.

Similarly, the WAA decided that athletic awards should reflect talent and achievement. One means of enhancing their value was to give them, literally, more weight. As the board complained in 1931, the standard emblems "are not pretentious enough and . . . everyone should be willing to pay a little more for better ones."[61] In 1934 the organization reformatted the trophy for the riding program; ending its democratic practice of inscribing the top three riders' names without place designations and prohibiting any student from being listed more than once, the group adopted a new plan that acknowledged rank of finish and perennial winners.[62] The biggest controversies centered on the WAA's top honors such as the Blue Blazer Girl, the program's outstanding senior. Although debates over the relative weight of athletic and personal qualities spanned more than a decade, with no clear resolution, the goal remained to recognize exceptional merit.[63]

Through the years, WAA board members were not of one mind about eligibility, points, and awards. They agreed, however, that a sports program should do more than promote democratic participation; skill and success also mattered. They believed that students wanted and deserved meaningful rewards for their accomplishments—to make a team, win a tournament, or earn an award was a valuable experience that should be encouraged and operationalized. Although the WAA did not renounce the faculty's orthodox philosophy of egalitarian recreation, members re-visioned active womanhood. Their version incorporated athleticism, competition, rewards, and glory—traits that Milwaukee-Downer's white, middle-class students did not consider unfeminine.

Many of their peers agreed. From Michigan to Massachusetts and California to North Carolina, white undergraduates became disgruntled with the Great White Mothers' dogma. While obeying their teachers in theory, student athletic associations often challenged them in practice. A survey in the late 1920s discovered that most WAAs around the country tried to accommodate exceptionally talented athletes as well as enthusiastic but casual "lovers of sport." Striking a balance between exclusive and accessible awards, many student groups made honors "difficult to get" but sufficiently graded "so that the majority have something to show for their efforts."[64] These issues spilled over from local campuses to regional and national meetings; the ACACW focused as much on students' grievances as their success as acolytes for the Old Guard.[65] By redirecting intramural programs, white female undergraduates asserted agency without nullifying their teachers' core principles.

Skilled Extramural Sports at White Institutions

More radical versions of active womanhood developed at white colleges and universities that approved extramural sports before mid-century. Some institutions experimented with "inter-class intercollegiate" contests that pitted teams representing the class years of one school against corresponding groups from another institution. Other schools restricted Sports Days to their most talented players. Elsewhere, varsity teams or exclusive athletic clubs competed against local colleges, preparatory schools, and amateur groups. By the late 1930s more than 20 percent of mainstream white institutions offered vigorous extramural events; by the late 1940s at least one-quarter had skill-based teams for Sports Days and more than one-fifth had intercollegiate varsity competition.[66]

No single variable determined which white colleges and universities sponsored women's intercollegiate competition between the 1920s and 1950s. Representing every region, examples span private and public schools, large and small, coed and single-sex, secular and religious, exclusive and second-tier, progressive and mainstream.[67] The group includes private women's colleges, such as Bryn Mawr near Philadelphia and Sweet Briar in Virginia, as well as teacher training programs, from small coeducational normal schools to public women's colleges. In Virginia, for example, the State Normal and Industrial School for Women at Harrisonburg (now James Madison University) and Farmville State Normal School for Women (now Longwood College) regularly competed against in-state and out-of-state opponents.[68] Hunter College, a free, nonresidential normal school in New York City, enrolled Protestants, Catholics, and Jews, and an unusually high proportion of blacks; its varsity teams competed against other schools in field hockey, basketball, swimming, fencing, and tennis.[69] The Washington Square branch of New York University, another nonresidential teachers program for young men and women of various races and religions, also sponsored female sports.[70] Athletics were available at relatively homogeneous single-sex institutions, such as Radcliffe and Pembroke, the "sisters" of Harvard and Brown, respectively. Pembroke organized intramural and varsity events in field hockey, basketball, swimming, bowling, archery, and tennis.[71] Coeducational institutions, from large public and private universities to small liberal arts colleges, are represented as well. State universities in the Southwest, including Arizona and New Mexico, sponsored women's intercollegiate sports, while Swarthmore College had varsity teams in field hockey, basketball, swimming, and tennis during the 1930s.[72]

One common impetus might have been convenience; arranging events with nearby competitors allowed physical education departments to economize while serving both athletic and less skilled students. Political and ideological factors were even more significant. If one or more campus constituencies successfully championed new perspectives on gender and difference, a school tended to endorse nontraditional activities, including women's extramural competition. Bryn Mawr illustrates the role of feminist administrators and teachers in redefining difference, equity, and sports at an exclusive women's institution. Meanwhile, female students at Stanford University lobbied for interschool competition by reformulating gender relations in the context of coeducation.

ELITE SPORTS AT ELITIST BRYN MAWR

At Bryn Mawr College, extramural sports flourished alongside academic innovation. A private liberal arts school, Bryn Mawr opened in 1885 intent on preparing young Quaker ladies for respectable lives as teachers and mothers. Senior administrators, especially M. Carey Thomas, the school's first dean and second president, soon raised Bryn Mawr's scholarly profile. Its admissions requirements, core curriculum, and postbaccalaureate programs came to reflect Thomas's feminist conviction that women were men's equals.[73] She did not, however, mean *all* women; before mid-century, Bryn Mawr usually rejected applicants who by virtue of poverty, race, or religion were not considered true ladies.[74]

Thomas also believed that young educated women should sample diverse extracurricular activities and sports. During the early 1900s Bryn Mawr athletes competed against their classmates as well as alumnae, amateur clubs, and local colleges in field hockey, tennis, swimming, water polo, basketball, and fencing. President Thomas promoted and regulated these opportunities throughout her twenty-eight-year tenure (1894–1922). Besides scrutinizing physical education facilities, staff appointments, gymnastics classes, and intramural events, she had a direct hand in the sports program; her internal memos applauded athletes' accomplishments, worried about their injuries, and monitored team rules, competition schedules, and athletic eligibility.[75] Given Thomas's personal history of physical disability and therapeutic exercise, she probably wanted to make sure that her students were strong in body as well as mind.[76]

The other force in Bryn Mawr athletics was Constance M. K. Applebee (1873–1981), an English field hockey expert whose demonstrations of her sport at American colleges in the early 1900s attracted wide attention. She served as Bryn Mawr's director of physical education from 1904 to 1928, earning a reputation as a strong advocate for her department as well as for undergraduate field hockey, swimming, and tennis. A strict but beloved coach, "The Apple" was uncompromising in her belief that every young woman, skilled or not, could and should play vigorous sports. She also helped run the college's elaborate May Day festival. Applebee's influence extended well beyond Bryn Mawr. She popularized field hockey at her famous camp in Pennsylvania's Poconos region and helped establish the United States Field Hockey Association. During the 1920s she also ran *The Sportswoman*, a magazine devoted to amateur and school-based athletics with a pro-competition slant.[77]

A formidable tandem, Thomas and Applebee did not allow sports to grow unchecked. To prevent athletics from becoming a distraction, the college prohibited on-campus contests before 4:00 p.m. as well as away games in team sports; before the Athletic Association added competitors to its extramural schedule, the board routinely consulted President Thomas.[78] Most importantly, Thomas and Applebee upheld Bryn Mawr's code of respectability by infusing sports with elite norms of white, Christian femininity.

For decades, amateur competition had been an acceptable pastime for well-to-do white ladies in the United States as long as decorum was preserved; this meant tennis, golf, and other exclusive sports in controlled settings, from colleges and country clubs to noncommercial national tournaments. Many white colleges and universities also favored individual and dual sports, such as golf, tennis, badminton, archery, bowling, and swimming, during the interwar period.[79] Symbolizing casual, lifelong exercise with the potential for co-recreation, these activities projected a white, heterosexual, middle- and upper-class aura. Team sports also gained popularity among college women. Although conservative institutions viewed basketball's masculine, working-class image with increasing suspicion, field hockey, an equally vigorous team sport, had been

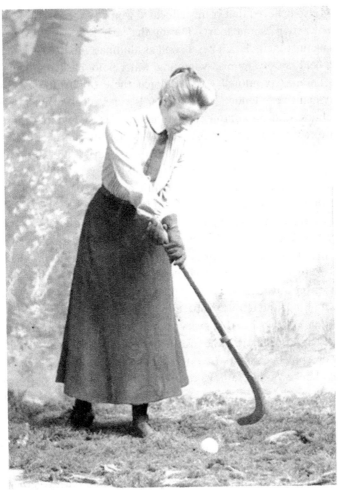

FIGURE 5.4 *Constance M. K. Applebee, ca. 1903. Courtesy of Bryn Mawr College Library, Special Collections.*

thoroughly domesticated by the 1920s; its rules, outfits, and all-female environment signified propriety.[80]

Bryn Mawr's program upheld this elite prescription for active womanhood. It featured field hockey, tennis, and other respectable games, while tolerating basketball and track and field. Although Applebee allowed some basketball teams to play by "men's rules," she normalized the game by having most intramural and intercollegiate squads follow "girls' rules." President Thomas drew equally sharp lines. She recommended that students with weak knees or other physical problems be excluded from basketball, and reprimanded track and field athletes when their events, especially the strenuous high jump, lasted late into the evening.[81] Because field hockey epitomized refined white competition, however, Thomas rarely criticized the school's premier sport, despite its physical demands.

In 1922 Marion Edwards Park, a Bryn Mawr alumna who had served as Radcliffe's dean, succeeded Thomas as president and led her alma mater for twenty years.[82] To foster a broader model of educated womanhood, Park lifted the school's smoking ban and took a more open-minded approach to enrolling African Americans.[83] Determined to keep the college an upright and studious place, however, Park tightened the reins on athletic competition by reorganizing various teams.[84] Overall, Bryn Mawr's sports program continued during Park's administration, but at a lower pitch than before.

During the first half of the twentieth century, Bryn Mawr's intellectual focus and feminist outlook represented women as men's equals. Extramural sports signified that the right to fair opportunities extended from the classroom into the gymnasium. As did most features of Bryn Mawr, athletics also maintained highly gendered distinctions of race, class, and religion: privileged white Protestant women played only respectable sports.

WOMEN'S SPORTS AT COED STANFORD

The calculus changed if men were present. At coeducational schools, men's numbers and influence often rendered female students "second-class citizens" who were "ignored, ridiculed, and isolated" in the classroom and campus community.[85] Women undergraduates responded by creating their own academic styles, social traditions, and extracurricular activities, including competitive sports.[86]

One example is Stanford University, a private institution that opened in 1891 with an endowment from Leland Stanford, a railroad tycoon who was California's governor during the Civil War. Committed from the outset to coeducation, Stanford University enrolled the sons and daughters of well-to-do California families. Although women comprised 44 percent of the student body by 1900, men still dominated campus life, especially its centerpiece, varsity sports. Female students sought equity by pushing for intercollegiate competition—a goal that Stanford's physical educators both resisted and obliged. Spanning several decades, this negotiation over active womanhood in a coeducational setting coincided with Stanford's effort to become an "entrepreneurial university" characterized by the masculinist ideals of research and innovation.[87]

Prior to World War I, student exercise consisted of voluntary gym class and extracurricular physical activities; male and female students largely managed their own sports, including extramural competition.[88] Under the auspices of the WAA, female undergraduates formed clubs for archery, bicycling, basketball, tennis, baseball, and track. Between 1891 and 1910 they competed against local schools and colleges in basketball and tennis. The most publicized event was a basketball game in 1896 against the University of California at Berkeley, held in San Francisco's Armory Hall before an estimated crowd of five hundred women (no men were allowed). Stanford prevailed by the score of 2–1, in a game involving nine-person teams playing on a nine-zone court.[89] Although Stanford's female athletes had fewer resources and less visibility than their male counterparts, their opportunities at the turn of the century compared favorably with those of women at other coed institutions.

This advantage was short-lived; in the early 1900s Stanford began regulating men's and women's sports more closely.[90] Administrators and faculty members had worried for some time that men's activities, especially football, were in disarray due to student mismanagement and rules violations. In 1906 the university established a Board of Control comprised of students, alumni, and two members of the existing Faculty Athletic Committee (FAC), which also supervised women's activities. The FAC had taken a dim view of women's extramural competition for several years; in 1903 it ruled that a proposed tennis tournament with Berkeley should not be "an intercollegiate event," but instead "would be conducted quietly and informally on the Stanford courts."[91] These decisions indicated that men's varsity sports would be systematized and women's competition would be curtailed. As if to confirm this official policy, "men students jeered when women dared take to the playing fields with their own athletics teams."[92]

The sharp gendering of physical activities in the early 1900s coincided with a comprehensive self-study at Stanford. Subscribing to the "California idea" of higher education, the school aspired to be both a college and a university—to cultivate moral, useful individuals through close professorial mentoring while also becoming a prominent center of professional training and original research.[93] When this goal proved elusive, Stanford undertook a broad review that soon converged on its masculine identity. During the Progressive Era, top officials at Stanford and other coeducational schools worried that their campuses were being feminized, literally and figuratively.[94] Stanford's leaders believed that the arrival of more female students, who typically were older and academically better than their male classmates, jeopardized its ascent as a premier institution devoted to the manly goals of useful knowledge and productive graduates. Prodded by Jane Stanford, the founder's widow, the school capped women's enrollment at five hundred and later mandated that its student ratio not fall below three males for each female—policies that stood until 1933. Having reduced its quandary over mission to a question of gender, Stanford differentiated its male and female students more sharply in the classroom, library, laboratory, and gym. In 1910/11, it separated the men's and women's divisions of the Department of Physical Training and Hygiene.[95]

The next two decades proved critical for these programs and the university as a whole. Stanford's steady growth to nearly four thousand students by 1925 could not mask its financial woes or nagging reputation as "a pleasant place that showed sporadic signs of scholarship."[96] To enhance its intellectual stature, the university undertook curriculum reform and renewed its emphasis on faculty research with real-world applications.[97] Most undergraduates, though, had other concerns. Preoccupied with campus life, school rituals, and varsity sports, they "considered the ability of Stanford's football team to challenge the University of California and the University of Southern California for selection to the Rose Bowl to be a top institutional priority."[98] Although this obsession might have weakened Stanford's academic ambitions, senior officials were convinced that varsity sports—alongside business-friendly curricula and limits on female enrollment—would bolster the school's male ethos.

To this end, Stanford further delineated physical activities by gender during the 1910s and 1920s. While men's varsity athletics enjoyed new facilities, ample coaching staffs, and formal competition, the university confined women to intramural activities and some low-key extramural events.[99] For some years, Stanford's WAA had arranged interclass-intercollegiate events involving teams of skilled and average participants from the intramural program.[100] To schedule outside competition, the WAA needed approval from the Faculty Committee on Athletics (FCA). Although the FCA usually sanctioned fencing and tennis matches, it became increasingly wary of basketball, especially if Berkeley was the foe. Despite students' many objections, the FCA abolished intercollegiate basketball in 1915 because of "repeated unpleasant experiences."[101]

Although top administrators welcomed this decision, they desired further oversight. Instead of managing women's sports through the Board of Athletic Control, the powerful new hybrid of the FCA and Board of Control that regulated men's sports, Stanford created a separate Faculty Committee on Women's Athletics (FCWA) in 1919 charged with determining "matters of policy, eligibility, and schedule concerning women's athletics." Wasting no time, the FCWA endorsed intramural events at its first meeting, emphatically opposing "varsity intercollegiate athletics for women." It approved, however, low-key "interclass-intercollegiate" events with "institutions of collegiate rank"—a position that stood through 1924.[102]

Headed by Helen Masters Bunting, recently hired in women's physical education, the FCWA consisted of Dr. Clelia Duel Mosher and other female faculty members. During the 1920s Bunting and Mosher presided (and quarreled) over women's instructional and extracurricular programs. A Stanford alumna in Zoology (B.A., 1893) and Physiology (M.A., 1894), Mosher had taught hygiene and gymnastic exercise and conducted physiological research as a student.[103] Following medical education at the Johns Hopkins University (M.D., 1900) and some additional training, she returned to Palo Alto and set up a small private practice. In 1910 she became Stanford's Medical Advisor for Women, Assistant Professor of Hygiene, and director of women's physical education and Roble Gymnasium. Believing fervently that "physical freedom" was a woman's birthright, Mosher argued that social expectations, not the physical body, restricted female interests and aptitude. Once liberated from cultural myths, women could enjoy health and self-confidence by understanding their bodies, following the laws of hygiene, and engaging in vigorous activity, including intercollegiate sports. Mosher defended these convictions through research on sex differences, including strength, respiration, menstruation, and sexuality. While debunking conventional wisdom, she also maintained that physical activity should be sex-segregated and females should not compete during menses. Helen Masters Bunting was hired in 1919 as Associate Director of Physical Training and Personal Hygiene for Women. A graduate of Wellesley's program in Hygiene and Physical Education (1912), Bunting staunchly advocated mass recreation and intramural games at Stanford as well as through professional organizations. She was active in regional and national societies of college physical educators and served on the executive board of the Women's Division of the National Amateur Athletic Federation.

On paper, their responsibilities seemed clear: Mosher focused on medical services, while Bunting supervised physical education. This structure, however, did not prevent professional conflicts; as Medical Adviser, Mosher could arrange modified exercise for students with special needs.[104] Their strong personalities

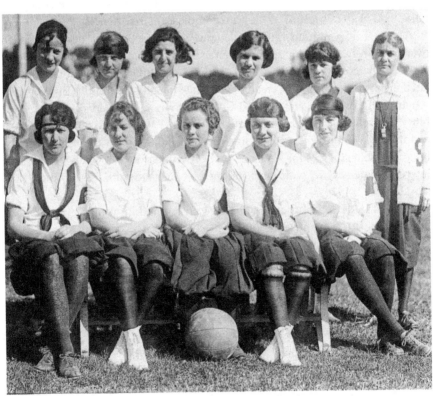

FIGURE 5.5 *Women's basketball team at Stanford University, 1924, with Helen Masters Bunting (back row, far right). Courtesy of Stanford Historical Photograph Collection, Department of Special Collections and University Archives, Stanford University Libraries, Stanford, California.*

also put the two women at odds. "On campus," Mosher's biographer notes, she "strove unreservedly to model the ideal of the active, self-reliant, sensible, unsentimental, productive, healthy, intellectual professional."[105] Mosher resented anyone or anything that interfered with her research and writing.[106] Bunting was a fussy administrator who clung tenaciously to her opinions on all matters, big or small—a stubbornness that irritated her colleagues.[107] Most importantly, their philosophies clashed; Bunting's conservative notions of women's health and sports soon overshadowed Mosher's liberalism.

When Bunting arrived, Stanford held most of its dwindling interclass-intercollegiate events with Mills College and the University of California at Berkeley.[108] Having formed a league in 1921, the three schools were conducting "triangle" as well as dual events by 1923. Pressure soon mounted, however, to reduce, even eliminate such activities. At its 1924 national conference hosted by Berkeley, the ACACW took a stand against varsity intercollegiate athletics. As affiliates of the organization, Triangle Conference members "went on record in support, for the present," of this strict policy, while politely asserting that extramural competition "has been successful" when conducted "under favorable conditions."[109] Over the next few years, the three schools organized field days, exhibitions, and Play Days with mixed teams, called "Triangle Sports Day" (TSD).[110] The new format appealed to Mills because it rarely had enough players or resources to field intact teams. Berkeley assented as well; since 1915–16, the school had staunchly favored intramural and low-key extramural events over varsity competition, a philosophy it maintained for decades to come.[111] Stanford's FCWA and physical educators also welcomed the switch to sociable Play Days; in February 1928 the department even recommended that competitive archery and swimming be replaced by "novelty" events and "amusing stunts."[112] After obeying for a few years, Stanford's undergraduates began criticizing the Play Day system, especially its "forced competition between arbitrarily chosen color teams" representing all three colleges. They sought alternate plans that would create more "unity" within teams and a "healthy, quite legitimate, and very ardent spirit of competition."[113] To quash this dangerous idea, Stanford's physical educators promptly reiterated their opinion that "mixed teams would foster more social contact which is the aim of Sports Day."[114] Reassured that no policy changes were forthcoming, the FCWA went into hiatus in 1929, while cautioning that the "need for Committee action might arise at any time," given "the present unrest in women's athletics."[115]

This warning proved correct. Over the next two decades, female athletes became more resentful of Stanford's habitual favoritism toward men. During the 1930s and 1940s the university responded to the rising stature and popularity of public institutions by concentrating anew on research and development. Academic departments were expected to acquire corporate and philanthropic funding, collaborate on projects, and produce useful knowledge. Reaffirming Stanford's masculine identity, this amalgam of scientific, economic, and military objectives transformed it into a nationally recognized entrepreneurial research institution.[116] By 1940 the university's "intense support of high-powered, utilitarian studies in the applied sciences," John Thelin notes, "coexisted with its traditional indulgence of an idyllic undergraduate social life and varsity sports program."[117] Social life meant fraternities and male culture (Stanford banned sororities in 1944), and varsity sports meant football. Objecting to the attention heaped on men's sports, female athletes pushed Stanford and its Triangle Conference partners toward gender equity.

The process began in the fall of 1929. Following Dr. Mosher's retirement, the university consolidated women's medical care, hygiene instruction, and physical education under one director.[118] Stanford's choice was Dr. Bertha Sabin Stuart Dyment, a graduate of the University of Michigan who had worked at Reed College and the University of Oregon. Departmental reorganization, though, meant little to WAA members; they kept protesting the mixed-squad format of TSD events, which undercut "team cooperation" and "stimulating competition."[119] By contrast, Berkeley students claimed to like Play Days with "positively religious fervor."[120] In 1931 Stanford coaxed its TSD partners to experiment with competition between intact teams of corresponding classes from each school with overall wins and losses tabulated by class year, not institution. By all accounts, the compromise worked. Stanford enjoyed the opportunity for team cohesion, while proudly noting that it would have won the overall competition had final scores been tallied by institution.[121] Despite a "few cases of school rivalry and tension," Berkeley had preserved mass participation and avoided the unthinkable, namely, intercollegiate competition with intensive practice and publicity.[122] Similarly, Mills College was content because the day-long TSD combined social activities and inclusive, nonvarsity contests.[123] Emboldened, Stanford's WAA suggested other TSD schemes, such as an annual series of Sports Days. Berkeley rejected the idea because it "would lead almost inevitably toward intercollegiate competition," creating "unpleasant feelings" due to Stanford's aggressive mind-set.[124]

While courting its TSD partners, Stanford's WAA also sought staff approval of new TSD arrangements along with more varsity competition against non-TSD opponents.[125] Most department members took the requests seriously. To determine if TSD events involving some type of intact school teams conformed to national standards, the staff consulted professional leaders in the WD-NAAF and ACACW and learned that occasional class-based games were permissible, as long as no major championship was being contested. Despite frowning on varsity competition, Stanford's physical educators also proposed limited intercollegiate events among TSD schools in archery, swimming, tennis, and golf. Finally, although the department vetoed events against distant schools, it approved some interclass intercollegiate games against nearby non-TSD institutions.[126] Except for Helen Bunting, who doggedly defended the status quo until her departure in 1934, the department concluded that moderate reforms would

stimulate interest in sports and afford "opportunities for keener and more sat-
isfying competition and practice," especially for talented students.[127] Although
this flexibility owed much to departmental reorganization and new personnel,
female students had set the pace and the agenda.

The WAA's paradigm was men's college sports; female athletes wanted to
compete as representatives of Stanford University on a varsity basis against
numerous institutions in multiple sports. No other arrangement seemed as exciting or rewarding to them. From the mid-1930s to late 1940s, Stanford's WAA
inched closer toward this goal. In 1934 the students proposed that TSD events
be scored by college, not class. Although Berkeley reluctantly consented, Mills
College vetoed the plan because it smacked of varsity competition.[128] Undeterred, Stanford's WAA approached non-TSD schools and also renewed its
campaign for intercollegiate, not interclass, TSD events.[129] Rebuffed by Mills
and Berkeley through the early 1940s, Stanford's WAA nevertheless effected
important changes at home. In 1947 the Department of Physical Education for
Women endorsed new policies for extramural sports that clearly acknowledged
intercollegiate competition as students' preference and entitlement.[130] Reform
soon spread to its TSD partners. When Berkeley's female athletes agitated
for more liberal policies in the early 1950s, the institution gradually modified
philosophies and practices that had been in place for decades.[131] These developments brought Triangle Sports Day to an end in 1952; it was immediately
replaced by the Bay Area Sports Day involving numerous contests for six area
schools.

These changes culminated several decades of negotiation between Stanford's female athletes, who wanted opportunities consistent with their talent
and competitive instincts, and the department's staff members, many of whom
gradually agreed. The athletes' position exemplified female students' general
response to Stanford's devaluation of their activities. As the university shored
up its masculine image during the first half of the twentieth century, women
undergraduates built a separate campus culture that supported their interests
and identity. When Stanford embraced men's varsity sports, female athletes
insisted on their fair share of competition. Constructing an alternate version of
active womanhood, women at a coeducational institution had successfully nar-
rowed the gap—both real and symbolic—between male and female athleticism.

Together, the stories of Bryn Mawr and Stanford illustrate the power of
feminist ideas in the realm of active bodies. In the former example, administrators and teachers believed that gender equality should include the body
as well as the mind. In the latter case, women undergraduates challenged the
privileges accruing to men under old ideologies and practices of gender; they
demanded parity on the athletic field as well as in the classroom. Although
neither institution disrupted elite white codes of class or race, female staff and
students used extramural athletics to blur traditional sex differences and reset
gender relations.

Historically Black Colleges and Universities

Undergraduates at Stanford and Bryn Mawr were part of white America's
march to college in the early twentieth century. A "culture of aspiration" convinced many families as well as government leaders, the business community,
and nascent professions that a college education was worthwhile, even essential
in a knowledge-based modern society. Widespread poverty and discrimination,
however, made this goal seem out of reach to many African Americans.[132] In
the mid-1930s, the total number of black undergraduates at predominantly
white colleges and universities averaged between fifteen hundred and two thousand per year.[133] Racism was especially strong at the country's most prestigious
institutions; between 1880 and 1960, only about five hundred black women
graduated from the Seven Sister colleges.[134] Barred from most white institutions, African Americans typically enrolled at private black schools in the early
twentieth century.[135] Between 1914 and 1925 the number of historically black
colleges and universities (HBCUs) increased 81 percent. Their combined enrollment rose from about two thousand in 1920 to fourteen thousand in 1930,
with women students becoming the overall majority. Although some single-sex
HBCUs gained prominence, most were coeducational. Extracurricular physical
activities for black female undergraduates were quite diverse. Despite meager
resources, most HBCUs organized broad intramural programs as well as May
festivals, gymnastic demonstrations, and other special events. Many participated in Play Days and Sport Days and a sizable number sponsored varsity-
style intercollegiate competition, but others soundly rejected such contests.

These varied opportunities were neither static nor uniform. Each institution's policies, especially about extramural sports, developed within a unique
context. Although some HBCUs were operated by black denominational societies, most relied on private white donors, including northern industrialists,
corporate foundations, and white benevolent and religious associations. At
many HBCUs, white trustees, administrators, and teachers dominated; elsewhere, African American faculty and staff held power. Some HBCUs emphasized vocational and industrial training; others featured liberal arts curricula to
prepare the "talented tenth"—W. E. B. Du Bois' term for America's black elite.
Together, a school's specific mission, financial base, religious affiliation, governance system, and racial composition influenced its decisions about women's
extracurricular physical activities.

These deliberations connected black campuses to broader discussions about
black womanhood. For decades, African American women had debated whether
to imitate middle-class white femininity, develop more authentic representations of their lives, or combine these two paths. While engaging white norms of
gender, black women also positioned themselves as African Americans. If black
women depicted themselves as identical to black men, they risked accusations
of mannishness; on the other hand, any suggestion that African Americans

differed sharply by sex might render racial progress more difficult. These issues were especially contentious in the domain of sports. Black activists and educators wondered if athletics would advance or hinder integration. While many white Americans believed that sports could help African Americans assimilate, the prospect of unfettered black athleticism alarmed them. Thus, whenever a black college or university contemplated women's sports, it entered a minefield of disagreements over gender, race, difference, and equality.

The following case studies examine three disparate HBCUs: Hampton Institute, an independent, coeducational, white-run school with practical curricula; Tuskegee Institute, a nondenominational, coeducational school with an industrial focus, black personnel, and close ties to white business leaders; and Spelman College, a women's school founded by white Baptists that maintained a fairly academic curriculum and predominantly white staff through the 1920s. Guided by unique characteristics, each institution pondered whether women's extracurricular sports should accentuate or minimize apparent differences between blacks and whites, males and females, elite and lower-class Americans. The strongest voices in the historical record are those of teachers, administrators, trustees, and benefactors; archival materials offer few direct clues about athletes' views.

HAMPTON INSTITUTE

Founded in 1868, Hampton Normal and Agricultural Institute was a quasi-public coeducational pre-collegiate school for young blacks, primarily from the rural South; Native American students arrived in 1878. The Institute's curricula, rigid discipline, and daily manual labor reflected the belief of its first principal, General Samuel C. Armstrong, and his fellow white administrators that Americans of color needed moral guidance even more than intellectual training. Rather than produce tradesmen or industrial workers, their goal was a corps of black schoolteachers who would "model particular social values and transmit them to the Afro-American South," thereby helping blacks adjust to their "subordinate social role in the [region's] political economy."[136] By the late nineteenth century, the "Hampton Model" of black education and racial subservience gained support from industrial philanthropists and some white religious organizations, as well as opposition.[137] During the Institute's first half-century, most of its trustees, senior administrators, and faculty members also were white.[138]

Initially, whites also prevailed among the physical educators who taught the Institute's female students and the children at Whittier, Hampton's elementary school where prospective teachers practiced. From the early 1890s until 1909, most female gym teachers were graduates of the Boston Normal School of Gymnastics (BNSG).[139] Although the schools' formal arrangement ended when Wellesley College absorbed the BNSG, Hampton still hired the program's white graduates during the 1910s. This racial preference apparently continued through the 1920s, when Hampton turned to other sources, especially the Central School of Hygiene and Physical Education in New York City. Hampton understood exactly whom it was hiring: white teachers of general recreation and sports, female experts in formal calisthenics, and disciples of the play-for-play's-sake philosophy promulgated by leading white professionals.

The resulting program clearly distinguished girls' activities from boys'.[140] In the 1880s Hampton conducted gymnastic classes for most female students and military drill for their male classmates. By the turn of the twentieth century, the girls' instructional program expanded to include a three-year requirement, anthropometric tests and medical exams, and occasional hygiene lectures. Because Hampton had long maintained that the "most effective physical training for boys [was] found in well-regulated athletics," few male students had physical education.[141] This changed in 1916 when physical training became mandatory for all students in most divisions, from preparatory and academic to business, trade, and agriculture. By this time, instruction for girls included games and sports; lessons in posture and dance were added shortly after World War I.

Girls' extracurricular activities also followed a conservative white model. Roller skating and croquet were available in the 1880s and 1890s. By 1910 the Institute required girls to participate in outdoor recreation on their own two afternoons a week. Hampton also organized intramural competition in tennis, basketball, baseball, croquet, volleyball, and field hockey. In 1911 these activities became the responsibility of the newly formed Girls Athletic Association, which eventually devised a system of points and awards to recognize participants' achievements in athletics, academics, health, and "spirit." By 1918 the Institute held an annual May Day festival as well as an intramural Field Day with interclass competition.

Besides imposing white standards on a black student body, the program also perpetuated racial stereotypes. Following the lead of Hampton's trustees and senior officers, white gym teachers inventoried black pupils' many shortcomings. According to Lucy Pratt, youngsters at the Whittier Training School suffered "pathetic physical neglect and inefficiency." Pratt hoped that proper exercise would relieve the children's "sluggish" minds and "unfairly equipped bodies."[142] Jessie Coope, who taught at the Institute for fifteen years, claimed that Hampton girls, like black females generally, showed little interest in outdoor recreation. With only a "latent" instinct for play, she declared in 1904, black children lacked a sense of imagination and "joyful amusement" during games.[143] Some physical educators attributed pupils' difficulties to their troubled backgrounds and lack of physical training.[144] At least one gym teacher worried that Hampton's rigorous schedule only worsened youngsters' problems.[145] For most instructors, though, the pupils were not so much disadvantaged as deficient; they belonged to "a race peculiarly handicapped, in certain respects, on the physical side."[146]

Regardless of how teachers answered the nature/nurture question, they set out to improve students' knowledge, skills, and values. Physical training embodied Hampton's central doctrine that blacks should emulate white America's high principles but also prepare to live and work as a segregated underclass. This adjustment began with fitness tests and medical exams that revealed students' health problems. Hygiene lectures then provided tools for the youngsters' unending "struggle against dirt and disorder." Games and organized recreation developed strong bodies and quick minds for the rigors ahead. Calisthenics and marching drills afforded practice in discipline, control, and responsiveness to commands. Structured exercise promoted the vigor, "poise and self-reliance" necessary for blacks to "take a firm, decided, and successful stand" in the world.[147] Training individual girls, white teachers believed, was comparable to influencing the entire black race. Echoing a familiar Institute slogan, Olive Rowell observed in 1920 that "every Hampton graduate is potentially and actually, if not nominally, a teacher" who would communicate to other blacks, "by precept or example, the art of living."[148] Practical roles lay ahead as well. When Institute alumnae "go out among their own people," another teacher explained, they will use the knowledge and strength acquired through physical education to organize neighborhood activities and advise families and communities on health, hygiene, and sanitation.[149]

Though necessary, these basic objectives were insufficient. White gym teachers believed that Hampton girls should aspire to nobler ideals, however unattainable. Intramural athletics and field days taught self-control, fair play, and inclusive recreation. Whereas boys' varsity teams emphasized victories, girls would come to understand that, win or lose, "'the game's the thing.'" Although "everything goes wrong," those who competed were always champions.[150] By participating in the Girls Athletic Association, students might learn "to handle their own [teams]—under some supervision," and regard athletic points and awards as symbols of diligence, not raw skill.[151] Finally, dance class and May Day festivals encouraged refinement and grace, offsetting black girls' coarseness. Together, these experiences were designed to lift Institute students toward more dignified lives.

In sum, Hampton's program constructed black womanhood along several axes of difference during the early 1900s. White gym teachers never doubted that African American females, by virtue of race, were destined for social subservience, with no hope of escaping a humble lower-class status. Physical activities also embodied white middle-class femininity, unsullied by masculine athleticism. This project did not signify assimilation, much less equality; although gym teachers envisioned Hampton's girls in traditional female roles, they expected alumnae to fall well short of white respectability. These overlapping ideologies of race, class, and gender precluded girls' competitive sports during Hampton's early decades.

Following World War I, Hampton matured as an institution of higher learning.[152] By the late 1920s nearly 40 percent of its students were at college level, coursework featured more liberal arts, and four-year B.S. degrees became available. This transformation mirrored general trends in black higher education.[153] When HBCUs prioritized postsecondary and professional studies, they attracted older, more qualified students; conversely, as more African Americans graduated from high school and sought college degrees, black institutions upgraded their admissions standards and curricula.

Campus life also changed. The experiences of black troops during World War I and the work of black intellectuals, artists, and writers in the 1920s heightened undergraduates' racial consciousness.[154] More interested in popular culture than political activism, other black collegians invented unique campus traditions and balked at their schools' dictatorial regulations.[155] This restiveness concerned W. E. B. Du Bois, who believed that black college men's preference for "selfish and even silly ideals" over the "hard grind of study and research" simply mimicked white student behavior.[156] Equally dismayed, Lucy Slowe, Howard University's dean of women, warned that frivolity was inundating serious academic work at black schools.[157]

Hampton put a local stamp on these national trends. In a widely publicized strike in 1927, students mobilized against the Institute's "low academic standards and repressive racial policies."[158] Some administrators agreed; during his eleven-year tenure (1918–29), James Edgar Gregg, Hampton's third white principal, implemented college-level studies, hired more black personnel, and introduced curricula and cultural programs featuring African American themes.[159] Opposing these steps toward racial equality, Hampton's white benefactors and trustees strengthened its conservative character and financial base. Although Gregg's resignation in 1929 "brought a temporary peace to the campus," notes the historian Raymond Wolters, two critical questions remained: "Was Hampton to be a vocational institute or a standard college?" Second, would it continue to be a black school run by whites?[160] The ensuing struggle over identity and power during Hampton's "troubled years" involved students, teachers, administrators, alumni, trustees, and donors, and affected department organization, faculty appointments, and curricular and extracurricular programs.[161]

In 1931/32 the Institute combined men's and women's physical activity programs into a single department headed by Charles H. Williams (1886–1978). A 1909 Hampton graduate and star athlete, Williams was studying at the YMCA International Training School when Hampton hired him in 1911 as physical director for boys.[162] Departmental consolidation, Williams argued, would promote "better cooperation and better efficiency" between general instruction, professional training, and intramural and intercollegiate sports. He recommended that the new unit's director be "responsible to the dean," while the "one teacher in charge of the work for the women [would report] to the head of the department."[163]

The new structure coincided with important staff changes.[164] The first leader of the women's division was Mary C. Baker, a white woman who held a professional diploma as well as a B.S. degree in Education.[165] Baker's apparent successor in 1937 was Grace C. Wood, who graduated from New York City's Central School of Hygiene and Physical Education and served at Hampton, with several breaks, from 1923 to 1944.[166] Concurrently, the program began hiring black women. From the early 1930s to the mid-1950s, more than three-quarters of appointments in women's physical education were African Americans, including many Hampton and Tuskegee alumnae.[167] One notable hire was Charlotte E. Moton, the daughter of Robert R. Moton, a Hampton graduate who succeeded Booker T. Washington as head of Tuskegee Institute.[168] By the late 1940s black women held most, if not all, positions in women's physical education at Hampton.[169]

This shift mirrored the Institute's changing racial profile.[170] By 1939 about 46 percent of its officers, instructors, and other workers were black. In 1940 the school appointed three African American senior administrators to serve under its new president (a white male). These numbers, however, did not appease Hampton's critics who insisted that power distribution, not head counting, constituted the true measure of racial equality at an HBCU. This controversy over racial composition and governance loomed over Director Williams and black female gym teachers throughout the 1930s and 1940s.

Williams's annual reports typically opened with an extensive review of men's intercollegiate and intramural athletics, followed by brief descriptions of men's and women's instructional programs and women's extracurricular activities, with occasional summaries by the female supervisor.[171] This format continued the primacy that men's sports had enjoyed at the Institute for several decades. In 1912 Hampton and four other black institutions—Howard, Lincoln, Shaw, and Virginia Union—established the Colored Intercollegiate Athletic Association. The CIAA arranged competitive events among members and developed rules about recruiting and eligibility. While adding members and enduring controversy in the 1930s and 1940s, the CIAA also "ran a modest program for women" in field hockey and track and field, but these efforts had little visibility or success.[172]

As a CIAA founder, Williams was keenly aware of the racial politics of sports. Properly conducted, he believed, athletics could foster "racial pride" and "create new friends for the race."[173] To this end, he expanded competitive opportunities for black boys and men. When the CIAA banned pre-collegiate students from varsity sports in 1931, Williams devised alternate forms of competition for upper-level boys in Hampton's Trade School.[174] In 1936/37 he proposed that men's intramural season conclude with games between the winning teams and other schools, thereby extending elite competition to nonvarsity athletes.[175] He also convinced the Institute to host tournaments for black high schools and national amateur groups, because segregation had limited their competitive venues.

These opportunities, however, had to be governed by high standards. By endorsing the CIAA's most stringent policies, Williams hoped to inspire equally strong "ideals of fair play and sportsmanship" among black high schools.[176] Perhaps white Americans, too, would notice the absence of "pitfalls and mistakes" in black sports programs and begin judging blacks "on their merit" as talented, decent individuals. Convinced that interracial activities could teach respect and understanding, Williams also took Hampton teams to athletic contests and social events at white colleges.[177]

Williams's reformist approach was not unique. During the interwar period, black educators and activists debated the implications of high-powered sports for race relations; whereas some believed that competition could foster black pride and racial assimilation, critics maintained that the athletic field was neither an appropriate nor viable arena for equality.[178] Holding the former view, Williams assured Hampton that its clean, high-minded program would replace white stereotypes of black physicality with positive symbols of skill and dignity. Institute leaders also anticipated that sports would further Hampton's transition from a pre-collegiate industrial school into an institution of higher learning. Given America's growing fascination with sports, Hampton decided to pursue credibility and burnish its image on the playing field as well as in the classroom.

The athletes, however, had to be male. While boys earned victories and acclaim, their female classmates learned noncompetitive femininity through inclusive instructional programs and extracurricular activities.[179] In keeping with national trends, women's gym classes gradually favored recreation and sports over basic exercise. When Mary C. Baker proposed in 1935 that Hampton's annual class demonstration include only the best performers, Director Williams demurred: the event was educational, he asserted, precisely because it involved every student, regardless of skill.[180] Similarly, most extracurricular activities for female students during the 1930s and 1940s emphasized mass participation and social interaction. The Institute organized intramural tournaments, festivals, and meets; it offered individual and dual sports as well as team sports, along with various recreational activities, from archery and roller skating to hiking, camping, and swimming. After grumbling that girls preferred socializing over physical activity, Williams tried enticing them with a "Women's Day," a noncompetitive festival consisting "of games, athletic events, dances and crowning a May Queen."[181]

The same philosophy governed extramural activities. In the early 1930s Mary C. Baker quietly arranged out-of-town tennis matches and other intercollegiate contests for the women's division—a practice that got her fired.[182] President Arthur Howe denounced Baker's "over-emphasis on the more strenuous athletic type of game" and her regrettable "lack of refinement." Although Williams applauded Baker's competence and efficiency, he objected that her preference for competitive games excluded less athletic girls, while her indifference to the "esthetic side" of physical education contradicted Hampton's values.[183]

   Shortly after Baker's dismissal, the Institute sanctioned an acceptably tame version of extramural sports. Beginning in 1938/39, Hampton, Howard University, and Virginia State College organized a series of Women's Sports Days, including volleyball, relays, folk dancing, basketball, ping pong, archery, and track and field.[184] These events soon evolved into the Women's Sports Day Association (WSDA) with Bennett College and other new members. A regular WSDA participant during the 1940s and early 1950s, Hampton endorsed the group's values of "cooperation, fair play, and high interest and appreciation for athletics."[185] The Institute's WAA climbed on board by arranging events and administering a conventional system of points and awards. The WSDA, Director Williams happily observed, sparked interest in Hampton's intramural program, introduced girls to various sports, and gave them "an opportunity to see other institutions, to study and compare life and programs, to get acquainted, and to develop real friendships among the girls from other schools."[186] In the gym and on the playing field, the stark contrast between black masculinity and black femininity was now set.

   Only the dance floor remained. During the 1930s and 1940s, dance became a regular feature of Hampton's cultural endeavors and physical education curriculum, with the acclaimed Creative Dance Group taking center stage.[187] These activities extended the Institute's performing arts tradition, from the Hampton Singers and other touring ensembles in the late 1800s to the incorporation of dance into gym class and campus concerts during the early 1900s.[188] Interest in dance as a distinct art form flourished at Hampton in the 1920s and early 1930s. Although a 1925 visit by the famed Denishawn dance company, directed by Ruth St. Denis and Ted Shawn, stirred racial tension, it also created a durable bond between Shawn and Williams.[189] Adding to the momentum was the growing expertise of Hampton's instructors and choreographers, who founded a student group with a repertoire of African and American dances.[190] Performing before black and white audiences throughout the South and Northeast, the ensemble gradually convinced skeptics that concert dance was an honorable activity for young blacks.[191]

   Williams and his colleagues regarded esthetic movement as a vital component of physical education and personal growth. It not only improved coordination, "posture and carriage," Charlotte Moton declared, but also produced "an increase in morale, in self confidence and out-going friendliness."[192] Only certain styles of dance, though, were edifying. Whereas social dance, cheap theatrical exhibitions, and wild, sensuous movements were degrading, the staff explained, dignified dance forms fostered self-respect among participants and allowed black and white spectators to witness young African Americans moving "with intelligent proficiency."[193] Besides affirming blacks' humanity, public performances could also safeguard and celebrate a distinctive black culture. The Institute's dance program thereby walked a fine line between the school's conservative roots and racial consciousness, between its founders' objectives and the "New Negro's" aspirations.[194]

At stake were the meanings of gender and sexuality as well as "blackness." Hampton's Creative Dance Group included male and female students directed by teachers of their own sex. Because black and white Americans alike associated rhythmic and artistic endeavors with femininity, women's participation was not controversial. During the 1930s, however, men's domination of the ensemble's membership and performances seemed problematic; dancing's expressive, even erotic character might conjure up white stereotypes of black sexuality.[195] For centuries, Western culture had portrayed blacks as hypersexual beings whose animalistic drives ruled their savage bodies; the primitive black man supposedly preyed on white women, while black females embodied lewd promiscuity. Feeding into anti-miscegenation laws and the eugenics movement in the early 1900s, these racist myths endured well into the 1930s and 1940s when Hampton's male dancers took the stage.

If uncontrolled heterosexuality might tarnish dance, the specter of homosexuality loomed equally large: Perhaps the Institute's male performers were "pretty boys" whose artistry betrayed effeminacy and sexual deviance? This suspicion dated from the mid-nineteenth century when middle-class Americans and Europeans differentiated more sharply between femininity and masculinity. One step was to deplore any form of male spectacle, from men in dramatic attire to male nudes in art; the male dancer's apparent softness and sensitivity now implied a feminine esthetic at odds with masculine power and rationality.[196] The failure to be a "man's man" seemed not merely peculiar but abnormal—a sign of homosexual pathology. Black homosexuality seemed especially dangerous; since the turn of the twentieth century, white doctors and scientists had asserted that black gays and lesbians threatened the nation's moral fabric by luring white Americans into degenerate, hedonistic lifestyles.[197]

The twin images of unrestrained heterosexuality and infectious homosexuality haunted Hampton's dance program during the 1930s and 1940s. To normalize the artistic black body, the Institute had to reassure white and black spectators alike that its male performers were "real" men. Single-sex dances displayed male bodies and character in isolation, free of the explosive suggestion of heterosexual contact. To avoid the taint of homosexuality, men's dances exuded power and muscularity. In his choreography based on African stories and ceremonies, Williams "took the African ideal of the warrior-athlete and turned it into an African-American ideal." Other pieces created masculine imagery by incorporating "high-energy athleticism and movement motifs drawn from sports activities such as boxing, sprinting, and shot-putting."[198]

Overall, physical education, sports, and dance at Hampton established a sharp gender duality, inflected by race, sexuality, and class. The model spoke simultaneously to white and black constituencies. By emphasizing ethical, well-managed competition for men and wholesome recreation for women, Hampton placated its white donors and trustees, while also asserting black dignity and solidarity. Whereas Hampton's white physical educators in the 1910s and 1920s had prepared alumnae for second-class citizenship, their black successors in the 1930s and 1940s envisioned graduates who could fit into white society while retaining their racial identity. The orderly, reserved style of the Creative Dance Group likewise suited the Institute's conservative origins and the cultural reality of white dominance; feminine grace and masculine power undercut white assumptions about black sexuality and degeneracy. Here too, however, Hampton's black teachers asserted a critical race difference; by celebrating the history and cultures that inspired its distinctive esthetic, the dance program fostered black pride and autonomy. Finally, active bodies furthered Hampton's class aspirations. From its founding through the 1920s, the Institute's milieu had been lower-class—a training ground for young rural blacks to become menial workers. During the interwar years, by contrast, the school delivered liberal arts curricula and bourgeois sports, recreation, and dance to college-level students. Hampton thereby hoped to associate itself with Howard and other academic schools rather than its original partners in industrial education.

TUSKEGEE INSTITUTE

By the late nineteenth century, the "Hampton Model" of black education became known as the "Hampton-Tuskegee Idea." The new name recognized Tuskegee Institute, the other exemplar of vocational training for young African Americans. Located in rural Alabama, Tuskegee was founded in 1881 by Booker T. Washington, an ex-slave and Hampton graduate who was the nation's foremost black advocate of industrial education and served as Tuskegee's principal until his death in 1915.

During its early history Tuskegee seemed to be Hampton's twin. Their social philosophies, moral focus, and rudimentary coursework reflected mutual ties to northern white businessmen. After World War I both evolved into full-fledged academic colleges. Two significant differences, though, also stand out. Tuskegee's teachers and administrators were black and, from the 1920s on, it sponsored competitive sports for female students, eventually producing world-class athletes in track and field. These two features were interrelated. The dynamics of an all-black coeducational campus affected how Tuskegee interpreted female physicality; conversely, women's athletics shaped the Institute's identity as a school of and for African Americans.

The Tuskegee State Normal School opened in a black church with one teacher, thirty pupils, and a modest public appropriation. Several decades later, it boasted substantial facilities and a healthy endowment. In 1915 about 60 percent of its 1,338 students were male, one-half hailed from Alabama, and most were enrolled in the elementary grades.[199] The administrative and instructional staff comprised several dozen black men and women, including graduates of other black institutions. During Washington's tenure, Tuskegee emphasized hands-on experience in agricultural, mechanical, and domestic trades as well as discipline and upright character.[200] It dictated pupils' schedules, chose their clothing, inspected their rooms, and monitored their behavior. The school expected staff members, especially single women, to be equally well behaved. If a pupil or instructor violated its code of conduct, Tuskegee promptly scolded, punished, or dismissed them.[201]

This educational system reflected Washington's accommodationist philosophy of race relations. Articulated most notably during a speech at the Cotton States and International Exposition in Atlanta in 1895, Washington's "Atlanta Compromise" focused on economic adjustment, not racial justice or political equality. To this end, Tuskegee Institute prepared graduates who would help other African Americans in the Deep South adapt to segregation and white domination.[202] The Institute also spread its ideology by operating a bank, dairy, hospital, and power plant for black townspeople as well as numerous outreach programs among black farmers and homemakers in rural Alabama.[203]

Washington's Atlanta Compromise appealed to the elite whites who financed Tuskegee Institute and served on its Board of Trustees. Although the private, nondenominational school received some state and federal aid, it relied primarily on donations from northern white businessmen and their philanthropic agencies, including the General Education Board, Slater Fund, and Carnegie Foundation. These benefactors assembled the "Tuskegee Machine," a powerful coalition of top educators, political figures, and members of the white and black press who promoted the school through well-orchestrated campaigns. By contrast, many black intellectuals, educators, and religious leaders criticized Tuskegee for undermining racial progress by surrendering to white interests.[204]

The school's conservatism permeated its physical activities. Initially, boys participated in military drill, while most girls learned calisthenics, practical hygiene, and Swedish gymnastics. Games and swimming were added for girls by 1905.[205] Although rigid schedules left little time for extracurricular programs, the Institute organized athletic teams for boys by the mid-1890s as well as exhibitions and intramural basketball for girls by the early 1900s.[206] Officials justified these activities on several grounds. Supervised exercise would "counteract the evils resulting from habitually incorrect positions" and poor breathing in the classroom as well as the imbalances associated with manual labor.[207] Physical training instilled positive habits and values; boys' drills taught "neatness and unquestioning obedience," while girls' Swedish exercise fostered "'ease, precision, and economy of force'" along with "'equanimity, patience, and self-confidence.'"[208] Finally, health instruction corrected the ignorance and poor hygiene that seemed prevalent among African Americans.[209]

Overseeing girls' activities before World War I was a small staff of black teachers whose appointments typically lasted only a few years, with two exceptions. In 1899 Tuskegee hired Azalie Thomas (1874–1935), a New Orleans native and Hampton alumna who was the BNSG's first black graduate.[210] When Thomas left after about five years, she was succeeded by Amelia M. Cromwell

(Roberts), who held a diploma from the Sargent School and spent her career at Tuskegee (1905–10, 1918–54).[211] Their program of formal exercise, group demonstrations, intramural sports, and hygiene instruction resembled that of many black and white schools in the early 1900s. The tone at Tuskegee, however, was unusually serious; by depicting exercise as more duty than pleasure, as training rather than culture, physical education brought the Atlanta Compromise into the gym.

During the early tenure of Washington's successor, Dr. Robert R. Moton (1915–35), women's physical education continued formal gymnastics and hygiene along with instructional and intramural athletics.[212] Between 1925 and 1935 extramural sports appeared. Secondary-level girls and, later, college students played basketball and tennis against black high schools, colleges, and YWCAs; interschool golf was short-lived because opponents were scarce.[213] The development of track and field was especially important not only for Tuskegee pupils but also for young black athletes throughout the South. The program's signature event was the Tuskegee Relays. Initiated in 1927 and open to girls in 1929, this annual meet featured track and field but offered tennis and golf matches as well. By 1933 the Relays drew more than five hundred competitors and coaches from more than sixty institutions. The Institute's participants were a select group of boys and girls; recruited from southern black high schools,

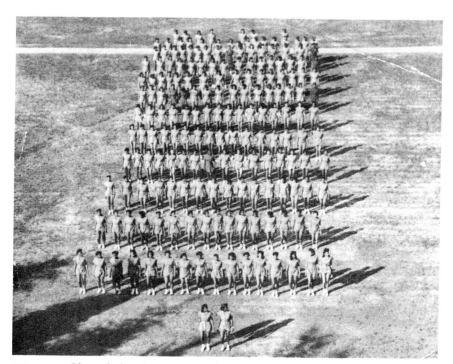

FIGURE 5.6 *Physical education students in formation at Tuskegee Institute. Courtesy of Tuskegee University Archives, Tuskegee University.*

the most talented girls often attended a special summer camp at Tuskegee, got work-aid positions upon matriculation, and trained with the boys' team.

Tuskegee's program was well known but not unique. Because custom and law excluded African American girls and women from white-controlled sports, they found high-level competition through black church groups, independent clubs, community centers, high schools, industrial and normal schools, and national sports organizations.[214] Although tennis, baseball, and basketball drew many participants, track and field was especially popular in school and non-school settings. Annual meets at Alabama State College and Prairie View A&M in Texas included women's events during the late 1930s. Fort Valley State of Georgia, Florida A&M, and other black schools sent female athletes to the Tuskegee Relays. Initiated in the mid-1940s, women's competitive track and field at the Tennessee Agricultural and Industrial State Normal School (later Tennessee State) gradually eclipsed Tuskegee as the nation's leading program. These opportunities, however, engendered debate. Although favorable reports of women's sports appeared in black newspapers, some African American writers and educators expressed misgivings: Would talented female sprinters and basketball teams encourage black pride and white respect or reinforce mainstream stereotypes of athletic black females as masculine and unrefined?

This controversy may have inspired the *Tuskegee Messenger*'s glowing images of campus athletes as "ebony Apollos" and "bronze Dianas."[215] The responsibility for developing these admirable competitors fell to Tuskegee's physical educators and coaches. At the helm was Cleveland L. Abbott (1894–1955).[216] A star athlete and graduate of South Dakota State College, Abbott taught at Tuskegee in 1916. After serving in World War I and working at a vocational school in Topeka, Kansas, Abbott returned to the Institute in 1923 and, until his retirement in the early 1950s, coached football, directed the Department of Physical Education and Athletics (a combined men's and women's program as of 1930), supervised the majors program (established in 1933), and organized the Tuskegee Relays. His wife, Jessie H. Abbott (1897–1981), was a key ally.[217] A native of Des Moines, Jessie studied business in high school and married Cleve just before he departed for war duty. Besides raising their daughter, Mrs. Abbott served at Tuskegee as a secretary for Mrs. Booker T. Washington, Mrs. Robert R. Moton, and Dr. George Washington Carver. A skilled athlete in her own right, Mrs. Abbott was a generous volunteer who coached golf and traveled with the girls' track and field team. Equally important were Tuskegee's female physical educators. Although Amelia C. Roberts, the most senior instructor, coached basketball and nominally headed the women's division through the 1940s, her roles diminished as Cleve Abbott strengthened the program through new appointments. Louise Atkins, who held degrees from Howard and Cornell, worked in the department between 1930 and 1934. Her successor was Christine (Evans) Petty, a Tuskegee physical education graduate and member of its first women's track team.[218]

Abbott and his staff created a nuanced model of femininity, athleticism, and black identity. To begin, they aligned Tuskegee's female athletes with white middle-class femininity and heterosexuality—a standard that, ostensibly, left little room for black females, much less sportswomen. Physical activity's function, the school insisted, was not to churn out star athletes but to complement the Institute's overall mission by developing character, enriching personal experience, teaching purpose and perseverance, and cultivating leadership.[219] To refute common impressions of black sportswomen, Tuskegee polished athletes' appearance and manners through lessons in clothes and etiquette.[220] The refined aura of golf and tennis also helped offset track and field's image of working-class masculinity. The final hurdle was extramural competition, which struck many white Americans as corrupting and unladylike. Tuskegee's version of varsity competition, the school responded, "tolerates only clean and wholesome sport, and aims to promote good sportsmanship among contestants and spectators."[221] In short, because Tuskegee's "bronze Dianas" were feminine and honorable, white Americans had little cause for disparaging them.

Abbott and his colleagues also described athletic womanhood in distinctly African American terms. Womanly, but not white, they observed, Tuskegee girls had a strength and resolve that black females routinely displayed in their families, jobs, and communities without compromising their femininity. While the two sexes held certain qualities and rights in common, they should not be regarded as identical. Apollos wrestled and played football, but Dianas did not. Institute boys played basketball by boys' rules, whereas girls' teams involved six players on a divided court.[222] As prospective teachers, Institute girls learned "elementary athletic games" along with "rhythms, singing games and folk dances," while boys practiced "conative contests adapted to large groups" and various "games of high organization."[223]

Overall, this portrait of active black womanhood incorporated similarities and differences across race and gender. Laying claim to femininity, the Institute granted black girls a measure of respectability usually reserved for white Americans. Tuskegee's ideal diverged from white middle-class norms, though, by affirming physical challenges and vigor as womanly and expanding students' opportunities during and after their time at school. To narrow the gender divide, the Institute asserted both sexes' right to be athletic. Equality on the playing field resonated with black Americans' custom, born from mutual struggle, of interpreting gender on more egalitarian terms than did most white Americans. But in valuing both sexes, the Institute did not regard them as interchangeable; just as most black leaders saw sex differences as asymmetric, Tuskegee's program in physical education and sports was gendered and unequal.

Despite the staff's careful efforts, this viewpoint met resistance. Initially, black townspeople and Tuskegee students, especially boys, expressed misgivings about, even opposition to girls' sports. By the late 1930s and 1940s, however, support from athletes' families and the campus was fairly broad.[224]

Many administrators, faculty members, and their spouses also approved both girls' and boys' athletics. They attended football games, tennis matches, and the Tuskegee Relays, helped officiate at events, and wrote sports articles for the black press.[225] They also served as role models.[226] Informal networks and organized clubs afforded Tuskegee employees, their spouses, and other black professionals in town many competitive opportunities. During the 1920s, Tuskegee's Diana Athletic Club played basketball against female faculty from other black schools before enthusiastic spectators. Groomed in local tournaments, some tennis players became well known regionally and nationally; in 1933, Mrs. Jessie Abbott and her tennis partner from Fort Benning, Alabama, ranked second in women's doubles at the ATA national tournament. In practical and symbolic ways, adults created a friendly environment for girls' sports at Tuskegee.

Ultimately, however, the Institute's policies and reputation were the responsibility of the trustees and the principal. A creditable tennis player, Dr. Moton supported intercollegiate competition and believed in racial assimilation through sports.[227] Welcoming participants to the Tuskegee Relays in the early 1930s, he described the event as

> a significant development in the aspirations and development of our race where youth makes test of its prowess and confirms itself in its ability to achieve. . . . It identifies the Negro with the common interests of our national life. Strong, clean bodies; fine, high ideals; strenuous, open, even-handed rivalry; modest pride in success; general self-satisfaction in defeat are the prizes which all contestants win regardless of the allotment of cups and medals.[228]

Although Moton rarely commented on female competition, his administrative style and priorities were conducive to its development. First, he surely endorsed the program's emphasis on decorum. Under Moton's leadership, Tuskegee students "were subjected to as strict a disciplinary regime as that in force at any college of the 1920s." Besides prohibiting tobacco, alcohol, and foul language, the historian Raymond Wolters notes, the Institute "proclaimed its right to open and censor students' mail, and no dances were allowed until the 1930s."[229] Because rebellious staff and students either left or were forced out, Tuskegee seemed quiet compared to campuses where the "New Negro" had joined America's boisterous student culture.

Educational goals went hand in hand with rigid codes of conduct.[230] During the 1920s, Moton added more academic coursework, upgraded graduation requirements, and started a college-level division. Extracurricular activities burnished this new image. Skeptics notwithstanding, Tuskegee's teams largely escaped the scandals that engulfed many black and white universities during the interwar years and usually generated favorable publicity. Even a prominent black critic of college athletics cited Tuskegee in 1932 as one of only a few commendable programs among African American schools.[231]

The combination of tough regulations, curriculum reform, and good press appealed to Tuskegee's white trustees and fundraisers.[232] After World War I, corporate leaders grudgingly accepted higher education for black Americans and enabled Tuskegee, Hampton, and similar institutions to evolve into degree-granting colleges. Lest black ambitions rise too high or race relations deteriorate, however, white businessmen welcomed systems of campus deference and restraint.[233] Their demands suited Principal Moton, who had a well-deserved reputation of placating affluent whites with his recommendation that blacks "make peace with segregation."[234] At the same time, Moton defended the "principle of black autonomy." He granted relative freedom to departments at Tuskegee and also insisted that African Americans staff the local VA Hospital for blacks.[235] A new "Atlanta Compromise" had emerged, one that defended black independence within the bounds of segregation.

In sum, broad disputes over racial equality and black self-determination influenced how HBCUs interpreted gender and physicality during the interwar years. The governance systems and racial composition of Hampton Institute and Howard University inclined them to bring black womanhood into line with white standards. Although white donors and trustees also held sway at Tuskegee, the presence of strong black administrators and teachers during the late 1920s and early 1930s opened room for independent philosophies and policies. In this narrow space, the Institute's black physical educators and coaches affirmed black female athleticism.

Tuskegee's transition from industrial high school to comprehensive college continued under its next president, Frederick D. Patterson, who served from 1935 to 1953.[236] A veterinarian educated at Iowa State, Patterson joined Tuskegee's agriculture division in 1928. A Ph.D. from Cornell University in 1932 made him Tuskegee's first instructor with a doctorate. Determined to build a genuine baccalaureate institution, Patterson expanded the school's liberal arts curricula and resisted its enthusiasm for sports (his passion for tennis notwithstanding).[237] Alumni pressure for football victories, he maintained, should not derail the principle of amateurism nor overshadow Tuskegee's educational mission.[238] Together with the financial crisis of the Great Depression, Patterson's academic agenda led to "a gradual but continued de-emphasis on intercollegiate athletics" during his eighteen-year tenure.[239]

Although these factors complicated Director Abbott's job of balancing general service courses, professional training, and intramural and intercollegiate competition, the women's sports program thrived. The varsity basketball team played about eight games per year. Tennis gained momentum in the late 1930s with the arrival of Lula Ballard, one of the country's premier singles and doubles players. The women's track and field team excelled in national and international venues.[240] The program benefited from the appointment of female instructors who, as skilled athletes in their own right, were dedicated to women's sports.[241] Christine Evans Petty, a Tuskegee graduate, served as the first female coach of the women's track and field team from 1934 until her death in 1942. Roumania Peters, another alumna, taught tennis and basketball from 1945 to 1956. The second female coach of women's track and field was Nell C. Jackson (1929–88), another graduate and renowned runner, who worked at her alma mater in 1953–60 and 1962–63.

The department justified varsity sports for women and men by pointing to its role in building diligence and determination.[242] Physical training, though, was not a competitor's only responsibility; Abbott also required the "bone-heads" and "bunnies"—his nicknames for male and female athletes—to perform manual labor. During the 1940s they cleaned the swimming pool, marked the tennis courts, prepared and laid cinders for the running track, cleared the baseball diamonds, ran concession stands, and recorded game-day statistics. Reflecting Tuskegee's time-honored philosophy, these chores taught the dignity of labor, the spirit of mutual assistance, and respect for one's community. Maintaining the Institute's facilities, one football player recalled, was comparable to cleaning one's house before visitors arrived; the only difference was you then tried to beat your guests.[243]

Initially, women's teams faced only African American "guests." Racial segregation and meager resources confined the Institute's female athletes to on-campus events and contests with neighboring black schools and clubs; until 1936 the Tuskegee Relays constituted their only intercollegiate competition in track and field. When the team ventured onto the national stage in the late 1930s, however, members began competing against white women. The team participated—as the only collegiate group, black or white—in the annual indoor and outdoor national championships of the Amateur Athletic Union (AAU); it won six consecutive titles in 1937–42 and a total of eleven senior championships in 1937–48. Entering international competition for the first time in 1948, several current and former Tuskegee students were among the nine blacks on the eleven-member U.S. women's track team at the Olympic Games, and Alice Coachman's gold medal in the high jump was the "only individual track-and-field medal won by U.S. women" and the "first medal ever received by a woman of African descent."[244] As a campus publication observed, Tuskegee had entered the "jungle of white competition."[245]

This site teemed with racial politics. In the 1930s and 1940s, notes the historian Susan Cahn, track and field was "a central component of African American college life and urban community recreation" and blacks dominated major competitions. Among white Americans, however, the sport lost popularity, and by the late 1940s, Cahn concludes, women's track and field "occupied a marginal, denigrated position within American popular culture." Condemning "the sport as undignified for women," middle-class whites and mainstream media generally ignored blacks' accomplishments.[246]

Tuskegee therefore positioned its female athletes carefully in terms of race and gender.[247] The athletes' "fitness and caliber," the school insisted, demonstrated

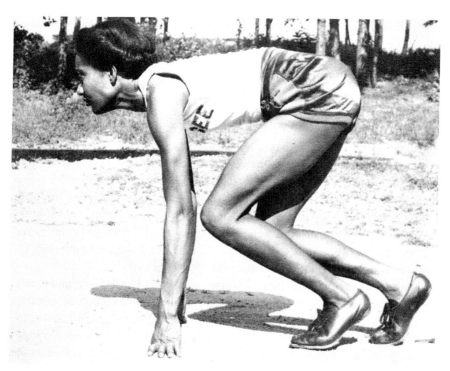

FIGURE 5.7 *Alice Coachman (Davis), Tuskegee Institute sprinter and high jumper (1939–46) and Olympic gold medalist (1948). Courtesy of Tuskegee University Archives, Tuskegee University.*

"what the colored woman can do, once she has the chance." Hard work, not racial characteristics, explained the speed and strength she displayed when defeating white opponents, just as track and field's growth as a "black sport" reflected equal opportunity, not biological destiny. Undercutting white prejudice, these arguments also affirmed power and skill as natural female qualities. Despite excelling in a "masculine" sport, Tuskegee's female track stars remained feminine and heterosexual. Exuding pride as its young women blazed "new trails into hitherto uncharted areas of the jungle of white competition," Tuskegee's coaches and physical educators drew a favorable picture of black female athleticism.

Embracing this model, most Institute athletes enjoyed testing their physical abilities and also learned how proper clothing, dining room etiquette, and feminine demeanor could negate white racism. Others, however, struggled to reconcile their athleticism, which the black community valued, with normative femininity, which white society demanded.[248] Trips to away meets were eye-opening, as the athletes visited historic sites, encountered diverse people and modes of life, and experienced discrimination firsthand.[249] Whites taunted and harassed them, and gas stations prohibited them from using restrooms.

The Abbotts had to "drive through the country and find a spot in the woods where the children could go." Because white restaurants refused service, team members bought food at grocery stores and made their own meals. To prepare an occasional hot meal, Mrs. Abbott recalled, she "would buy canned baked beans, and . . . set them on the hot radiator of the car." The lack of black motels forced the team to travel day and night, unless they found a black school that could house a large group. These experiences taught the athletes to be dignified and resilient in a white-dominated world.

After fifteen successful years, however, women's sports at Tuskegee began to falter.[250] In the early 1950s its famed track and field team no longer ranked first in the country. Other schools, especially Tennessee State, offered good opportunities (and usually more aid) to promising female athletes. Moreover, Abbott's successor as department head was less enthusiastic about women's sports and increasingly uneasy about the program's costs. The Institute terminated the women's track and field program after the 1964/65 season.

The decision involved matters of money, gender, race, difference, and equity. Some Tuskegeans worried that the publicity and resources accorded women's sports threatened men's programs.[251] In the late 1930s, projected athletic expenses rose sharply as female track and field athletes entered national competition. By the late 1940s, the anticipated cost of women's participation in the AAU outdoor track and field meet and Olympic Trials exceeded the sport's total budget of previous years; meanwhile, football—Tuskegee's most expensive sport—outspent both men's baseball and track and field (men and women combined) by nearly sixfold. For some administrators, strained budgets made the investment in women's sports seem increasingly burdensome. These financial qualms masked gender politics, and by mid-century, the school's leaders decided that affirming women's athletic rights and abilities was less important than the unquestioned prerogatives of men's sports.

Women's forays into the "jungle of white competition" disrupted racial politics as well. Although the wealthy northern businessmen who still dominated Tuskegee's Board of Trustees generally supported Patterson's fiscal and curricular reforms, they may have balked at any endeavor that inserted African Americans directly into white domains.[252] Patterson was not inclined to object. Convinced that he had to "tread carefully" in dealing with powerful whites, Patterson often "bow[ed] to the exigencies of race relations" and accepted equal opportunity, not full integration, as the measure of racial progress.[253] He probably joined white leaders in regarding sports events that breached the racial divide as both unnecessary and incendiary.

Tuskegee's athletic program had always posited that black women both resembled and differed from white women and black men. This interlacing of gender and race served the Institute well from the 1920s through the 1940s. Skillfully navigating institutional politics, white prejudice, and disagreements over gender and race, advocates created a positive, independent model of female athleticism. Their formulation held firm until black female athletes began defeating their white counterparts and overshadowing their black brothers. As gender norms hardened and debates over racial equality escalated in the United States before mid-century, support for strong black womanhood wavered even at an all-black institution.

SPELMAN COLLEGE

At Hampton and Tuskegee, women's physical activities developed alongside those of men in departments where female teachers typically worked under a male director. By contrast, few men were in sight at Spelman College, which opened in 1881 as the Atlanta Baptist Female Seminary under the auspices of the Woman's American Baptist Home Mission Society (WABHMS) based in New England. After surveying conditions among southern blacks, the organization's leader, Sophia B. Packard, and a fellow teacher, Harriet E. Giles, convinced the WABHMS to establish a school for black girls and women in Atlanta. Despite close ties to industrial philanthropists, Spelman differed markedly from Hampton and Tuskegee. It was a single-sex institution and remains so today. During its first half-century, most administrators and faculty members were white women. As proclaimed in Spelman's motto "Our Whole School for Christ," campus life and educational programs centered on spiritual rebirth and preparation for service.

The goals of "spiritual regeneration and societal reform" characterized many projects undertaken by northern white Baptists after the Civil War.[254] Their purpose in establishing churches and schools for African Americans was acculturation, not integration or equality; if all Americans adopted white, middle-class, Protestant values, northern Baptists reasoned, racial strife would diminish and social stability become possible.[255] White churchwomen in particular believed that only a broadly educated black elite could lift up the poor, illiterate members of their communities. By training the "head, heart, and hand," Spelman Seminary promised to turn young African American females into "self-disciplined, hardworking, order-loving Christian women" whose contributions as mothers, teachers, church members, and community leaders would elevate the black race.[256]

The school's diversity probably made this goal seem daunting.[257] Drawn primarily from poor families in the rural South, most students entered at the primary grades, one-half were nonresidential, and about one-third were between twenty-five and fifty years old. Beginning in the early 1900s, Spelman attracted more secondary-level students, including the daughters of black middle-class families from Atlanta and nearby areas. Because of Jim Crow laws and the dearth of black public schools, its student body remained largely working class and under-educated through the 1920s. Constant supervision seemed necessary to mold the pupils into dignified women.[258] To develop "habits of thoughtfulness, self-control, obedience, and courtesy," the school policed every detail of their daily sched-ules and personal lives. Pupils rose, ate, studied, attended classes, prayed, and retired at prescribed times. Besides caring for their clothing and rooms, they also performed domestic chores for the school, from waiting tables to dusting and sweeping. Although some regulations faded during the 1910s and 1920s, students still had to account for their whereabouts throughout the day.

For their academic model, Spelman's white leaders chose the curricula of northern liberal arts institutions, especially the Seven Sisters, and offered reli-gious, academic, and vocational instruction to qualified upper-level students.[259] Almost 90 percent of early graduates became teachers. Its highly regarded nursing program operated from 1886 to 1928, and the Department of Home Economics earned a strong reputation for coursework in dietetics, microbi-ology, and "household management." Nevertheless, the school's collegiate as-pirations proved impractical; as late as 1926/27, the primary and secondary grades constituted more than 80 percent of total enrollment.[260]

Spelman's character suited its system of funding and governance. Although northern white Baptists and Georgia's black Baptists supported the school, its key benefactors were industrial leaders, especially the oil baron John D. Rockefeller.[261] Between 1882 and 1902 Rockefeller's donations totaled around $200,000; thereafter, his contributions came through the General Education Board, a philanthropic instrument for wealthy businessmen. A related group, the John F. Slater Fund, also made substantial donations. The infusion of cor-porate money not only kept Spelman solvent but also reinforced its conserva-tive milieu and practical curricula.

Along with weathering serious financial problems, Spelman and other Bap-tist missionary schools confronted questions of gender and race. Should they admit both men and women or be single-sex institutions? In 1883 advocates of coeducation proposed merging Spelman and the Atlanta Baptist Semi-nary, a men's school that became Morehouse College. The plan faltered (as did later schemes) when Sophia Packard, Spelman's first president, declared that coeducation would hinder women's special interests.[262] The issue of racial control also preoccupied the American Baptist Home Mission Society (ABHMS), the male-dominated national organization, as well as the denomi-nation's segregated black "convention." Should missionary schools employ primarily white or black administrators and instructors? Major battles over black self-determination forced most ABHMS institutions to become more interracial; by 1915 almost one-half of faculty members at the nine ABHMS colleges were black, as were three of their presidents.[263] Spelman was a striking exception; as late as 1928, only three members on its sixteen-person board of trustees were black, and no African American served as president until the mid-twentieth century.[264] By contrast, its record of female leader-ship was noteworthy; during Spelman's first four decades, most teachers were white women, as were its first five presidents.[265]

Between 1881 and 1924 physical activities reflected Spelman's moralistic regimen and white control.[266] To regenerate the black body as well as save minds and souls, instruction emphasized formal calisthenics. Although practicing around the many support posts in the makeshift gymnasium of Giles Hall's basement was difficult, the intent seemed worthy. As the material home of the soul, the logic ran, the human body was subject to divine rules; disobeying the laws of health—"by eating improperly, [or] by intemperance in drinking, or by laziness, filthiness, etc."—was comparable to any other sin.[267] By preventing such vices, structured drills and marching would transform Spelman girls into "emblems of purity" who radiated discipline, obedience, cooperation, and other habits of "noble character."[268] Calisthenics also built the knowledge and vigor that students would need later as they guided fellow blacks toward physical and spiritual well-being.[269]

Extracurricular activities were confined to intramural games and casual recreation. Beginning in the early 1900s, students from different grade levels, as well as teams representing the faculty and campus YWCA, competed in basketball and baseball and, later, tennis, dodge ball, and captain ball. Founders Day, the annual spring celebration to mark Spelman's history (and raise funds) became an occasion for interclass games, races, and various "feats for entertainment and amusement."[270] Although the student newspaper eagerly reported such exploits, the seminary did not formally honor the participants. As President Lucy Hale Tapley explained in 1918, "permanent character training," not public acclaim, was activity's true value. "All games which demand good team work, concentration of the mind, control of the muscles, and generosity of treatment of opponents have a real place in education."[271] This menu of wholesome, noncompetitive recreation embodied Spelman's white middle-class standard of womanhood.

Physical activities also had to accommodate the school's religious and racial profile. The prohibition against dancing respected both Baptist precepts and racial difference; as a "younger civilization," African Americans were not "ready for that yet."[272] By contrast, informal exercise seemed both feasible and uplifting. Campus strolls renewed harried scholars and built friendships, as "grave dignified seniors, ambitious juniors, [and] happy-go-lucky grade girls" walked and talked during their free time.[273] Evoking the mythology of Old South plantations, this image commended black girls' wise use of their "leisure hours," while ignoring the strictures of student life.

Overseeing physical education were white female teachers.[274] Between the 1880s and early 1920s, the school's small faculty included only one or two teachers of physical culture who often handled an academic subject as well. Although the first instructor stayed for twenty-four years, most appointments were short term. Regardless of background or tenure, gym teachers were expected to uphold Spelman's missionary philosophy. In the early 1920s the school asked job applicants about church membership and religious service, their willingness to "enter heartily into the religious life of the school," and their attitude about the "work that is being done for the elevation and education of the Negro."[275] One applicant in 1921 assured the administration that she was a young woman "of a deeply religious nature" who, given her "interest in the colored problem," could "be of great good" to Spelman girls.[276] Similarly, former employers and instructors were asked to evaluate a candidate's effectiveness as a teacher and disciplinarian, her personal appearance and Christian character, and "ability to work harmoniously with others." Having crossed these hurdles, a successful applicant often received a no-nonsense letter from the dean or president reminding her of Spelman's expectations. Besides teaching in their specialty, many faculty members handled extracurricular activities and supervised a group of boarding students. As the nominal "mother" of a "family life" unit, a teacher was responsible for "assigning her students daily tasks, instructing them in manners, neatness, orderliness, and healthy ways of living, and fostering their moral development."[277] Of course, a mother could not lead unless her own behavior and grooming were above reproach; Spelman teachers, no less than students, were subject to surveillance and censure. While most students and instructors acquiesced, others apparently resisted.[278]

Dedicated to preparing black females for lives of Christian service, Spelman's initial model of gender both disrupted and reinforced mainstream attitudes. On the one hand, the seminary undercut white stereotypes about black degradation; liberally educated and morally upright, alumnae would improve their race's condition—not by imitating black men, much less white men, but in distinctly feminine ways. At the same time, the school regarded its black students as works-in-progress. Although graduates left with a moral sensibility, they would remain black; although alumnae would work, play, and serve much as white women did, they would do so in a segregated world. Simply put, Spelman girls were female not male, black not white, and remediable but never equal. To instill obedience and self-control, the school's white physical educators stressed formal gymnastic drills, whereas other institutions began diversifying their curricula. Emphasizing recreation and cooperation, intramural activities contrasted sharply with programs at the all-male Atlanta Baptist Seminary; except for watching their black brothers play sports or borrowing their facilities, Spelman girls did not stray into the world of masculine athleticism between the 1880s and early 1920s.

Spelman's next chapter was delimited by 1924, the year it became a four-year college, and 1953, when President Florence M. Read retired. During this period Spelman elevated itself as an intellectual and cultural institution, its faculty became more interracial, and the students were more qualified and independent. Curricular changes signaled this evolution.[279] Although practical coursework continued after World War I, a shift to postsecondary general education was underway. The process accelerated under Read, a white Mount Holyoke graduate and Reed College professor who became president in 1927. Besides closing Spelman's elementary school and teacher education course, Read discontinued certificates in household arts and missionary work, ended the nursing program, and converted the high school into an institution jointly operated with Atlanta's other black colleges. Smaller donations from the WABHMS made Spelman's cozy relationship with corporate patrons increasingly vital. These benefactors agreed with Read that large vocational programs were out of character and too costly for a liberal arts college. Spelman also enhanced its collegiate identity by becoming a cultural hub; students and faculty members enjoyed an array of plays, musical events, art exhibits, and lectures and performances by distinguished African Americans.

Further changes secured Spelman's identity as a place not simply for, but of black Americans. Whereas the eighteen-member teaching corps in 1928 included only one African American, black instructors outnumbered non-blacks by two to one in 1937 and by three to one in 1952/53.[280] The same trend occurred in physical education.[281] During the 1920s and early 1930s, the staff consisted of two or three white women, typically graduates of the Sargent and Posse training programs in Boston. In the mid-1930s the department began employing graduates of Spelman, Hampton, Howard, and Tuskegee. By the 1950s the staff was predominantly African American, and a black female director arrived in 1957.

Spelman's more refined image and black workforce attracted students with stronger academic backgrounds as well as independent spirits. They socialized with the opposite sex and, despite limited means, donned "flapper-style dresses and fur coats" and experimented with new products for their hair and skin.[282] Rather than simply mimic white culture, however, personal styles incorporated African American themes.[283] To some extent, the college tolerated this youthful exuberance. After all, President Read observed, intense involvement was a hallmark of the "New Negro" who was pushing black and white Americans toward a more open society.[284] At some point, though, passion could slide into impropriety; for instance, flamboyant attire might evoke stereotypes of black hypersexuality. To contain students' impulses in the 1920s, white administrators stiffened Spelman's rigid dress code, along with other regulations.

This tension between autonomy and discipline inspired new concepts of educated black womanhood. Between the 1920s and 1950s, Spelman's white leaders, increasingly multiracial faculty, and black undergraduates explored disparate versions of the "New Negro." Negotiations took place in the gymnasium as well as the classroom, library, and performance hall. In both instructional and extracurricular activities, students pushed for more freedom while teachers and administrators generally clung to tradition.

Basic coursework in physical education included "marching tactics, formal gymnastics, organized and unorganized games, and apparatus."[285] This scheme of regimented exercise persisted through the 1940s—long after most schools had shifted to elective sports, recreational games, and swimming. Although

Spelman's inadequate facilities precluded much variety, the main factor was the department's steadfast preference for discipline and self-awareness over skill and spontaneous expression. This tradition made sense to Marguerite Simon, a Spelman alumna (1935) who taught physical education at her alma mater from 1943 to 1980. Simon firmly believed that fostering respect for oneself, one's body, and other people was more important than athletic ability.[286] For some undergraduates, however, gym class represented autocratic rule, not personal enlightenment. In the late 1940s, students reported, their teachers' favorite sayings were "Are you chewing?" "Please take those earrings off!" and "Just go back and get your white shirt, miss."[287]

Perhaps extracurricular activities would prove more liberating. Between the 1920s and 1940s, Founders Day still served as a popular athletic meet and fund-raiser during which students participated in softball throws, relays, and other track and field events; groups gave demonstrations of stunts, mimetic drills, and apparatus work, while intramural teams competed in various sports. When some students requested formal recognition for their achievements, the college consented, with little fuss. By the late 1920s Spelman awarded numerals to girls who walked one hundred miles during the spring months (approximately three hundred trips around the campus quadrangle). "Tramping" was now a favorite pastime, one student exclaimed, instead of a "punishment inflicted by the Physical Education teachers for the loss of keys, for class cuts, etc."[288] In 1928 the college began presenting a silver Athletic Cup to the best performer on apparatus during the annual meet.[289] Lest ambition run amok, though, the student Athletic Council dutifully bestowed medals regardless of win-loss records, rewarded "scholarship, character, and interest in athletics," and prohibited excuses, gloating, and cheating in its "true sportsman's code."[290] As was true at other conservative institutions, athletes' plea for recognition evolved into a bureaucratic system that downplayed performance.

Nevertheless, intramural events whetted students' competitive appetite. After Spelman's Thanksgiving Day soccer match in 1927, one undergraduate declared that her classmates' running and kicking equaled that of Morehouse boys playing Howard. She urged the girls to "play on," because they someday might "have the chance to challenge another school."[291] Such opportunities proved hard to come by because the faculty controlled athletic policy and rarely approved intercollegiate contests.[292] After a brief but exciting foray into high-level competition in the early 1930s, Spelman College shut the door on extramural events. In 1931 eight students from Spelman and its affiliate, the Atlanta University Laboratory High School (AULHS), participated in the Fifth Annual Tuskegee Relays, without winning either the 50-yard or 100-yard dash. One year later, representatives had reason to celebrate: an AULHS pupil set a national record in the high jump for high school girls, and her team placed fourth overall. Although the *Spelman Messenger* and campus newspaper beamed with pride, elite competition ended abruptly.[293] In 1933 the student

Athletic Council bowed to institutional norms by organizing its first Play Day, including a baseball game, tennis matches, and various "comical games and jolly stunts" that stressed "fun and enthusiasm."[294] Dignified black womanhood once again meant sociable recreation, not individual prowess.

The college kept an equally tight rein on its dance program. With the repeal of Spelman's long-standing ban on dancing, the physical education department organized a May Day Festival in 1935 with "Danish exercises, shadow waltz, and the Virginia reel" as well as sports contests.[295] After the General Education Board funded President Read's request for an "experiment in dance," the college appointed Florence Warwick, an alumna who used GEB money to attend Bennington College's famed summer dance school.[296] Thereafter, the department typically had a dance specialist, and its basic curriculum included "fundamental techniques in the modern dance" alongside traditional calisthenics and drills. Dance performances also became a regular feature of Founders Day, dramatic productions, and special campus events.[297]

To prevent such activities from encouraging self-expression or harming the school's image, top administrators occasionally intervened. In 1937 President Read and the college dean dismissed a black dance instructor for unacceptable habits and hired Julia R. S. Denham, a graduate of William Smith College in Geneva, New York, who had studied and taught in reputable dance programs in the Northeast. President Read undoubtedly felt confident that a young white woman of such "character and poise and ability" would steer the dance program along the right path, and she worked hard to retain Denham beyond five years.[298]

The next long-term appointment in dance (a black woman) did not come about until 1953—one of several changes in physical education as Read prepared to retire. In 1951 the college opened a new health and recreation building, with a gymnasium and swimming pool that allowed new types of exercise and sports. At the same time, the building harked back to Spelman's Christian roots. Regarding human bodies as "the abode of our souls, and the temple of [God's] spirit," the college consecrated its new gymnasium to developing "graceful growing bodies, social poise, and spiritual power."[299] Religious themes and personal growth still permeated campus life, and physical education continued to emphasize "appreciations, understanding, attitudes and personal development rather than mastery of special activities."[300]

This philosophy captured Spelman's official view of active femininity between the 1920s and 1950s. Administrators counted on exercise, sports, and dance to distinguish the college as a center of black education and culture. It was, first and foremost, an institution for women, not men. Whereas male athleticism was public, black female physicality should be quiet and self-reflective; while Morehouse teams competed (in front of the opposite sex), Spelman women participated in Play Days and intramural meets, collecting modest rewards and, more importantly, self-awareness. Physical activities embodied class and racial identities as well. Lest Spelman be confused with Tuskegee, its ideal student was a proper middle-class lady, not a supposedly crude, working-class athlete. Mandatory formal calisthenics taught her self-discipline, while dance projected the dignity and culture of a feminine "New Negro." These standards assured white trustees and benefactors that Spelman's aim was racial assimilation, not equality. The dividends of middle-class respectability in a white-dominated society were clear also to black donors, parents, and faculty members. Various campus constituencies, though, rejected white expectations and asserted alternate versions of black womanhood. Some undergraduates believed that competitive sports were compatible with middle-class femininity, while black dance instructors explored African American history and culture with their students. We are black, not white, they declared; this is Spelman, not Mount Holyoke.

Women, Competition, and Difference

Between the 1920s and 1950s, institutional identity determined women's physical activities at American colleges and universities. Some contrasts seem self-evident; for instance, extracurricular programs at rural, working-class Tuskegee differed from those at urban, middle-class Howard. Other pairings, however, yield surprises. Although both Hampton and Tuskegee were coed, industrial schools for young African Americans, they reached different decisions about women's sports. Smith and Bryn Mawr, two elite colleges for white women, also had dissimilar athletic policies. At coed, academic Howard University, black women participated in mild forms of extramural recreation, whereas white female students at coed, academic Stanford pushed for competitive opportunities.

Single factors such as race, class, locale, or educational mission cannot explain the complex historical patterns within extracurricular programs for undergraduate women, especially the extent of skilled competition. Predominantly white institutions did not uniformly oppose varsity contests nor did historically black schools always support them. Elite colleges and universities did not dutifully ban women's sports nor did schools with less privileged students routinely sponsor competition. Coeducational institutions were not automatically hostile or friendly to high-level women's athletics. Nor did female-only schools invariably regard extracurricular sports as either appropriate or antithetical to femininity. Some male directors promoted skilled competition, but others, white and black, soundly rejected it. If programs were diverse, they also were fluid. Between the 1920s and 1950s most institutions altered their policies, in large or small steps. Some virtually eliminated intercollegiate events, while others experimented with various formats, from benign Play Days to high-powered contests.

Whatever direction a school chose, the process was contested. Decisions about women's sports involved many stakeholders, including donors, trustees, senior administrators, academic faculty, male and female physical educators, students, and alumni. Their interactions took place in specific historical and institutional contexts. The robust 1920s were neither the anxious 1930s nor the turbulent 1940s with respect to educational controversies, resources, or campus life. A school's origin, purpose, demographic profile, and power structure also influenced policy negotiations. At issue was not simply which female students would play which sports against which opponents. Extracurricular recreation and athletics embodied a school's vision of active, educated womanhood. Physical activities delineated how female undergraduates resembled or differed from men of the same or a different race as well as from women of another race or class. Concepts of difference, however, were more than ideological structures; they helped institutionalize power relationships and resource distribution. A school could deploy its personnel, facilities, and image to expand women's athletic opportunities or constrain them; a college or university could promote equity or obstruct it.

Institutions that resisted gender parity generally frowned on women's competitive sports. During the interwar years, disparate schools—white and black, coed and single-sex—sought order amid the upheavals in American culture and higher education. Conservative institutions imposed dictatorial schemes of *in loco parentis* and enforced mainstream femininity through curricular and extracurricular programs. Although more centrist colleges and universities dealt with student assertiveness less harshly, they too welcomed the wholesome, heterosexual New Woman. As America's young women flocked to college and entered male spaces, conservative and centrist schools alike relied on their gymnasia to draw clear gender boundaries. Restricting female undergraduates to mild recreation and sports served both symbolic and material purposes. Such programs contrasted men's innate athleticism with women's sociable pastimes; this difference, in turn, justified concentrating institutional capital—physical, financial, and human—on men's programs. Active bodies also clarified how the ideal female student related to women of other races, classes, and sexual orientations—how her character surpassed their unnatural masculinity. When women and other marginalized groups approached some college gyms before mid-century, they heard a broader message about American life—about who may or may not enter, who mattered and who did not.

Among the gatekeepers were physical education's Great White Mothers, who championed white, middle-class, heterosexual womanhood. Their protégés upheld this standard at Agnes Scott, Smith, and Milwaukee-Downer, despite white undergraduates' quiet resistance. At Hampton and Spelman during the 1920s, white teachers required black students to emulate mainstream norms, while expecting them to fail by virtue of race and class. Believing that high-level competition negated black femininity, many African American teachers also endorsed the central dogma. Led by male and female directors during the 1930s, black instructors at Hampton and Spelman agreed with Howard's Maryrose Allen that extracurricular activities should develop gracious, heterosexual womanhood—a model that represented their students as both equal to and different from white women and black men. Together, these diverse examples demonstrate the capacity of "difference" not only to outline behavioral codes but to constitute (and sometimes challenge) hierarchical relationships of gender, race, class, and sexual orientation as well.

While many colleges and universities stifled women's athleticism before mid-century, a substantial number embraced it. Opportunities were especially common whenever a key constituency advocated gender equality. At Bryn Mawr, white administrators and teachers pushed a feminist agenda in the gym. Outnumbered and overshadowed by Stanford's men, white female undergraduates regarded intercollegiate sports as both the symbol and substance of fairness. At Tuskegee, African American educators, male and female, looked upon competition as an authentic expression of black femininity; in their view, athleticism and refinement, personal achievement and racial progress were synergistic. Together, these examples illustrate how "difference" became a wedge for contestation and change before mid-century. In the critical domain of active bodies, some college students and educators consciously interrupted traditional systems of gender and race. Some lines of difference, though, seemed sacrosanct. Bryn Mawr ensured that sports befit the school's elite white status. Despite empowering young blacks, Tuskegee's coaches accommodated white middle-class expectations and fended off accusations of sexual deviance by cultivating heterosexual femininity. Limited by institutional dynamics and social conditions, most educators never considered completely overhauling "difference" for the sake of full justice in the gym.

{6}

Separate and Unequal

THE PUBLIC SCHOOLS OF WASHINGTON, D.C.,
1890s–1950s

The challenges that college physical educators faced probably looked mild to public school instructors. Whereas many postsecondary institutions could handpick their students, the nation's public schools had to admit youngsters of diverse ages, aptitudes, and social backgrounds. While broad questions of curriculum and governance preoccupied college teachers, their counterparts in elementary and secondary schools contended with the practical difficulties of public education and the constant din of popular opinion.

In 1903 a doctor in Washington, D.C., wrote the local Board of Education to complain that "'forcing pupils to march up and down the stairways'" was a form of "'cruelty.'"[1] Such objections were not uncommon as physical education took shape in the District's large, racially segregated school system. Physical culture was officially introduced for white primary schoolchildren in 1889, followed by black elementary pupils in 1891. Mandatory exercise for older white and black girls arrived in the late 1800s and for older boys in 1901, supplementing intramural and varsity athletics. Because formal instruction was relatively new, school authorities politely explained to the physician that marching was "really a part of the physical training." Far from being harsh or worthless, they elaborated, exercise was essential to a child's intellectual growth, personal character, and physical well-being.

As the program's scope and costs expanded, isolated criticism gave way to full-blown disagreements. Between 1900 and 1950 no school year passed without a key constituency voicing concern over instructional exercise or extracurricular sports. Some District residents wanted gym class to be more frequent, but others believed it detracted from academic subjects. Athletic boys scoffed at compulsory calisthenics, while girls' competitive drill teams struggled to gain recognition. Parents and administrators weighed the purpose of boys' varsity sports and argued over arrangements for white and black teams. The Board of Education tried to resolve daily problems while developing general policies for boys' and girls' programs in white and black schools. The Department of Health, Department of Recreation, and other municipal agencies quarreled with school officials over jurisdiction. Gym teachers pleaded for more funds and staff. Black personnel objected to second-rate equipment and facilities. The National Association for the Advancement of Colored People (NAACP) and other groups also demanded equity for black pupils.

As controversy swirled, various board members, superintendents, principals, and gym teachers articulated physical activity's role in comprehensive education. According to Rebecca Stoneroad, the program's first director, regular supervised exercise enabled muscles to stretch and grow while developing the brain, the "supreme center of the nervous system" that controlled thought, sensation, and volition; the result would be grace and economy of movement, along with "subordination of the body to the will."[2] Black teachers also underscored the vital "connection between strength of body and power of mind" that fostered a sense of purpose and discipline while training students' bodies.[3] Our duty, Anita J. Turner declared, must be "to protect, conserve, and insure the health of school children, making them mentally alert, active, and vigorous, and at the same time make them happy." Over time, she predicted, the "building of better and healthier human beings" would "produce a stronger and better nation."[4]

Generic goals notwithstanding, no facet of public education treated the city's pupils as interchangeable. Racial segregation was the schools' most entrenched mode of "difference." When the U.S. Congress mandated in 1862 that all District children, white and black, six to fourteen years old, receive three months of education per year, the enabling legislation implied, but did not stipulate a dual structure. Extending the city's general practice of discrimination, public education was divided by race, with parallel, but unequal systems of administration, finances, facilities, and instruction. No curricular or structural reform between the 1860s and 1940s altered the basic separation of white schools (Divisions 1–9) and black schools (Divisions 10–13).

Within this dual system, white and black physical educators tailored their programs to suit pupils' age, gender, and ability. Simple drills, marching, and other low-organization activities for young children eventually gave way to basic games, fitness contests, public exhibitions, and health lessons. Physical activities for older pupils were divided by sex. Although academic coeducation was common when American high schools developed in the late 1800s, peripheral subjects such as physical education and some extracurricular programs were routinely sex-segregated.[5] The District also differentiated upper-grade activities by perceived skill; athletic boys competed, "average" boys occasionally exercised, and all girls learned recreation and hygiene.

Their instructors were also organized by race and, to some extent, sex. White teachers worked primarily in Divisions 1–9, and black instructors handled Divisions 10–13. In the lower grades, girls and boys learned the three Rs and exercised together usually under the direction of women of the same race. Over time, these regular classroom teachers received help from itinerant trained physical educators, who were assigned to schools based on race. Resident female specialists became fairly common for girls in the upper grades, as did male coaches and eventually physical educators for older boys.

Administration paralleled instruction. Given the District's emphasis on young pupils, its first director of Physical Culture in 1889 was a white female. Two years later a black woman joined as an assistant director, reporting to the black superintendent; she and her successors focused on physical education for black children but gave some attention to upper-level black girls.[6] Systemwide consolidation in 1900 brought all units of physical education into one department under the program's original director. Further reorganization in 1924 established the first directorships in white and black secondary school physical training, filled by two men. In 1934 the District appointed a white male to head health and physical education throughout Divisions 1–9 and a black male as his counterpart in Divisions 10–13.

Few white leaders considered these arrangements illogical or discriminatory; in their view, dividing instruction and staff by sex and race simply applied common notions of difference to public education. School policies and operations, though, were far from benign. Under the guise of fairness through difference, school systems in Washington, D.C., and other segregated cities deliberately privileged certain activities, pupils, and personnel, while disadvantaging others. Although racial and sex discrimination pervaded D.C.'s schools, physical education and athletics were especially potent forms of inequity. Since "bodies matter schooling," authorities relied on exercise and sports to convey blunt lessons about gender, race, sexuality, and class, and to regulate how youngsters moved, interacted, and used space.[7] Conversely, physical activities denoted which bodies mattered—which pupils had to take gym class, who could participate in sports, and which programs deserved resources.

This chapter analyzes physical education and sports for boys and girls in the white and black divisions of the segregated public schools in Washington, D.C., from the introduction of formal physical training in 1889 to racial integration in the mid-1950s.[8] The District's school system is an instructive case study: its student population was diverse, physical education and sports were well developed, and school politics were intense and well documented. Leaders' regular use of difference to marginalize certain pupils and teachers allows for an analysis of the multiple, often subtle mechanisms by which inequity operated and the conflicts it engendered. Two examples are especially informative: the privileging of athletic boys through sports and the subordination of black pupils and staff through segregation. Although this might suggest that gender and race were independent, both examples demonstrate how physical activity embodied hierarchies of gender and race simultaneously. Finally, by examining disfranchised groups, the chapter explores the potential of difference to alter the politics of gender, race, and active bodies.

Athletic Skill and Male Privilege

Between the 1890s and 1940s, most school leaders believed that activities for older girls should be gentle, whereas boys relished physical contests; only exceptional boys, though, displayed superior skill and competitiveness. Because these ideas seemed self-evident, officials rarely justified them. Only Rebecca Stoneroad, the program's first director, wrote extensively on sex differences. In 1889 the D.C. superintendent invited Stoneroad, a fifth grade teacher with training in English, to head the new physical culture program, based on her reference to Delsarte exercises (a system of movements and gestures developed by François Delsarte in the mid-nineteenth century) during one of the superintendent's classroom visits. She expanded her knowledge by attending Dudley Allen Sargent's summer school at Harvard and William G. Anderson's Chautauqua program, supplemented by a European tour to observe various gymnastics systems. In 1903 Stoneroad received a medical degree from the National Medical School in Washington, D.C. Though nominally in charge of all pupils, Stoneroad focused on the lower grades and white divisions, a priority reflecting the schools' racial hierarchy as well as her latent prejudice.[9]

Due to girls' innate frailty and future responsibilities, Stoneroad asserted, they need more physical training than boys do.[10] To lay the groundwork for strong motherhood, physical educators should encourage a love of activity and sense of purpose in pubescent girls, while compensating for their weak bodies and "emotional nature." Not only were activities that "develop great strength" unnecessary, but bursts of physical energy or nervous strain were risky; strenuous or jarring movements, such as the standing broad jump, might disrupt a young girl's internal organs, especially during the first years of menstruation. Among older girls, though, "lighter forms" of baseball and other team games could develop sociability and an ethic of fairness. Although Stoneroad's colleagues would not have disagreed, they cared more about lesson plans than general theories: What did sex differences mean in the gymnasium or on the athletic field? School programs revealed their answer: white and black boys' activities differed from girls' in type, importance, and purpose, with competitive sports serving as a rite of passage into manhood.

Intramural and varsity athletics had long dominated D.C.'s program for older schoolboys.[11] In the late 1800s, white and black youngsters participated in football, baseball, basketball, track and field, and competitive military drill. Students usually initiated these activities, with help from faculty volunteers and outside coaches. Seeking more control in the early 1900s, the District established a Board of Faculty Advisers to Athletics, comprising representatives from white high schools who arranged interscholastic contests. In later years, the Board of Education granted partial authority to principals and then to its

Committee on Athletics and other ad hoc and standing committees. This jurisdictional muddle stemmed partly from the board's uncertainty over whether athletics was a curricular entity or sui generis activity.[12]

This conundrum did little to slow athletics' momentum. From the early to mid-1900s, administrative decisions—and sometimes neglect—privileged boys' varsity sports at the expense of activities for girls and "unskilled" boys. High school athletics, especially white programs, commanded a disproportionate share of resources, thanks to student-solicited funds, athletic association fees, gate receipts, and donations. Physical education was not eligible for such revenue precisely because it was instructional. As Anita J. Turner, the assistant director for black schools, observed, funds for girls' activities were scarce because "we do not believe in girls coming together in public places and exhibiting for money."[13] Instead, physical education limped along with small budgets and student contributions.

Boys' teams also monopolized equipment and facilities, especially in white secondary schools.[14] Despite their many advantages, white schools had only modest facilities for boys' and girls' interscholastic teams in the early 1900s; to alleviate the pressure, practice spaces were open to girls' teams only infrequently and at inconvenient times. When interscholastic competition for white

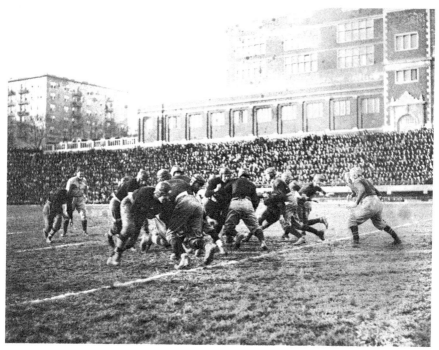

FIGURE 6.1 *Football game between Central and Tech (two white high schools), at Central's stadium, Washington, D.C., 1919. Courtesy of the Library of Congress, Prints & Photographs Division, LC-DIG-npcc-00840.*

girls was eliminated in 1906, boys' domination of gymnasia and playing fields increased.[15] In the 1920s and 1930s, when land development and building construction expanded white schools' options for indoor and outdoor activities, the District continued favoring sports over recreation and boys over girls. Despite its ample facilities, McKinley High School acquired additional space for boys' varsity sports through rentals and municipal permits. Central High girls played field hockey at a public playground three miles away because boys' teams controlled the school grounds. Forced to practice off-site, Western High girls often used vacant lots for field hockey in the 1920s until neighborhood boys reclaimed their traditional playgrounds and drove the schoolgirls away. These examples illustrate widespread gender discrimination that persisted long after white high schools gained spacious new quarters.[16]

Rather than acknowledge and correct such inequities, school leaders concealed them. In 1946 several Central High teachers and parents requested that the "deplorable situation . . . regarding [outdoor] play facilities for the girls" be rectified.[17] Opened in 1917, Central had arguably the best facilities in the school system, including two gymnasia, a swimming pool, and a stadium for varsity sports. Given the expense and technical difficulty of any new construction, the superintendent asked school officials to "work out some plan" that solved girls' problem "in a more economical manner." Although a board member proposed an obvious solution—that girls could simply use part of Central's large stadium, the group sidestepped the matter by referring it to committee.[18]

School officials also privileged boys' athletics through personnel decisions, especially senior appointments. In 1934, on the eve of Rebecca Stoneroad's retirement, the board decided to evaluate the entire program in health, physical education, and athletics, responding partly to a widely publicized fracas at a football game between two white schools. The purpose was to "investigate and devise ways and means to establish a broad and efficient plan with reference to all school athletics and contests, and to investigate also the physical training department."[19] The top priority was more effective governance of interscholastic competition, leaving physical education as an afterthought. The superintendent and Special Committee on Athletics (SCA) recommended that the new director's position encompass sports, health, and physical education in all white elementary and secondary schools. Given the job's broadened scope, the superintendent declared, "a man should occupy the office," and the SCA readily agreed.[20] A few months later, the District hired Birch Evans Bayh.[21] A student-athlete at Indiana State Teachers College (later Indiana State University) from 1914 to 1917, Bayh became the college's director of physical education before he even graduated. Besides coaching baseball, basketball, and track and field, Bayh revitalized Indiana State's football program and officiated high school sports. He then directed health and physical education in the Terre Haute public schools. District officials probably expected that Bayh would be an ally of athletics, while modernizing physical training as well.[22] Rather than also hire a new female assistant director of girls' programs for Divisions 1–9, the superintendent and board split the job between three current staff members; although administrative efficiency was the stated rationale, this cost-saving measure simply increased women's workload.[23]

In 1940, the board also consolidated health, physical education, and sports in the city's black schools under one director. The first appointee was Edwin B. Henderson (1883–1977).[24] Having joined the staff in 1904 and overseen physical activities in black secondary schools since 1924, Henderson's seniority in Divisions 10–13 was unquestioned. His record as an innovative physical educator and advocate of rational athletics was equally clear.[25] By appointing Bayh and Henderson, school officials looked forward to efficient, centralized management of all programs in grades 1–12; both men were seasoned professionals with executive experience who, the board anticipated, would be good stewards of athletics.

As resources, facilities, and leadership gravitated toward boys' sports, the program sparked controversy. Rather than blindly support athletics during the first half of the twentieth century, board members, superintendents, principals, teachers, and parents argued frequently. They discussed whether postseason and intercity competition should be allowed, how misconduct at athletic events could be regulated, whether eligibility rules were fair and enforced, and if officiating and insurance were properly managed. Stakeholders voiced their opinions, board members voted, policies were implemented, and more disagreements arose.[26]

By contrast, other physical activities seemed less consequential, even distracting. Mandatory physical education for older white and black girls dated back to the late nineteenth century. Interscholastic competition for upper-grade white girls also became common, with basketball generating as much "interest and enthusiasm" as boys' games did.[27] When girls' contests were banned around 1906, the decision received little attention at board meetings or in administrators' reports; only a few student newspapers and principals commented on the change.[28] Although some competition continued into the 1910s, white and black secondary schools began favoring field days, athletic exhibitions, intramural games, and Play Days for girls, along with recreation, dance, achievement tests, and lessons in hygiene and first aid. Free of intense rivalry and male athleticism, girls' programs were successfully domesticated by the mid-1920s.[29]

The fate of one other group remained: the average boys who "would never make team membership" because they gave no "promise of special power."[30] The issue of physical education for older schoolboys surfaced sporadically during the first half of the twentieth century. Noting imbalances between athletics and exercise and the neglect of boys compared to girls, some principals, superintendents, board members, and gym teachers called for full-time staff and more resources for boys' physical education.[31] Results were, at best, modest. The first instructor for older white boys following the gym class mandate in

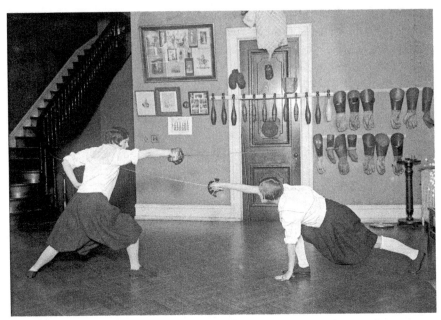

FIGURE 6.2 *Western High School fencers, Washington, D.C., 1925. Courtesy of the Library of Congress, Prints & Photographs Division, LC-DIG-npcc-13660.*

1901 was a track and field coach who visited each white high school once a week to conduct twenty-five-minute sessions of free-hand exercises. In reality, one boy observed, the "only exercise which those with narrow chest and weak muscles" got was their "frantic yelling for the football team or baseball nine."[32] Dissatisfaction led to longer, more frequent periods of exercise, namely, forty-three-minute sessions of group calisthenics or free play twice a week under the supervision of a resident instructor, often a former athlete or coach.[33] In the late 1930s, though, McKinley High boys could fulfill their gym class requirement by serving as hall monitors, while seniors were excused altogether.[34] Instead of counterbalancing athletics, instructional reform sometimes solidified it. In 1909, Principal Edith C. Westcott of Western High School requested the appointment of "a male teacher specifically charged with the physical welfare of the boys" whose duties should include "supervising practice, directing sports, [and] organizing and coaching teams." Every school should have such a director, at District expense, she continued, because athletics "have become so vital an interest in the high schools of Washington."[35] In more ways than one, most District boys could not compete with their athletic brothers.

Though excluded from elite teams, "average" schoolboys and girls could aspire to join D.C.'s cadet program. Originating in the late nineteenth century as military training for white boys, cadet drills were available to black boys by the early 1900s and then to girls; they quickly became a prominent feature of high school culture. The cadet program, though not athletics in a traditional sense, had all the trappings of a varsity sport and was regarded as such: membership was selective, teamwork and discipline were essential, uniforms and awards were highly prized, and interschool exhibitions and contests were intense. Gender inequities also prevailed. Despite the program's popularity, neither white nor black schools formally recognized girls' cadet units until 1945. While applauding the corps' value to schoolgirls, the District was reluctant to award even a half-credit to female participants, although boys earned a full credit. The two programs, officials contended, differed substantially. This argument drew a distinction where none existed: both programs involved competitive admission and promotion, rigorous practice schedules, regular community service, and similar motives and benefits.[36] As the descendant of military training, however, cadet drills struck school officials as prototypically male; they could not grant equal status to girls' units without disrupting the masculine connotation of skill and teamwork.

Overall, the convergence of resources, personnel, and attention on boys' activities created clear winners and losers between the 1890s and 1940s. By displaying high-level talent and competitiveness, only exceptional schoolboys could achieve true masculinity and earn its rewards; no typical boy or any girl met this standard. These presumed disparities in ability were a pretext for unequal treatment based on gender and race. The distinction between elite competition and mass instruction protected white, middle-class norms of masculinity and femininity. It cast suspicion on "unskilled" boys and athletic girls: Were they normal youngsters or gender anomalies? White notions of physical proficiency also established a racial standard that black teachers and pupils were expected to emulate. From its varsity teams to quasi-athletic cadet drills, D.C.'s activity program marked gender boundaries, marginalized pupils deemed unskilled, and instituted as well as disguised material inequities in the District's public schools.

Conditions in Washington, D.C., were not unusual. Broad social changes in the early twentieth century prompted many school districts to differentiate between boys and girls through athletics. Gender imbalances in American education were one perceived problem. Girls outnumbered boys as high school students and graduates; most teachers in urban elementary schools were female; a slight majority of secondary school teachers were women, while men taught in the upper grades and served as administrators.[37] Although these disparities stemmed from deliberate efforts in the nineteenth century to make public education more economical and male-controlled, some officials worried in the early 1900s that their institutions had been "feminized."[38] This trend seemed symptomatic of larger dislocations. As immigration, urbanization, and industrialization increased, many middle-class whites mapped their anxieties onto issues of gender. As new economic and family structures upset women's roles, masculinity also seemed threatened because, some observers claimed, American culture afforded boys and men so few outlets for their inborn talents and energy. These twin crises became known as the "Woman Question" and the "Boy Problem."

Many Progressive Era educators and civic leaders identified public education as the best solution. First, however, schools' inefficient structure and one-size-fits-all curricula had to be overhauled.[39] Using intelligence tests and other ostensibly scientific tools, school districts began organizing pupils more systematically by age and ability. Curricula became sequential and, in the upper grades, differentiated along academic and vocational tracks. Diverse extracurricular activities allowed older students to explore personal interests and relieve the school day's increased discipline. The answer to the "Woman Question" now seemed straightforward: gender-specific activities and courses in home economics, sex education, and pink-collar vocations would prepare schoolgirls for their modern responsibilities.[40] Because schoolboys underachieved and dropped out more often than girls, the "Boy Problem" was more perplexing. To stem the tide of feminization and create a more virile environment, high schools experimented with boy-friendly courses, new pedagogical methods, and the appointment of male teachers.[41] Extracurricular programs for boys and girls also expanded. School authorities believed that voluntary activities could teach the habits and values of corporate society, maintain order by making school more pleasant, and allow students to pursue their natural (that is, gendered) interests.[42]

As job prospects shrank in the 1920s and 1930s, young Americans, especially working-class teens, flocked to public schools just as their social function was being reassessed. During the interwar period, secondary schools became custodial institutions focused on personal growth.[43] To hold students' interest (and attendance), districts introduced "life adjustment" courses and more extracurricular activities, which became the most sex-segregated of all high school programs. By the 1930s and 1940s, girls dominated academic clubs and literary societies, while boys chose student government, science clubs, and interscholastic athletics.[44]

Initiated by students themselves in the late nineteenth century, varsity sports quickly grew in popularity. In the early 1900s, "sports competition was a common feature in the life of secondary schools," as institutions big and small fielded boys' teams in football, baseball, and basketball. By the 1920s, "high school athletics enjoyed a wide and fanatical following."[45] Special funds, independent personnel, and student management enabled sports to flourish even in schools that lacked adequate facilities and physical education programs.[46] The dearth of regulation prompted school authorities to wrest control from students in the 1920s through various state and national organizations governing interscholastic competition.[47] Confident that varsity athletics had been cleansed, many educators hailed sports as the epitome of "manly character." One need look no farther than "the boys on the gridiron or the diamond and the men who coached them," authorities claimed, to see that "high schools were not 'feminized.'"[48] By equating sports, masculinity, and modernity, this agenda left no room for girls' athletics. In Washington, D.C., and other cities, both the "Woman Question" and "Boy Problem" had been solved.

Surviving in the Shadow of Athletics

The supremacy of boys' sports presented gym teachers with the difficult options of acquiescing, adapting, or resisting. Most chose the middle path. The simplest means of rescuing pupils left in athletics' wake was to appeal for more resources. While acknowledging that girls' physical training at Central High was "better than [work] with the boys," the school's principal, Emory M. Wilson, pointed out that a small, poorly lit armory, with no bathing or dressing facilities, was "in every way unfit" as a gymnasium. Moreover, one lone teacher could "not satisfactorily look after the physical well-being of over 600 girls."[49] Reports from black administrators and teachers were more insistent. In 1910 the principal of M Street High reiterated his school's desperate need for exercise space and equipment. Given current handicaps, Edward C. Wilson noted, the "good that is accomplished" in physical training "is due entirely to the zeal and earnestness" of M Street's regular teachers and physical educators.[50] When personnel called the glass half empty, the Board of Education inferred that the glass was half full. This indifference probably discouraged white and black employees from pushing their case too vigorously, lest they fuel board members' doubts about physical training's effectiveness.

Given athletics' cachet, gym teachers also decided to protect instructional activities by converting them into "games." During the 1910s and 1920s, competitive formats invaded many aspects of physical education, from exercise class to health programs. Exercise-as-sports arrived in the form of achievement tests. Known as physical efficiency or athletic badge tests, these annual events involved performing various skills, such as running, jumping, and throwing, along with an assessment of posture, weight, and health habits. Athletic managers helped their classmates practice the skills beforehand. On test day, pupils received scores in each area plus a cumulative total representing overall fitness. They earned color-coded pins, certificates, and other awards for meeting specific standards, thereby becoming eligible for more advanced tests (and more points and prizes) the following year.

In a classic case of teaching-to-the-test, standardized fitness events soon became the instructional centerpiece for all pupils. The District introduced tests for white elementary schoolboys and black primary and secondary schoolboys around 1910, followed by tests for upper-grade black girls. Within a few years, the program was available to all boys and girls in white grammar schools and, thereafter, to boys in several white secondary schools.[51] Director Stoneroad issued directives and encouragement. "Practice should begin at once," a memo to staff advised in 1918, because "[s]uccess in each school building depends greatly upon organization."[52] Stoneroad happily reported participants' high turnout, achievements, and enthusiasm, as well as the introduction of more rigorous events.[53]

In their heyday, fitness tests signified that competition now constituted instruction, and athletics epitomized competition. The program reflected sports' familiar trademarks, such as physical feats, quantitative assessment, and recognition of success. To avoid any negative connotations, advocates referred to physical efficiency tests as "rational athletics" because they averted competition's risks while democratizing its benefits. As one principal explained, the tests grabbed students' "interest through the element of competition" but channeled their energy toward healthy goals.[54] "The inspiration," Director Stoneroad concurred, "is that of self-improvement or an ideal to be attained rather than that of merely beating a classmate." While the "consciousness of achievement" might be sufficient "reward" for some pupils, others needed the lure of proficiency awards, because "now a purpose is added to the power of achievement." Although fitness tests emphasized success, Stoneroad defended them as egalitarian, not elitist. "The benefits of the exercise generally enjoyed by the skilled few who need them least," she noted, "are extended over the whole school, even the weaklings being inspired to effort."[55] Convinced—at least conceding—that competition had become the accepted way to motivate, train, and evaluate children, physical educators transformed gym class into "rational athletics" for the masses.

The masses included girls. Less than a decade after banning varsity sports for older girls, the school system endorsed fitness tests as constructive female competition. "Girls, even more than boys," Stoneroad reasoned, "need encouragement to exercise and improve their physical powers."[56] While readmitting girls to the world of competition, the program differentiated events by sex. Girls executed stunts on a balance beam and ran the potato race (a short run during which participants picked up and deposited objects in designated areas of the course). By contrast, boys did chin-ups and the standing broad jump. Performance standards were sex-coded as well; the target in the girls' 50-yard dash was 8.6 seconds, while boys were expected to finish a 60-yard dash in the same time.[57] Fitness tests thereby identified poise and agility as feminine, while associating masculinity with the more valued traits of power and speed.

The competitive ethos also permeated the District's health programs. During the 1910s, health education became more common, especially for younger pupils; talks on posture, dental hygiene, and other daily habits were designed to improve children's knowledge and practices.[58] In 1919, under the auspices of the National Tuberculosis Association and Junior Red Cross, the white and black elementary schools embarked on a "Health Crusade." The program turned health education into a "tournament."[59] Upon earning points for following various hygiene rules, pupils were rewarded with social ranks and insignia from the Middle Ages, such as page, squire, and knight. After comparing results from different schools and divisions, a central office conferred pennants, banners, and publicity on groups with the highest averages, while giving "special encouragement" to schools where "interest was lagging."[60] The program also included health plays and pageants for young children, while older pupils earned monetary prizes through essay contests on such topics as "'How much good health depends upon our own effort.'"[61] Believing that youngsters not only enjoyed but needed special incentives to learn, the Health Crusade accepted sports as its model of reward-based motivation. As the "Crusade Leader" observed, the children "were keenly interested, not in being scrupulously clean but in scoring their charts and winning emblems and ranks of knighthood."[62]

The competition motif was not unique to Washington, D.C. During the first half of the twentieth century, school districts around the country converted physical education into sports by emphasizing athletic skills, intramural games, and fitness tests.[63] By the 1920s, tests of motor ability and physical achievement were commonplace in American schools and colleges, fueled by scientific developments along with concern about physical shortcomings among World War I draftees. Seeking reliable tools, physical educators applied contemporary science to classify fitness activities and criteria by age and sex.[64] Instruction in health and hygiene also became linked to physical education and sports in many public schools. Despite some professionals' objections, the functions of physical education and health education merged through overlapping curricula, personnel, and administration.[65] Bringing information and activity to many youngsters, regardless of age, sex, or race, the sportification of gym class and health education enabled instructional programs to stay alive as boys' interscholastic athletics expanded. By imitating athletics so closely, gym class replicated the very cause of its secondary status. While chafing at sports' preeminence, physical educators in Washington, D.C., nonetheless accepted its formula in order to survive.[66]

Racial Inequities and Resistance

Racial disparities also belied the school system's rhetoric of equality. Although the District's curricular templates made its physical activities look race-neutral, actual programs for black and white pupils were neither identical nor fair. Segregated gym class and athletics entailed deliberate inequities in facilities, finances, and personnel decisions that disadvantaged black schools. "Our work," Anita J. Turner acknowledged, "is as good as the conditions permit."[67]

Between the 1890s and 1940s, facilities for black pupils were substandard. A case in point was M Street High, an academically based school opened in 1891 that became legendary for rigorous programs and exceptional staff and graduates.[68] Its physical plant, though, was second-rate. With a low ceiling and meager ventilation, the basement was a poor substitute for a gymnasium.[69] Local streets served as the playground.[70] In 1910 pupils still had "no lockers, no gymnasium, no swimming pool, no running track, and practically no yard." Alluding to discrimination, the principal noted that M Street teams could not rent athletic sites that "may be obtained on favorable terms by other schools in the District."[71] In 1916 Dunbar High School replaced M Street High.[72] Despite its swimming pool, two gymnasia, and other upgrades, Dunbar suffered in comparison to Central High, a white school completed in 1917. As Edwin B. Henderson noted, "Central was set on an inspiring height surrounded with beautiful grounds. Dunbar was built right on the curb in a slum section. Central was furnished with the best stadium in the city. Dunbar's rear yard was a stonemason's work place with drilling of stone assailing the ears of students all day long."[73] Rising black enrollments after World War I strained existing facilities. By the late 1930s, the average playground space per pupil at some white elementary schools was four times that of black primary schools.[74] In the late 1940s, the District's three black high schools occupied dilapidated buildings within eight blocks of each other in the city's Northwest section, a virtual slum.[75] Dunbar High shuttled one thousand girls through exercise classes in a 40' x 60' gymnasium.[76] The "crowded old building" of Cardozo High sat "on a triangle between highly travelled arteries" offering no space for outdoor activities, while its track and field coach "trained national high school champions in a hallway" on tile and wood flooring.[77]

District law mandated an equitable allocation of funds between Divisions 1–9 and 10–13, based on the city's relative proportions of white and black children, six to seventeen years old. In reality, per capita expenditures favored white pupils by more than 25 percent.[78] Disparities were especially glaring in athletics. Unlike most programs, sports could generate extra funds through ticket sales and other sources. The Board of Education deliberately opened many such revenue streams for white programs while denying comparable opportunities to black teams. For example, although the board prohibited postseason competition in all schools during the mid-1930s, it approved end-of-season championship football games for white schools, with the competing teams sharing the gate receipts.[79] In the late 1940s, the board allowed the championship football game in Divisions 1–9 to be a charity event, benefiting both the white sports program and an outside organization; the game often raised between $2,000 and $10,000 for equipment purchases and for the white Interhigh School Athletic Council. The annual game between vocational and senior high school teams also supported white football programs.[80] As these opportunities multiplied, some school authorities asked if black teams also could hold championship series or charity events. Board members even considered a white versus black championship game, but with such an explosive idea afloat, the board quietly deferred action on all options for black teams.[81]

Initiatives favoring white programs, though, continued. In 1948 the board approved a revenue-generating game between the white public school football champion and the leading team from the District's private schools—a move that required an exemption to the ban on postseason play; board members did not extend the waiver to black schools.[82] To dramatize the mounting inequities,

Edwin B. Henderson noted that Divisions 10–13 netted less money in a year from all athletic events combined than white schools took in during a single charity football game. "Although our boys put up a good game of football or basketball, their uniforms cost just as much,. . . [and] officials and travel expenses are as costly," black programs were trapped between scarce revenue and hidden outlays. Gate receipts were small because gymnasia in black schools did not accommodate many paying spectators, but discrimination made renting larger facilities impossible or too expensive.[83]

The Supreme Court's 1954 ruling that dual education was unconstitutional posed difficult questions for public school athletics. Because football remained segregated through 1954, D.C.'s Board of Education was uncertain whether the top-rated white or black team should play the Catholic school champions. In fact, members acknowledged that the best white team could no longer automatically represent the public schools.[84] Charity events also came under review. In 1955 and 1956, the income from a basketball game involving black and white all-stars was earmarked for a white-only organization. A black board member objected that black youngsters "would be playing in a game for money-making purposes, the proceeds of which will go for a club to which they do not have entrée." After another member reassured his colleagues that the organization in question performed "good work" in the black community, the majority approved the arrangement—in effect condoning discrimination even as the schools began to desegregate.[85]

Saddled with inferior resources, the District's black teachers also faced professional hardships. In 1935 thirty individuals handled health and physical education in Divisions 10–13; all but four had college degrees, seven had master's degrees, and several had undertaken doctoral studies.[86] Despite strong credentials, African American teachers and directors had to fight for the respect accorded so readily to white staff members. In 1926 Anita J. Turner requested compensation for her extra work in the District's black normal school. After a negative initial ruling, the Board of Education took Turner's follow-up appeal more seriously and referred it to the District's auditor.[87] One year later, Edwin B. Henderson's status was called into question when the District Attorney of Washington, D.C., accused him of illegal conduct, including outside compensation, connections with sham institutions, and mail fraud. A formal indictment on the latter charge prompted the Board of Education to suspend Henderson. Realizing that dismissal without a conviction might be improper, they reinstated Henderson, whom most members believed was an honorable person.[88] One might argue that racial bias did not affect these personnel matters; not only did both cases end favorably but white staff members also became embroiled in disputes over salaries and responsibilities. Teachers in Divisions 10–13, however, began from a subordinate position. As employees whose rights and status were contested, not implicit, they contended with inequitable appointments, salaries, promotions, and course loads as well as direct harassment.[89]

Substandard facilities, inadequate resources, and mistreatment of staff formed a web of disadvantage in the District's black schools. Dual education depicted black students and teachers as different and inferior; the privileging of white schools and marginalization of Divisions 10–13 turned this representation into concrete reality. School-based physical education and sports also extended the city's general practice of segregated recreation. The racial division of municipal playgrounds and swimming pools, private arenas, commercial pastimes, and neighborhood games meant that blacks and whites did not play as equals in the nation's capital.

Injustice engendered both silence and protest. Because segregation upheld their social power, most white authorities either ignored the many privations in Divisions 10–13 or rationalized them through illogic and doublespeak. When called upon to equalize physical activities, white Board of Education members declared that reforms were underway, and critics were misinformed and quarrelsome.[90] This indifference reflected a common mind-set among prominent white educators around the country that public schools should help black children rehearse and accept their supposed inferiority.[91] Attitudes among African Americans in Washington, D.C., varied. Holding considerable influence over appropriations, programs, and personnel in black schools, the District's black elite both accepted and exposed the plight of Divisions 10–13. Many lower-class blacks, however, believed that the city's fair-skinned black aristocracy made decisions and granted favors to schools based on color and wealth.[92]

As these inter- and intraracial disagreements unfolded, some black citizens and educators in the District pressed for justice. Their efforts mirrored a national pattern, as African Americans effected critical reforms in many segregated urban school systems throughout the North and South.[93] Intensifying between the 1930s and 1950s, the battles in Washington, D.C., and other cities involved black civic leaders, community groups, parents, school administrators, and teachers. Although segregation made every black educator a second-class employee subject to white scrutiny and control, it also created space for subversion and innovation. The strategies of the District's black physical educators illustrate the complex mix of adaptation and resistance that typified black educational reform before mid-century.

Edwin B. Henderson argued that dual education was unjust, uneconomical, and unwise. Segregation, he declared, not only violated the American principle of fairness but also wasted valuable resources.[94] Recreation and sports, he continued, could promote racial harmony as well as curtail delinquency and crime.[95] By saying that good athletes made good citizens, he did not mean that healthy blacks were submissive blacks. Nevertheless, Henderson's logic probably appealed to white school authorities and political leaders who regarded sports as one arm of racial management.

Knowing that actions spoke louder than words, Henderson and his peers set out to make physical activity for black youngsters varied and egalitarian. To counter discrimination, he helped found the Inter-Scholastic Athletic Association (ISAA) of the Middle Atlantic States (1906) and the Public School Athletic League (PSAL, 1910). The ISAA sponsored events primarily between black high schools from Washington, D.C., Baltimore, and Wilmington, Delaware, along with Howard University's preparatory division. Activities included track and field, basketball, football, and swimming, with occasional events for high school girls.[96] Modeled after a New York City organization, the PSAL sponsored interclass and interscholastic games for boys and girls in the District's black elementary and secondary schools. Although the objective was to develop character and citizenship through inclusive competition, regardless of skill, most PSAL activities were varsity-style rather than mass participation.[97] Other programs were more genuinely democratic. Henderson and fellow teachers adopted athletic badge tests in 1910, probably before such programs began for white schoolboys.[98] Black schools also sponsored field days, cadet drills, and May festivals that allowed hundreds of African American pupils to display their skills before large public audiences. In the mid-1940s Henderson developed a novel sports program for elementary pupils; using homeroom classes as the team unit, the activities combined intramural and extramural competition

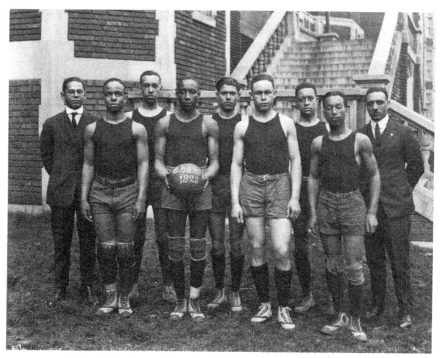

FIGURE 6.3 *Edwin B. Henderson (far right) and the Dunbar High School basketball team, ca. 1922. Courtesy of Scurlock Studio Records, Archives Center, National Museum of American History, Behring Center, Smithsonian Institution.*

for boys and, to a lesser extent, girls.[99] Finally, Henderson strengthened general instruction, especially in secondary schools, by extending requirements and broadening the curriculum.[100]

Since white schools conducted similar programs, the activities in Divisions 10–13 probably struck white authorities as inconsequential, even puzzling. They might wonder, Henderson noted, why so many black children participated in military drill and why annual cadet competitions attracted such large black audiences. "Is it because [African Americans] like the showy phases of life?" he asked, mocking white myths. "Is it because colored children are more subject to authoritarian control in education?"[101] The real explanation, he insisted, was discrimination, not racial difference. As Henderson understood, dual education gave black pupils few opportunities to develop skill or demonstrate their accomplishments. Annual field days, ISAA and PSAL competitions, and other public events countered the demoralizing effects of segregation by building self-esteem and school cohesion. The activities also showcased students' talent, teamwork, and discipline for their parents and friends, thereby fostering racial pride and displaying respectability in a society that systematically denigrated African Americans. Black athletes, amateur and professional, often became social symbols in the early twentieth century.[102] For fellow blacks, they represented racial solidarity and the promise of assimilation. For whites, they proved blacks' allegiance to mainstream values while confirming or refuting prejudices about black physicality. The District's school athletes probably were more interested in playing the game than serving a cause; nevertheless, their efforts on the drill field and basketball court had broad social significance for blacks and whites alike.

However imperfect, efforts to democratize physical education also conveyed a racial message. Given black children's limited options in and outside school, teachers in Divisions 10–13 recognized the importance of inclusion. Anita J. Turner advocated corrective exercise because no social agency in the District provided the service to black youngsters. Similarly, the schools' Health Crusade taught lessons about personal health and hygiene that some children might not otherwise have learned. By filling a void, black teachers believed, their work contributed to self-determination and racial uplift.[103] By embodying new knowledge, skills, and values, physical activities in Divisions 10–13—from competitive leagues and public exhibitions to democratic exercise and health instruction—reconfigured the racial politics of active bodies.

Delineating gender proved more difficult. While defending girls' right to be active, some black physical educators questioned if high-level competition was appropriate for them. In the early 1900s Anita J. Turner welcomed the revival of public exhibitions because girls deserved the same chance as their brothers to display athletic skill.[104] She puzzled, though, over how closely girls' activities should mimic boys' sports. On the one hand, she did not want exhibitions to become large fund-raising spectacles that excluded girls of average ability; hard work and interest among the majority, she argued, were more important than quality performances by a select few. At the same time, Turner understood that girls in Divisions 10–13 faced special obstacles. Compared to PSAL events for boys, girls' activities hobbled along with minimal attention and funds; moreover, the smallness of black facilities prevented girls' exhibitions from involving numerous pupils from different schools. Combining middle-class norms with a critique of inequity, Turner promoted mass participation and feminine decency while addressing schoolgirls' unique problems.

Henderson joined his colleague's discussion of gender and race. In terms both conservative and progressive, he advocated healthy recreation for all black girls and women as well as high-level competition for exceptional athletes. He began by acknowledging common misgivings about female competition.[105] Some people worried about injury and emotional strain, especially during puberty and motherhood. Others were convinced that active women would "lose some of their charm and possibly what is more important, health."[106] Many feared that the abuses infecting men's sports would spread to women's activities. Because these concerns had been so strong, Henderson noted, leading physical educators replaced competition with less intense options. While not questioning that female activities should emphasize "physical development, healthy living and recreation," he objected to critics' exaggerations of competition's dangers and their extreme solutions.[107] Ample evidence proves, he said, that sports and womanhood are compatible. He pointed to athletics' increasing popularity among average American females, including black girls. He cited black female physical educators who got their start on neighborhood playgrounds. Most of all, he recommended looking at the roster of black female champions, including national and Olympic stars, for inspiring examples of "strong virile womanhood."[108]

Realizing that his adjectives sounded oddly masculine, Henderson elaborated. He did not mean that true female athletes were manly, biologically or personally. Some "famous so-called women athletes" certainly "have been border-line men."[109] In fact, a "great Russian allegedly woman athlete" underwent surgery and became a man "after winning over the women of the world."[110] Dismissing such cases as anomalies, Henderson declared the black women representing the United States at the Olympic Games, such as Tuskegee's runners, to be "normal girls. Whatever they win will be done as real female women and not as men temporarily masquerading as women."[111] Moreover, intensive training and competition did not compromise reproduction. "I doubt that any of the Tuskegee-trained girls have been the worse for wear as wives and mothers."[112] If Henderson's logic was biological, his message was cultural; since athleticism and femininity were congruent, the black community "should not be too squeamish" about female competition.[113]

While noncontact games are the best outlets for average girls and women, Henderson continued, talented athletes should be able to "display their skill and natural sport ability to a wider extent."[114] He beseeched teachers and coaches to support these future champions. "Get some of the girls out of the bleachers ruining their delicate throats for the boys on the gridiron. Put them on the track, over the hurdles and the jumps."[115] First and foremost, female athletes were entitled to pursue their interests. "So long as women of other races and other nations engage in these sports with no proven evidences of detriment," Henderson asserted in 1951, "our girls have reason and right to compete." More broadly, their accomplishments would advance racial progress. "Victory in physical contests, as with high rating in mental or spiritual measurements, helped to kill off the Nazi-inspired doctrine of inferiority or superiority of groups of people classified as races."[116] In short, female athleticism was a matter of justice for women and the race.

This view was alien to most white educators and officials in the District. Seeing competition and womanhood as contradictory, they expected black schoolchildren to absorb white middle-class beliefs about body and gender. By contrast, Henderson publicly engaged questions of gender, race, and athletics. His conclusions reflected the double-sidedness of being black and American; while confronting white norms of gender and race, he also depicted female athleticism in the framework of middle-class black values. From the pupils in Divisions 10–13 to Olympic stars, he declared, active black females are strong, decent, and feminine. Henderson's concessions to respectable, heterosexual womanhood resembled those of other black and white proponents of elite competition; they opened the door to female athleticism but made admission contingent.

Difference and (In)Equity at Mid-Century

Developments in the District's black schools reveal the seemingly paradoxical capacity of "difference" to both disable and empower. On the one hand, white authorities in Washington, D.C., belied their separate-but-equal rhetoric by deploying dual education to restrict the opportunities and aspirations of black pupils. Racism permeated every policy and program. Sports and physical education were especially powerful ways of managing students and institutionalizing inequity. The reach of difference, however, extended well beyond the white/black divide. To mark boundaries of gender and sexuality, the school system also differentiated between pupils deemed talented or unfit as well as between athletic boys, unskilled boys, and all girls. Drawing these lines was neither arbitrary nor abstract. By specifying who could exercise where, in which ways, and with what resources, the District's activity programs systematically benefited some groups while marginalizing others. Some constituencies, though, appropriated notions of otherness to contest discrimination and assert self-determination. Confined to "race work," black teachers and administrators gained some autonomy and self-definition, exercising significant power over the curricula, appointments, and milieu of individual schools. Despite their uncertainty over how to balance compliance and agency, few African American educators doubted that a dual system could empower as well as oppress. From their second-class gyms, Anita J. Turner and Edwin B. Henderson protested inequities, fostered racial pride, and interrogated the meaning of black womanhood.

By mid-century, dual education in Washington, D.C., was contested on many fronts. African American leaders and their allies filed petitions and lawsuits that targeted the run-down buildings, overcrowded classrooms, and inadequate resources in Divisions 10–13. Congressional reports underscored the schools' problems and proposed controversial remedies.[117] As pressure for educational reform mounted between the 1930s and 1950s, racial segregation in jobs, housing, recreation, and public accommodations also came under scrutiny. Despite legal and political progress, full equality in education and other domains of life, however, remained an unfulfilled promise in the nation's capital.

{7}

"It's just the gym"

FEMALE PHYSICAL EDUCATORS, 1950–2005

> I have pride in the facilities and surroundings and am embarrassed for
> the college and the department when the appearance of both [is] far less
> than one should expect. I am tired of some workmen who chide me by
> saying "It's just the gym," which has been and still is a prevalent attitude.
>
> —Professor Kate McKemie, *Agnes Scott College, 1974*

During the second half of the twentieth century, American physical education matured as a profession. Its internal structure and public presence seemed more stable than before. Training programs became more rigorous and standardized. Prospective teachers typically earned a baccalaureate degree, and a growing number pursued a master's or doctoral degree. Job opportunities were diverse; Americans encountered physical educators at elementary and secondary schools, colleges and universities, community agencies and youth centers, municipal and state bureaus of recreation, sports leagues and summer camps, athletic clubs and fitness centers, churches and retirement homes, rehabilitation clinics, the armed forces, veterans' hospitals, and factories and businesses. Professional organizations sponsored conferences and journals, connected members to resources and networks, regulated the field, and promoted its interests throughout American society.

Despite these gains, both the leadership and rank and file were concerned. Many Americans still regarded gym class as "glorified recess." Paying so-called experts for "bouncing a ball and working up a good sweat" in order to make children "busy, happy and good" seemed wasteful.[1] Physical educators suffered tangible slights as well. After the 1970s, mandatory gym class became less common at schools and colleges; as the number of students declined, so did employment for instructors. By contrast, the rising popularity of competitive sports in and outside academe made coaches' prospects seem bright. Meanwhile, experts in sports management, exercise science, sports medicine, and recreational services came to dominate university faculties and professional curricula. Many institutions reorganized their departments, combining physical education and athletics as well as programs for males and females. These dramatic changes exacerbated teachers' qualms about their purpose and reputation. Their constant hand-wringing prompted one leader in 1985 to diagnose the field "a hapless neurotic" beset by isolation, insecurity, and dysfunction.[2] Although the psychological metaphor seemed strained, most physical educators probably recognized the symptoms.

Developments in American law and society after mid-century recast the field's long-standing concerns. Federal legislation and court rulings stipulated that physical activity programs accommodate students formerly deemed "different" based on race, sex, or physical and mental ability, with significant consequences for female physical educators. New notions of health and fitness also emerged. Exercise, diet, and other "lifestyle behaviors" dominated popular culture and public health campaigns. Shifting their attention from infectious diseases to chronic systemic conditions, doctors, scientists, and other experts argued that managing personal risks through sound nutrition and regular physical activity could prevent disease and promote health. As Americans puzzled over whether and how to be active, they got advice from numerous sources, including public health leaders, sports medicine doctors, exercise scientists, fitness gurus, and health entrepreneurs. These groups now bombard average citizens with recommendations via the Internet and mass media. Physical educators have struggled to find a niche in this dizzying array of information and specialists. They have tried to distinguish their roles, validate their effectiveness, and solidify their place in educational institutions and other settings. These goals resonated particularly for women in health, physical education, and recreation (HPER). For decades, their professional identity and authority had revolved around serving the "special" population of girls and women in sex-segregated programs, a function that became less clear after mid-century.

This chapter examines the status of white and black female physical educators, coaches, and administrators in academic institutions between 1950 and 2005. As the counterpart to chapter 1, the discussion focuses on teachers in grades K–12 and postsecondary programs. At first glance, women's opportunities and setbacks in HPER might look unexceptional. Educational access and anti-discrimination laws increased female participation in many occupations after mid-century, especially medicine, law, business, and other professions; likewise, women in diverse fields encountered glass ceilings, locked doors, low pay, and second-class status. The chapter asks whether female physical educators faced unique problems and, if so, why their field's history of marginalizing "different" members continued.

The analysis spans several generations. Between the 1950s and mid-1970s, in-service teachers and professional leaders included third-generation women (born 1900–20) approaching the end of their careers as well as older members of the fourth generation (born 1920–40). From the 1970s through 1990s, the field comprised younger fourth-generation women and members of the fifth generation (born 1940–60). Current teachers, coaches, and administrators are older fifth-generation women as well as members of the sixth generation (born 1960–80). The discussion addresses these generations' backgrounds, training, employment prospects, and professional responsibilities and status.

Backgrounds

White physical educators in the third through fifth generations typically grew up in middle-class families.[3] African American teachers born before mid-century had less privileged upbringings; their fathers and mothers tended to work in trades or service. Later cohorts of black personnel came from various social strata; many young black coaches and administrators in the late 1980s had educated middle-class parents, while others came from families in which high school diplomas were uncommon and blue-collar jobs were the norm.[4]

Regardless of socio-economic status, most teachers discovered their love of physical activity at an early age. As youngsters, they enjoyed outdoor pastimes and pick-up games with siblings, classmates, and friends; they may have participated in organized sports through clubs or recreation centers. In some cases, activity was not only enjoyable but also therapeutic for childhood ailments. Physical education at school was another chance to be active. In earlier decades, as today, gym class varied widely by region, school, and grade level. In elementary school, a girl probably had simple exercises in her regular classroom each day or structured drills and games at a playground or gymnasium. Secondary school often entailed more formal instruction and organized sports supervised by a specialist. For white and black girls alike, a gym teacher or school coach was usually the first person to suggest physical education as a vocation.

Their families were often skeptical but supportive. Although white and black parents wondered if physical education was a viable career, they approved the field's emphasis on education, service, and health; for black families especially, physical education represented a middle-class rather than menial way of helping others while earning a good income. Other parents, though, were mystified; they were unsure what a gym teacher did and whether respectable jobs were available. The answers became both easier and more complex after mid-century. On the one hand, new careers opened as the field grew, and by the 1970s a young woman could envision becoming a gym teacher, college coach, athletic trainer, fitness expert, recreation leader, or exercise scientist. At the same time, changes in American education and society made job prospects in particular specialties uncertain.

Training and Credentials

Whatever their ambitions, young women understood that postsecondary training was expected, even required, especially for employment at a school or college. To help candidates meet this higher standard, the field sought to improve teacher education through more rigorous admissions criteria, curricula, and degree requirements, as well as more systematic evaluation and accreditation of professional programs. Although similar issues had arisen in the early 1900s, a new breed of leaders spearheaded reform from the 1940s through the 1990s. Their initial focus was undergraduate training. In 1948 a National Conference on Undergraduate Professional Preparation in Health Education, Physical Education, and Recreation was held at Jackson's Mill in Weston, West Virginia. By setting standards for teacher education, the conference consolidated changes that had been quietly underway for two decades. Most private normal schools closed, became colleges, or affiliated with an established institution of higher education. During the 1950s many colleges and universities, especially state schools, introduced or expanded their professional programs in HPER, while raising their curricular and degree standards. In 1954 the National Council for Accreditation of Teacher Education (NCATE) assumed responsibility for reviewing training programs in physical education; the profession's national organization accepted the NCATE ratings in 1960. Leaders also pushed for improvements in graduate training. Following various surveys and modest reforms during the 1940s, top professionals organized a conference at Pere Marquette State Park, Illinois, in 1950 to discuss accreditation and other aspects of graduate education. After mid-century, prominent physical educators applauded their predecessors' achievements but sought further progress. Accreditation, specialization, and undergraduate requirements and curricula remained central concerns in the 1960s and 1970s. The issue of teacher credentials also came to the forefront, as state regulations became more demanding. By 2000, 80.6 percent of American public and private schools required "newly hired physical education teachers to have undergraduate or graduate training in physical education or a related field, and 73.2 percent of schools require[d] newly hired physical education teachers to be state-certified, licensed, or endorsed in physical education."[5]

While some leaders considered whether prospective teachers were well trained, others asked if they were representative. For decades, the graduates of professional programs had been disproportionately male and white. In 1950 women constituted only 22 percent of new college graduates in physical education, while 22 percent of master's degrees and 16 percent of doctorates were awarded to women.[6] Although female candidates gained considerable ground over the next twenty-five years, they remained underrepresented. In 1974, 42 percent of the country's bachelor's degrees in physical education went to women, as did about 34 percent of master's degrees and 30 percent of doctorates.[7] At the end of the century, women's share of advanced degrees had grown, but the distribution of undergraduate degrees was unchanged.[8]

Stark racial disparities also persisted. During the 1940s and 1950s discrimination at white institutions forced most black trainees to attend historically black colleges and universities (HBCU). By 1951 more than thirty HBCUs offered a

PROFESSIONAL EDUCATION FOR WOMEN

SCHOOL OF PHYSICAL EDUCATION

STUDENT AIMS
1. Professional preparation for (a) teaching Physical Education; Dance; or Health Education;(b) Recreation leadership; or (c) pre-Physical Therapy training.
2. Preparation for family living and community responsibility.

	Physical Education	Dance	Health Education (women and men)	Recreation (women and men)
BASIC GENERAL COURSES	Rhetoric and Composition Hygiene Psychology American Government American History Speech Humanities electives Social Science electives	Rhetoric and Composition Hygiene Psychology American Government American History Speech Philosophy Poetry Drama Acting Stagecraft	Rhetoric and Composition Hygiene Psychology American Government American History Introduction to Social Work Child Development Child Welfare Psychology of Adjustment Physical Education	Rhetoric and Composition Hygiene Psychology American Government Speech Sociology Social and Group Work Sociology of the Community
BASIC SCIENCE COURSES	Biological Science Anatomy Physiology	Anatomy Physiology	Biology Anatomy Physiology Chemistry Bacteriology Foods and Nutrition	Biological Science Public Health
MAJOR COURSES	Team Sports Individual Sports Body Mechanics Tumbling Contemporary Dance Social, Square, and Folk Dance Rhythmic Analysis Games for Children Teaching of Sports Kinesiology Prescribed Exercise Tests and Measurements First Aid School Health	Creative Dance for Children Teaching of Dance Production Workshop Theory and Philosophy of Dance Musical Composition for Dance Square, Social, and Folk Dance Social Recreational Activities Swimming and Individual Sports Kinesiology Prescribed Exercise Contemporary Dance Technic Rhythmic Analysis Composition History of Dance Percussion	Public Health Safety Education First Aid Prescribed Exercise Physical and Health Inspection Driver Education Principles of Health Education School Health Programs Tests and Measurements Field Work in Community Health	Social Recreation Activities Square and Social Dance Physical Education Activities Games for Children Camp Counseling Teaching of Swimming Organization of Sport Programs Recreational Crafts Recreational Music Recreation in Rural Areas Dramatics for Teachers Principles of Recreation Organization of Recreational Programs Design for Recreational Areas Planning of Towns and Cities Recreation Field Work
EDUCATION COURSES	Professional Orientation Foundations of American Education Principles of Secondary Education Educational Psychology Technic of Teaching in Secondary School Practice Teaching	Professional Orientation Foundations of American Education Principles of Secondary Education Educational Psychology Technic of Teaching in Secondary School Practice Teaching	Professional Orientation Foundations of American Education Principles of Secondary Education Educational Psychology Technic of Teaching in Secondary School Practice Teaching	Professional Orientation Educational Psychology
ELECTIVE COURSES	Electives may be selected from any University courses including those offered by the School of Physical Education.	Electives may be selected from any University courses including those offered by the School of Physical Education.	Electives may be selected from any University courses including those offered by the School of Physical Education.	Electives may be selected from any University courses including those offered by the School of Physical Education.

FIGURE 7.1 *Information sheet for women physical education majors, University of Illinois, 1950. Courtesy of the University of Illinois Archives.*

major in physical education, but only a handful conferred advanced degrees.[9] Although many programs were accredited, their curricula and student services suffered from limited resources, facilities, and staff. From the 1960s through the 1990s professional training among African Americans increased, then stagnated.[10] Desegregation enabled some black men and women to enroll at predominantly

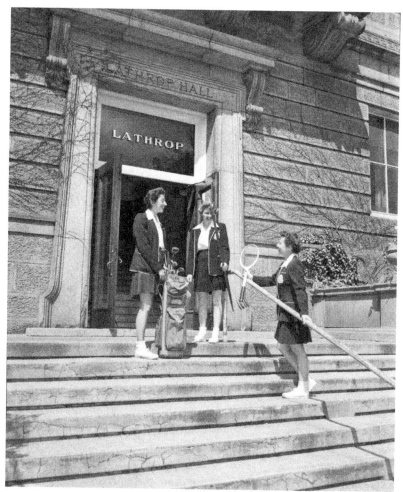

FIGURE 7.2 *Physical education majors at the University of Wisconsin, ca. 1950. Courtesy of the University of Wisconsin–Madison Archives, Image #S04622.*

white institutions, especially for advanced training, but most still earned their undergraduate degree at an HBCU, where opportunities and standards steadily rose after the 1960s. Despite these gains, imbalances continued. Between the 1970s and early 1990s the overall gender ratio among black undergraduate majors as well as candidates for higher degrees averaged about 1.5 males for each female.[11] African Americans also remained a distinct minority among HPER candidates and degree recipients overall, leading some to wonder if black physical educators were an "endangered species."[12] The bleak outlook in HPER mirrored general trends in higher education.[13] Although academic opportunities in many fields increased for black students at both HBCUs and predominantly white institutions during the 1960s and 1970s, economic and social forces soon depressed black representation among postsecondary students, college graduates, and candidates for advanced degrees generally, and fewer black Americans chose teaching as a profession as the century closed. Overall, physical education instructors, faculty, and researchers remained distinctly white but slightly less male during the late twentieth century.

On the Job after Mid-Century

To some extent, women physical educators who retired in the 1950s or 1960s would have recognized the dilemmas facing their successors; each generation worried about securing good jobs and earning respect for themselves and their profession. In other ways, however, women's work changed fundamentally after mid-century. Most notably, the enactment of Title IX in 1972 accelerated processes already apparent in earlier decades, especially the growth of competitive sports for girls and women. Title IX is a short, but powerful law: "No person in the United States shall, on the basis of sex, be excluded from participation in, be denied the benefits of, or be subjected to discrimination under any education program or activity receiving federal financial assistance." The impact was most evident in academic institutions, as departments of physical education and athletics used Title IX to alter their mission, structure, and membership. Although Title IX was hardly the sole catalyst behind these developments, the law marked a watershed for female personnel.

It therefore is appropriate to analyze women's careers after mid-century in two parts: the 1950s to early 1970s, and the mid-1970s to 2005. Dividing personnel by workplace is equally important; the experiences of teachers in elementary and secondary schools differed from those of college and university staff. The following sections examine women's status, responsibilities, and problems within these two cohorts, first, between the 1950s and early 1970s and, second, during the post–Title IX decades. The discussion emphasizes how female teachers, coaches, and administrators—white and black, gay and straight—fared as their profession and American society preached equity but failed to practice it.

Schoolteachers: 1950s–Early 1970s

The story of women physical educators after mid-century begins, ironically, with newly minted teachers who were not employed. Female leaders cited marriage as the main reason for women's apparent scarcity in the postwar workforce.[14] Although verifying this claim is difficult, available information suggests that many female graduates in the 1950s either did not enter the workforce or soon left because of marriage; by corollary, many career women in HPER remained single. A 1958 survey of graduates of the women's department at the

University of Illinois elicited 217 responses, primarily from individuals who received their degrees in the 1940s or the 1950s. Although the questionnaire did not ask specifically if alumnae were married and teaching, returns implied that these two choices were often mutually exclusive. About 58 percent were married or had been married; among the graduates "not teaching, 64 percent were homemakers and 54 percent indicated that they had left the teaching profession to be married and/or to raise a family" and had done so quite early in their careers.[15] Combining marriage and employment probably was more common among women of color, but data on K–12 teachers are scarce. The number of in-service physical educators, gay or straight, who entered committed relationships outside marriage in this period is even harder to gauge.

New physical educators who got full-time positions were employed primarily at elementary and secondary schools. During the 1950s and 1960s few novices, male or female, initially worked at a college or university, went into recreation work, continued their studies, or were "unplaced." School jobs were plentiful partly because compulsory gym class was common. Individual states had authority to require physical education or at least mandate that some program be offered, while local school districts specified curricular content, a requirement's scope, and exemptions. During the 1950s most states required some form of physical education for most pupils, although many programs fell short of experts' recommendations about duration and frequency. In the 1960s requirements increased somewhat, especially in the lower grades.[16]

Being a gym teacher was arduous.[17] In primary grades a physical educator usually served as an observer and consultant for regular teachers who were responsible for gym class and recess. Secondary schools were more likely to hire full-time specialists. Instruction, though, constituted only a fraction of their responsibilities. Female gym teachers also handled intramural programs, special interest clubs, the Girls Athletic Association, and interscholastic sports, along with supervising cheerleading squads and chaperoning at athletic and social events. These noninstructional duties expanded after mid-century due mostly to the growth of girls' athletics. Women's multiple duties, however, did little to enhance their status. Their initial salaries typically were lower than men's; moreover, female staff usually did not receive extra pay, reduced teaching loads, or other compensation for noninstructional activities.[18]

Conditions among black personnel were even more difficult. For decades segregation made African American men and women the primary teaching corps in black institutions.[19] Many physical education graduates from HBCUs in Georgia, for example, worked in the state's rural school districts; although some left their jobs in search of better pay, others reported being "displaced in [the] school integration process."[20] Far from eliminating discrimination, the consolidation of dual systems allowed white officials to close many black neighborhood schools and favor white personnel over African Americans. From the mid-1950s to the late 1960s, black high school physical educators and coaches were fired, reassigned to other fields (such as driver education), or transferred to elementary schools. Between 1965 and 1970 the number of African American head coaches across fourteen states fell by more than 90 percent.[21] "In Mississippi alone," one critic noted, "over 150 [black] coaches and physical education teachers were displaced when desegregation began in 1969."[22] Arguably, the plight of black personnel as well as white female teachers should have grabbed their field's attention. Mainstream reports, however, typically bemoaned the supposed shortage of white male physical educators.[23] Except for vigorous critiques by black personnel and white women, the profession overlooked the plight of its most marginalized members working in grades K–12.

College Teachers: 1950s–Early 1970s

One might expect that women at postsecondary institutions fared better due to higher prestige and more established programs. Between the 1940s and 1960s most American colleges and universities—public and private, coed and single-sex, predominantly white or black—mandated two years of physical education for all undergraduates; many granted academic credit for gym class and factored students' grades into their GPAs.[24] This favorable situation, how-ever, concealed widespread skepticism. Wondering if institutions of higher learning should support, much less require, gym class, senior administrators and academic faculties debated if such activities warranted academic credit, whether students' knowledge, not skill should determine their grades, and whether requirements should be kept, reduced, or abolished. Although some institutions eliminated compulsory gym class with one blow, most chipped away at it over a decade or two.

Because requirements for female students tended to be extensive and long-standing, the job of defending gym class usually fell to women's departments. At the University of Nebraska, various academic units attempted to lessen or abolish mandatory gym class for their female students. As the colleges of Arts and Sciences, Agriculture, and Business Administration asserted ownership over their separate curricula, they questioned physical education's value; one critic asserted in 1960 that only intellectual subjects that are "absolutely necessary" warranted a requirement, and gym class failed the test. The women's physical education department and its alumnae strenuously objected; higher education must include physical training, they insisted, because a fit body is essential to health and personal development. This argument was only partially successful, and compul-sory physical education at Nebraska gradually shrank after mid-century.[25]

Physical educators regarded such challenges as symptomatic of America's confusion over their contributions and rightful membership in academe. Colleagues in other fields often dismissed physical educators and coaches as

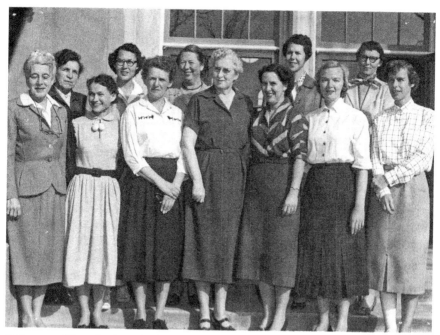

FIGURE 7.3 *Women's physical education staff, Stanford University, 1956. Courtesy of Stanford Historical Photograph Collection, Department of Special Collections and University Archives, Stanford University Libraries, Stanford, California.*

"knuckleheads" because they trained the body, not the mind; health educators seemed slightly more respectable because they were "do-gooders."[26] Even faculty members who valued physical education were tempted to view gym teachers primarily as capable organizers who could be enlisted to plan big campus events or serve as marshals at commencement ceremonies.[27] Some female physical educators sought other means to establish their academic credentials and intellectual heft. Conducting research, for example, not only suited some teachers' interests and aptitude but also earned respect on college campuses; moreover, such work could boost one's career through promotions, administrative positions, or graduate program appointments.[28]

Whether focusing on teaching or research, a university employee might wonder if her status matched her qualifications and responsibilities. At coeducational institutions, departmental organization complicated the answer; as was true in earlier decades, neither the merger nor separation of women's and men's programs ensured gender equity. A combined department under male leadership had inherent disadvantages. After forty years of consolidated administration, the women's division at Hampton University petitioned (unsuccessfully) for independence, asserting that the existing system hindered effective programs for female students and fair treatment of women faculty.[29] Women's frustration was equally high if men's and women's departments were separate, since "independence" did not guarantee self-governance. When the University of Nebraska placed physical education under the jurisdiction of the Teachers College in 1948, it split the men's and women's programs. The lines of authority remained so murky, however, that prominent female physical educators declined offers to lead the women's division, fearing that their supposed autonomy "with respect to budget, policy, personnel and promotions, facilities and equipment" would be illusory.[30] Invariably, any proposal to reorganize physical education and athletics stirred conflict, and the stakes were high. From unification to separation, and every arrangement in between, departmental structure affected how decisions about women's programs were made, by whom, and on what basis. No scheme guaranteed female physical educators control over their budgets, curricula, resources, or personnel. Regardless of women's position on the organizational chart, men's programs and university politics impinged on their authority, rendering female staff subordinate and neglected, while men's varsity athletics flourished.

Disparities in facilities and equipment were a common sore point. Women's programs often contended with buildings, fields, and gear that seemed woefully inadequate. The situation at Duke University's coordinate college for women was typical. In 1954/55 physical educators criticized the maintenance of the department's primary athletic field. Because it had not been rolled after resurfacing, the field suffered "deep ruts, large depressions where water stands after a rain, and no place . . . where a court of any sort can be laid out." The "stand of winter grass," though lovely, was "so thick that the golf balls and archery arrows would get lost." Mowing machines simply created more "ruts in the soft ground." Like many buildings on campus, the department continued, our indoor facilities also show a disturbing "shabbiness." "Woodwork is rotting around windows and in pool; the pool roof leaks; one floor is very badly eaten by termites; the reception and meeting room needs new furniture; pressure in water pipes is not good; [and] a ceiling radiator fell recently." After requesting a new building for more than thirty years, the department's patience ran out. How can we run a quality "modern program," the chair protested in 1960/61, in such "antiquated and inferior" facilities?[31]

Staff members at the University of Nebraska had waited even longer. Upon returning to the Lincoln campus in 1960, an elderly former departmental assistant was appalled by the decrepit condition of the women's gym. Writing to a university trustee, Mrs. Charles I. Taylor offered analysis as well as examples:

> I was shocked to find that no improvements had been made in all the fifty-seven years since I left the Department. The building was cleaner and the janitor work done far better then than now. Actually state law permits no motel to offer the unsanitary and inadequate facilities women must put up with in those showers. . . . Probably there would be more enthusiasm over the needs of the Department if it enjoyed even a fraction of the publicity and excitement lavished on men's competitive sports.[32]

No longer associated with the university, Mrs. Taylor had few qualms about naming a culprit. Her claim that Nebraska allowed men's athletics to eclipse women's programs was well founded. Far from being detrimental, turmoil in Nebraska's beloved football program had sparked more interest among fans and sportswriters, a new fund-raising system, and administrative reform that put men's athletics directly under the chancellor and board of regents.[33] Nebraska's priorities were clear: win or lose, tainted or clean, men's teams mattered. Meanwhile, women's physical education and intramural programs persevered in rundown facilities, with little notice.

The situation at traditionally black colleges and universities was even tougher.[34] Compared to white institutions, HBCUs had minimal resources for academic or extracurricular programs. Their physical education and sports facilities in the mid-1950s rarely met professional standards; although most schools had a gymnasium, few could afford a regulation swimming pool, dance studio, recreational game rooms, corrective rooms, or adequate outdoor facilities. These shortages were especially burdensome for women; whereas most white institutions reserved certain outdoor spaces (however shabby) for female students, men and women at HBCUs typically shared their school's limited outdoor courts, diamonds, and athletic fields.

Individuals suffered along with their departments. Being in a low-status field hurt every college-level physical educator; at all ranks, their salaries generally fell below those awarded to academic faculty.[35] White women incurred an extra tax for being female, and black women paid doubly by virtue of gender and race. Although no study between the 1950s and early 1970s was comprehensive and well designed, available data indicate that women's status at predominantly white colleges and universities changed little during this period. In 1950 teaching loads in departments with graduate programs were fairly gender neutral, but women were concentrated in the lower ranks despite strong credentials.[36] Two decades later, women's status had not improved. At four-year public institutions, male physical educators enjoyed newer facilities, held higher rank, had fewer class contact hours per week, taught more graduate courses, were promoted more quickly than women, and earned higher salaries, even "when rank and degree were equal."[37]

Racial discrimination was equally tenacious during the third quarter of the twentieth century. Despite steadily increasing qualifications, male and female staff at HBCUs received only modest pay, job benefits, and resources.[38] Black women found themselves at the bottom of the pile with numerous responsibilities. At public HBCUs, female physical educators averaged nearly twenty-one hours of instruction per week, while also handling several extracurricular activities; at both private and state black institutions, women's workloads typically exceeded the profession's recommended standard by 30 percent.[39] Although a bachelor's degree, even master's work, had become standard among black female teachers, their male colleagues nevertheless enjoyed higher rank and pay, served primarily as coaches, and had more opportunities for research.[40] Most black women were well aware of these inequities. As one pioneer recalled, dealing with both racial and gender discrimination was "'just like having a *log* across your neck. And you have *both* of those things to deal with. . . . There was no way out.'"[41] Despite strong backgrounds and heavy workloads, both white and black women typically ranked below male physical educators in terms of salary and other signifiers of status. Simply put, they did more but got less.

Homophobia: 1950s–Early 1970s

While sexism and racism could be quantified and exposed, homophobia remained physical education's unspoken prejudice, and many gay and lesbian teachers stayed securely in the closet. Postwar conditions added to their apprehension; although some developments could have liberated physical education, other forces drove the field more deeply into silence. On the one hand, sexual attitudes and expression in the United States had changed considerably since the early twentieth century, and homosexuality became more visible. During World War II, sex-segregated civilian jobs and military units allowed gays and lesbians to explore their identities, form intimate relationships, and create relatively safe networks that continued after the war. Moreover, Albert Kinsey's famous studies on men and women, published in 1948 and 1953 respectively, demonstrated in dry but startling terms that sexual activity in the United States was remarkably diverse. Among Kinsey's most surprising findings was the extent of same-sex desires and experiences among both men and women. Awareness of homosexuality, however, did not signify acceptance. In the 1950s leaders of many religious, legal, and political groups condemned homosexuality as a perversion, while various doctors, sexologists, and mental health experts produced ostensibly scientific evidence that same-sex attraction was pathological.

Social conditions fueled this hostility. The postwar campaign of intimidation and repression launched by Senator Joseph McCarthy targeted domestic Communists and then other so-called subversives, especially homosexuals. Rooting out gays and lesbians, McCarthyites argued, would reestablish the country's moral foundation and "normative gender roles and stable heterosexual relationships."[42] The pressure to conform was more than rhetorical. Homosexuals were purged from military service, barred from government employment, and dismissed from civilian jobs. Mainstream media depicted them in increasingly pejorative terms. From small towns to large cities, in public spaces and private homes, gays and lesbians faced surveillance, arrest, and punishment on an unprecedented scale. As repression continued through the 1960s, America's gay community fortified itself through cultural networks and created political organizations that promoted social justice.

Given this turbulence, physical education's unyielding heterosexism during the 1950s and 1960s was predictable, albeit disheartening. To protect the field's reputation, leaders chose not to acknowledge, much less correct its deep-rooted homophobia. To be safe, many gay and lesbian teachers remained silent and private, and women's calculations were especially tricky. Being easy targets for suspicion and harassment, many female teachers, coaches, and administrators—whether gay or straight—adopted "apologetic" strategies, namely, clothes, grooming, and behaviors that projected normative hetero-sexuality. Hoping to banish "'muscle-builders' and 'masculine-appearances'" from the women's gym, professional leaders monitored the dress and de-meanor of physical education majors and young staff members.[43] During oral histories, women who trained between the 1940s and 1960s all men-tioned the "feminine uniform" of hats, gloves, and sensible shoes. At the same time, many female physical educators protected their professional colleagues. Although members of the third and fourth generations rarely broached the issue, they often knew which friends identified as lesbians and insulated them through a code of silence. Nonetheless, mentors and employers who regarded a prospective or in-service teacher as "abnormal" could sabotage her career through expulsion, firing, or other measures.

Come the Revolution: Early 1970s–2005

During the last quarter of the twentieth century, women physical educators revisited old dilemmas. At the forefront was the question of priorities: Should programs emphasize general instruction, intramural activities, voluntary recreation, and/or competitive sports? This problem intensified after 1970 as schools reduced their gym class requirements, departments downsized instruc-tional staffs, and interscholastic and intercollegiate sports grew, especially for girls and women. Although competitive opportunities had been expanding for several decades, by the 1970s the trend seemed less objectionable and probably inevitable. Critical issues remained, however, about the governance, principles, and official practices of women's athletics, both locally and nationally. Seizing the moment, female leaders founded the Commission on Intercollegiate Athletics for Women (CIAW, 1966–72) and its successor, the Association for Intercolle-giate Athletics for Women (AIAW, 1972–82), which devised policies, provided services, and sponsored championships. Various forces ultimately doomed these groups and enabled the male-dominated National Collegiate Athletic Association (NCAA) to gain control over women's intercollegiate sports.

No single event caused these developments. Instead, many interlocking factors—political, financial, legal, and philosophical—were at work.[44] Among these was the passage of Title IX of the Education Amendments Act in 1972. Uncertain what the new law meant in theory or practice, the AIAW generally favored it, while the NCAA and other interested parties debated whether to ignore, support, or sabotage it.

The concise thirty-seven-word text of Title IX does not include the terms *athletics*, *physical education*, or *recreation*, and few proponents or legislators anticipated that the law would be applied to these domains.[45] Nevertheless, Title IX affected who competed in which sports and at what level, as well as how women's athletics were administered, by whom, and with what resources in educational institutions and other settings.[46] Applied to school-based physical education, Title IX "requires equity in grading, testing, facilities, equipment, assignment of teachers, locker rooms, and other areas of support and application of the curriculum. Title IX requires coeducational experiences in all activities except contact sports." Intramural programs also fall within the law's scope "if the institution that hosts them [does]. Community club and recreation programs, however, pose a greater jurisdictional challenge," because the "connection to federal financial assistance" may be less clear or direct.[47] Although Title IX stipulated fairness in gym class and athletic programs, it neither defined equity nor set practical benchmarks. These omissions complicated the interpretation, implementation, and enforcement of Title IX.[48] After decades of clarifications, court cases, and study groups, however, some analysts now regard Title IX as "clear, enforceable, applicable, and unchanged."[49] By law, active girls and women are entitled to fair opportunities as well as redress for inequities.

Although Title IX focused on participants, it had major consequences for the women professionals who devised curricula, ran activity programs, coached teams, and harnessed resources. Secondary school teachers adapted to coeducational gym classes and girls' interscholastic sports. At the college level, women's varsity athletics mushroomed, along with publicity, money, and expectations. These developments transformed women's work—from their daily responsibilities to administrative relationships, from practical concerns to philosophical debates, from professional status to on-the-job challenges.

Teachers and Coaches in Grades K–12

Because women had traditionally supervised girls, their job prospects in athletics seemed likely to improve under Title IX. Virtually every report, however, has shown a shrinking number of female head coaches, sports officials and trainers, equipment managers, and athletic administrators in secondary schools.[50] In just one decade (1972–82), the proportion of female high school coaches was cut in half in many states; women's share dropped from 100 to 45 percent in Wisconsin and from 69 to 33 percent in Kansas.[51] High schools often hired men to replace female coaches for existing girls' teams or to head the many new interscholastic teams created under Title IX. At the helm of minor sports, rather than flagship teams, women fared poorly in salaries and resources, and teenage girls lost role models.[52] Women also held few leadership positions in local, state, or national governance. Although females might head their school's division of girls' sports, they typically were subordinate to male directors who controlled athletic budgets, personnel, and policy.[53] Pervasive discrimination and men's consolidation of power stripped female coaches and administrators of jobs and authority.

As interscholastic sports grew, instructional programs declined. During the 1970s and 1980s, children in grades 1–4 were more likely than older pupils to be enrolled in physical education, but many elementary schools substituted recess for formal instruction. By the late 1980s less than 40 percent of all U.S. pupils, regardless of grade, had daily physical education.[54] Despite claims during the 1990s that physical education remained "an established component of the educational program in virtually [all] states, districts, and schools," such generalizations overlooked the continued erosion of basic instruction.[55]

Although most states still mandate physical education to some extent, many programs do not meet national standards of frequency, scope, or duration. As a 2006 report indicated, daily gym class is increasingly rare and requirements shrink by grade level:

> The percentage of students who attended a daily physical education class has dropped from 42 percent in 1991 to 28 percent in 2003. The percentage of schools that require physical education in each grade declines from about 50 percent in grades 1 through 5 to 25 percent in grade 8, to only 5 percent in grade 12. Eight percent of elementary schools, 6.4 percent of middle school/junior high schools, and 5.8 percent of senior high schools provide daily physical education or its equivalent . . . for the entire school year for students in all grades in the school.[56]

Gym teachers have long complained that their programs suffer the most when schools cut budgets or reorder priorities. Recent federal legislation, especially the No Child Left Behind Act of 2001, exacerbated the situation, as tests and performance standards in "core academic subjects" have left fewer class periods and resources for subjects deemed nonessential. Even states that protect physical education encounter problems. Although Maryland lists gym class as "one of seven mandatory subject areas," tight schedules, inadequate facilities, and meager staff development hinder effective teaching.[57]

As requirements declined, so did the number of instructors. Between the late 1970s and early 1990s, the number of gym teachers in the nation's schools dropped nearly 25 percent, despite an expanding student population.[58] Teachers' losses were especially evident in the upper grades, where requirements are weakest. Between the mid-1960s and mid-1980s, the proportion of secondary health and physical educators "within the total teaching force . . . dropped from 8.2 percent to 6.5 percent."[59] By 2001 the figure had fallen to 3.9 percent, with fewer than 46,000 health/physical educators working in public secondary schools, compared to about 80,000 in 1976.[60] Unsurprisingly, women physical educators fared the worst.[61] As the teaching corps became increasingly male, particularly in the upper grades, gender gaps continued in workloads, compensation, and professional opportunities. To this day, women are still underrepresented as department chairs, district supervisors, and state directors of physical education. Although data by race are scarce, fewer men and women of color apparently entered the teaching profession in recent decades, and their presence as in-service physical educators in grades K–12 has continued to decline.[62]

While their numbers shrank, teachers' qualifications and duties steadily rose. In the early 1970s most middle and junior high school gym teachers were college graduates in physical education; nearly one-third also held master's degrees. In the 1990s secondary school gym teachers often had baccalaureate degrees in physical education or related fields as well as state certification in their specialty.[63] Besides teaching several periods of physical activity each day, a typical high school physical educator, male or female, handled another instructional subject, coaching and other extracurricular activities, administrative work, consultations with staff members and parents, and general duties, ranging from safety patrol to supervising the school lunchroom.[64] By the late 1990s some states expected new hires to be certified in one or two fields besides physical education.[65]

Teachers' strong credentials and diverse responsibilities did little to improve their standing. Pupils often viewed gym class more as recess than a "real subject," and some parents believed its easy content and dubious grading rendered "Phys Ed" pointless.[66] Primary school instructors who had to supervise gym class reported that they would "'rather chew on some aluminum foil.'"[67] Instead of valuing physical educators as agents of fitness and skill, many school administrators saw them simply as disciplinarians who turned out "well-behaved children."[68]

Many American schoolteachers, regardless of subject area or grade level, experienced similar disrespect and disempowerment in recent decades; as bureaucratic rules and routinized duties multiplied, diverse instructors wondered if their job's burdens outweighed its rewards. Physical education's plight has been especially severe. Gym teachers have not received the "same status, rewards, or support accorded to teachers in general," and their subject is "located at the bottom."[69] Female personnel have suffered the most. Saddled with multiple duties, low status, and fewer resources and rewards than males enjoy, women physical educators stand at the periphery of their increasingly marginalized field. Men's growing monopoly in school-based athletics and physical education sends a clear message—girls may compete, but (white) men lead. The historical record demonstrates the structural constraints and persistent inequities that female teachers, coaches, and administrators must—and have—overcome to be successful professionals in the wake of Title IX and other social developments.

Collegiate Personnel: 1970s–2005

Significant changes also occurred at postsecondary institutions. Collegiate physical educators who were mid-career or near retirement in the early 1970s would barely recognize today's programs. Four decades ago, a shift from comprehensive undergraduate mandates to limited requirements, even elective programs, was underway.[70] In 1978 only 57 percent of four-year institutions had compulsory physical education, lessening the need for full-time instructors.[71] Although requirements continued at many small schools, HBCUs, and women's departments, they often covered fewer students over a shorter period, and academic credit and letter grades became less common. Colleges and universities also wondered how the burgeoning interest in women's athletics might affect resources and staff; through the 1970s, however, Title IX remained a new law with little bite. Despite wide variations in administrative structures for physical education, athletics, recreation, and teacher training, most institutions still had separate men's and women's departments in the early 1970s.

By the turn of the twenty-first century, the mission and organization of most programs had changed dramatically. Mandatory physical education was rare at large institutions but continued, albeit tenuously, for some undergraduates at smaller institutions.[72] As traditional gym class and full-time instructors disappeared, departments served the general student body through voluntary recreation and lifetime physical activities.[73] Intercollegiate sports also flourished. Social approval of women's athletics and stronger implementation of Title IX enabled more female undergraduates to compete at the varsity level; regardless of size, most institutions of higher education maintain numerous varsity teams for men and women—with five times more female participants today overall than three decades ago. Teacher training and graduate programs became more specialized, reflecting the diverse subfields of HPER. Departments with baccalaureate degrees in physical education retooled to meet the need for coaches, fitness coordinators, recreation leaders, physiotherapists, and athletic trainers. Departmental makeup changed accordingly. While fitness specialists handle general services for undergraduates, various administrators, coaches, and affiliated experts run intercollegiate athletics. Among larger institutions, the academic marketplace increasingly favors graduate faculty in exercise physiology, biomechanics, and sports management who conduct research while training candidates for advanced degrees.[74] Most institutions now house these diverse experts in a single administrative unit encompassing physical education, athletics, and recreation, and by the late 1980s the majority of coeducational schools had merged their separate men's and women's programs into one division under one (usually male) director. These developments represented a sea change, at once exciting and difficult, for female personnel at both single-sex and coed institutions. Women faced new responsibilities, more diverse colleagues, and unfamiliar administrative schemes. Although consequences varied by age, race, specialty, and institution, equity remained elusive for most postsecondary professionals.

One indicator is women's multiple duties without commensurate status or benefits. During the 1970s female personnel typically handled more contact hours than men, worked in older facilities, were concentrated in the bottom ranks with lower salaries, had slower rates of promotion, and accumulated other responsibilities, from mid-level administrative and committee work to teacher training and intramural programs. Strong credentials made little difference, as women with doctorates were more likely than men with advanced degrees to be hired as "activity teachers, rather than researchers, theory course professors, or administrators."[75] As instructional physical education declined in the 1980s, women continued juggling instruction, coaching, and/or mid-level administration, while their male colleagues typically had only one primary role. Women's workloads often ruled out other opportunities, such as conducting research, producing scholarly publications, or serving the wider profession.[76] Although disparities were most pronounced at large schools with extensive athletic programs (Division I), they also occurred at smaller institutions (Divisions II and III).[77] Despite gains for African American professionals in the 1970s and 1980s, racial inequities persisted. Older black women usually spent their careers at black schools managing limited resources, while younger cohorts, often graduates and employees of predominantly white institutions, earned higher salaries but held low-rank positions.[78] Between 1990 and 2005 many departments of athletics and recreation, especially at small institutions and HBCUs, assigned multiple duties to both male and female staff, but sex discrimination, job insecurity, and scarce resources complicated women's prospects for success in unique ways.[79]

Women's disadvantages have been especially glaring in intercollegiate athletics, the powerful center of resources and prestige. As varsity sports for female undergraduates expanded between 1970 and 2005, women steadily disappeared as head coaches and senior administrators, while predominating in unpaid and mid-level positions. From the standpoint of Title IX and Title VII (which regulates workplace practices), a coach's or Athletic Director's sex is irrelevant "as long as no discrimination occurred in the hiring, pay-scale determination, or conditions of employment."[80] Despite its seeming neutrality, Title IX nevertheless facilitated a radical makeover. With women's sports heralding career advancement and visibility, more men entered the arena, aided by well-established professional networks and favorable hiring practices.[81] The consolidation of men's and women's departments also contributed to the centralization of power and the marginalization of female athletic leaders.

Women's losses occurred early and rapidly. Although the number of head coaches for women's varsity teams nearly tripled between 1972 and 1978, women's share of these positions dropped from 90 percent to 58.2 percent, with black women's representation being only 5 percent.[82] During the 1980s the overall proportion of female coaches of women's teams fell another 10 percent, with high-powered Division I programs having the weakest representation. Male coaches not only commandeered women's sports but also kept their 98 percent share of men's teams.[83] By 2004 women held only 44.1 percent of head coaching positions for women's intercollegiate teams, a figure "close to the lowest representation of females as head coaches of women's teams in history."[84] As men accumulated new and existing coaching jobs, female coaches often worked without full-time assistants while also covering a second sport, intramural programs, or administrative jobs such as rules compliance or financial oversight.[85] These imbalances vary by sport, division, and race.[86] Though common in field hockey and lacrosse, female coaches are rare in track and field. Division III institutions are more likely than larger schools to hire female coaches. Despite some progress, African American women are severely underrepresented as head coaches of women's teams, regardless of sport or division; between 1995 and 2005 they held between 1 and 3 percent of top positions, excluding HBCUs.

Women's salaries and benefits reflect their marginalization. "Only in fencing, volleyball, and tennis, the sports paying the lowest salaries to coaches of male teams, do coaches of women's sports receive equal or greater pay than coaches of the equivalent male sports."[87] Since men frequently coach women's teams, gender inequities in salaries surface more clearly in highly sex-segregated sports;

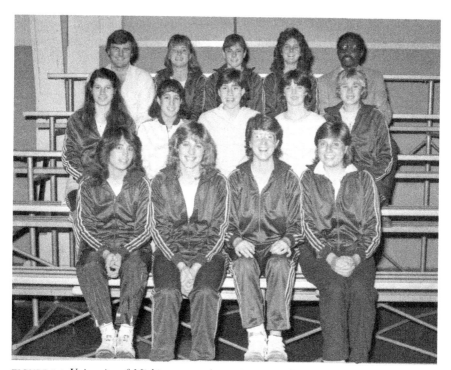

FIGURE 7.4 *University of Michigan women's tennis team and male coaches, 1984. Courtesy of the Bentley Image Bank #BL009946, Bentley Historical Library, University of Michigan.*

the salaries of head coaches (nearly 92 percent female) of women's Division I lacrosse teams are about 26 percent lower than the salaries of head coaches (exclusively male) of men's Division I lacrosse teams.[88] Although salaries for both male and female coaches rose in the late 1990s, women's increases were less than a third of men's.[89] Other than the compensation packages available to prominent women leading flagship sports in Division I, female coaches generally have not kept pace with their male peers.

As coaching opportunities dwindled, women also lost their traditional leadership positions. In 1972 females governed more than 90 percent of the country's athletic programs for undergraduate women; a few years later they ran only 15 percent.[90] Black women constituted about 5 percent of athletic directors (AD) and 2 percent of assistant ADs.[91] The disappearance of female directors coincided with the consolidation of men's and women's instructional and athletic programs at coeducational institutions. "Typically, the former head of the men's department assumed the primary authority over both the men's and women's programs, and the previous head of the women's athletic department was relegated to a secondary, non-decision-making role."[92] Not surprisingly, the process stirred further tension between male and female personnel. When Purdue University's programs quarreled over merging in 1975, an exasperated dean told members to simply "do it."[93] Female professionals themselves, though, were far from unanimous. Some national leaders and rank-and-file teachers endorsed mergers, believing that joint administration would be more efficient and economical for everyone. Others predicted that mergers would destroy the relative autonomy that women's separate programs had enjoyed for decades; female staff and students alike, the argument ran, would fare better if women administrators kept the reins of power.

By 1980 consolidation was a fait accompli at most coeducational institutions, large and small, and more women administrators vanished. In combined departments, the top woman typically served as Assistant Director of Women's Programs under a male director. Most strikingly, more than one-third of women's intercollegiate programs had "no female at all involved in their administration."[94] By the late 1980s women of color were "rapidly becoming invisible" among the ranks of coaches and athletic administrators.[95] Despite enjoying their work, African American women became impatient with "dead-end positions, inadequate salary," limited support, heavy workloads, and the double burden of racism and sexism. Administrators discriminated against them; male colleagues, black and white, questioned their competence in men's "'hallowed ground'" of athletics; co-workers "resented women being in key positions." One longtime coach recalled that her institution offered a head coaching position to an inexperienced white man at a higher salary than hers. Did such injustices come about "'because you're black, or because you're a woman,'" or—as most veterans believed—because they were both?[96]

These disparities continued through the 1990s and early 2000s. The most common administrative structure became the triumvirate (a male AD, a female associate or assistant AD, and a male associate or assistant AD); next was a two-person arrangement (a male AD plus a female Senior Woman Administrator). Together, these two configurations account for one-third of departments of athletics and recreation at colleges and universities.[97] In 2004 only 18.5 percent of ADs were female, with the proportion in Division III being three times that of more prestigious Division I departments.[98] Virtually all Senior Woman Administrators at non-HBCUs are white women.[99] Athletics programs also entail many mid- and low-level positions. When these bureaucracies grew 40 percent, top to bottom, between 1988 and 2004, women gained jobs but lost clout as they collected in the lower ranks or disappeared altogether. Simply put, "as the status and salary of . . . positions increase, female representation decreases" and racial disparities multiply.[100] These imbalances matter. Senior administrators determine resource allocation, hiring practices, and other policies—and many outcomes are gender-related. "In all three [NCAA] Divisions," two experts note, "when the athletic director is a male, the percentage of female coaches is lower than when the athletic director is a female."[101]

Power arrangements and sex discrimination also affected the relative health of men's and women's varsity programs in recent decades. Paying only lip service to Title IX, many postsecondary institutions failed to support women's teams and their leaders with consistent or adequate resources. In the early 1970s institutional size and reputation had little effect on compliance.[102] Although the women's program at the University of Texas was top-rated, female head coaches typically had part-time appointments and earned less than assistant football coaches, and female athletes had few scholarships and inferior benefits.[103] During the 1960s and 1970s, Nell C. Jackson, the renowned track and field star, coached at Tuskegee Institute, the University of Illinois, and Michigan State University. One institution, she recalled, provided resources with one hand, then snatched them away with the other: "Equipment ordered by the coaches of men's sports were maintained by them for their sport. Equipment ordered by me for women's teams became property of the entire department (i.e., stop watches)."[104] Problems also arose at single-sex institutions. When male administrators and professors at Agnes Scott College pushed enthusiastically for competitive sports in the 1970s, physical educators wondered how such a program could survive given the school's "buckled basketball court," "cracked tennis courts" with loose wire fencing, debris, and puddles, and a rarely mowed "athletic field with uneven turf and poor drainage."[105]

Four decades later, difficulties still abound. Budgets for intercollegiate teams, men's and women's, typically cover recruitment, scholarships, game-day expenses, equipment and facilities, and salaries. Extra support comes through fund-raising, perks, and special services. Title IX does not require institutions to spend identical dollar amounts on men's and women's teams; instead, the standard is whether student athletes receive equitable benefits in such areas as coaching, equipment, facilities, and travel.[106] Benefits are measured across an entire athletic program, not on a team-by-team basis or between major and minor sports. Even institutions that ostensibly comply with Title IX still privilege male athletes. In 2005–06 total expenses for Division I men's athletics averaged 66 percent, with women's sports receiving the other 34 percent; Division I institutions typically spent more money on football programs that year than on all women's teams combined.[107] Although national averages obscure differences between sports as well as institutions, they nevertheless reveal a disturbing pattern. Despite assurances that mergers would allow pooled resources to be distributed fairly, the long-standing gap between men's and women's programs has continued.

Court cases expose the local impact of such disparities. Consider the 1993 case of *Favia v. Indiana University of Pennsylvania*, a Division II athletic program:

> The coach of the field hockey team wore two hats. She was a full-time physical education teacher as well as a coach. She received no monetary compensation for her coaching duties. . . . The coach kept the team's uniforms in the trunk of her car along with other equipment because no on-campus storage was available. For every $8 spent on male athletes, IUP spent only $2.75 on its female athletes. Several male coaches of men's teams received complimentary cars and golf club memberships. No coach of a women's team enjoyed such perks. Male athletes garnered 79 percent of the scholarship dollars. IUP encouraged spectator support for men's teams by offering raffles for a full semester of tuition at each men's basketball and football home game. IUP did not offer similar enticements to spectators at women's competitions.[108]

The court ruled that tight budgets were no excuse for IUP's stark "favoritism." At many coeducational schools, legal decisions and institutional goodwill have reduced, but not eliminated, the gender inequities that persist after participation opportunities for male and female students have been balanced.[109]

While female athletes went to court, their mentors also mobilized. In the 1970s professional organizations voiced women's concerns and defended their rights at the regional and national levels; the AIAW sought to govern intercollegiate sports, while the National Association for Girls and Women in Sport (a unit within AAHPER) served primarily as an advocacy group. At individual colleges and universities, women physical educators wrote position papers for or against departmental mergers, sought redress for long-standing problems from equipment shortages to unfair salaries, served on innumerable task forces and committees, and tapped their field's venerable "old girls" network to get advice and plot strategy.[110]

As setbacks mounted in the 1980s, white and black women pushed their field to address gender and racial inequities. Although most women attributed their declining fortunes to discrimination and the powerful "old boys' club," many men believed that personal, not structural, causes were at work; in their view, "qualified women coaches and administrators" were in short supply and in-service women seemed unwilling or unable to manage varsity athletics.[111] Women routinely disproved these assumptions. Having joined the profession expressly to be college coaches, young women persevered, despite predictable and unforeseen obstacles. Having begun their careers as physical educators, many senior women found satisfaction in coaching and other leadership roles—difficulties notwithstanding. Antagonistic workplaces and athletics' eclipsing of general education, however, led some older women to seek different jobs or retire.[112]

Today, some women enjoy lucrative, high-profile careers, especially in Division I sports. For most teachers, coaches, and administrators, though, career tracks can be rocky; despite new opportunities, their salaries, resources, and authority rarely reflect their multiple contributions. Most notably, white and black women are underrepresented in key decision-making positions, and numerous female teams are underresourced. Many colleges and universities adapted to Title IX by continuing to privilege male personnel and men's activities.

HPER's "Open Secret": 1970–2005

Over the past few decades, professional organizations took some steps to address gender inequities among physical educators and athletic personnel. Efforts to acknowledge and rectify racial injustice were more tentative. The field did little, though, to counter the deep-seated homophobia that it shared with American society at large. The presence and struggles of lesbians remained the field's "open secret"—the issue was everywhere and nowhere. During the past fifteen years, however, some HPER professionals along with scholars in other disciplines confronted the topic more directly. Their studies documented what female gym teachers and coaches already knew: navigating prejudice is a daily project.[113]

Women's personal experiences are a useful starting point for understanding HPER's open secret.[114] Whether gay or straight, gym teachers and coaches are aware of constant surveillance; colleagues, administrators, students, and parents regularly judge their behavior, scrutinize their bodies, puzzle over their identities and lives, and worry about the intimate physicality of their job, especially when working with youngsters. For gym teachers and coaches, everything feels public and nothing seems private.

In homophobic cultures, conjecture about someone's identity invariably converges on sexual orientation. Female coaches and physical educators particularly describe living under a cloud of suspicion.[115] Most Americans, they believe, "stereotype women physical educators as more likely than most women to be single, childless, feminist, and lesbian, to dress in pants and go without makeup." Simply put, "'If you're over thirty and you're a PE teacher and you're single, you're a lesbian.'"[116] In many circles, this label is pejorative, rather than neutral or affirmative. Once stigmatized, a teacher or coach might be harassed, threatened, shunned, or fired. A college athletics department might "reassure prospective athletes and their parents not only that there are no lesbians in [its] program but also that there *are* lesbians in a rival school's program," a tactic known as negative recruiting.[117] Discrimination can also be direct and personal: "At some schools, a new coach's heterosexual credentials are scrutinized as carefully as her professional qualifications. Coaches thought to be lesbians are fired or intimidated into resigning."[118]

The fear of persecution affects all women, regardless of sexual orientation. Many heterosexual teachers and coaches carefully protect themselves from the taint of deviance. They remain silent and complicit about homophobia, steer clear of lesbians in their departments and professional groups, and project unambiguous heterosexual femininity, while hiring assistants and recruiting athletes who seem equally proper.[119] Lesbians' options are far more difficult. Being out is honest but risky; being closeted seems safe yet isolating and hypocritical. To navigate this minefield, many lesbian teachers and coaches compartmentalize their lives; they present a conventional self in public, while maintaining an authentic private self. If being out at work seems unsafe, lesbians must deny and conceal their true identities, distance themselves from personal conversations and gay issues, be "hypervigilant" about how they act and talk, and invent "cover stories" for their private lives. As the pain grows, many lesbian teachers and coaches feel alone, afraid, invisible, silenced, and oppressed. As one intercollegiate coach remarked, "'I'm constantly thinking, I'm constantly monitoring, how I am, how I behave, what I say, how I react, what I stand for, what I represent, in a way that I know I wouldn't if I were straight.'"[120]

Broad social changes both eased and complicated physical educators' dilemma. In the 1970s America's highly sexualized culture emboldened many homosexuals to come out of the closet; while some created vibrant, more public forms of gay culture, others sought full rights through political action. A strong, well-coordinated backlash, though, limited the movement's successes. This climate reinvigorated debates among doctors, psychiatrists, and other professionals about the origins and meaning of homosexuality. Denouncing some experts' reductionist theories and promise of biomedical "cures," gays and lesbians helped effect new policies, most notably the American Psychiatric Association's 1973 decision to "remove homosexuality from its official manual of mental diseases."[121]

During the 1980s the fight for basic rights intensified as did resistance. With religious fundamentalism and the New Right holding sway, some gays and lesbians despaired by moving deeper into the closet; others mobilized to defend their cultural networks, political gains, and very lives. These struggles continued through the 1990s and into the twenty-first century. From the local to national levels, conservative politicians championed anti-gay laws and rallied their electoral base with inflammatory wedge issues. Nevertheless, America's sexual revolution may have become "too deeply embedded in the fabric of economic life" and Americans' private behavior to be reversed.[122] Furthermore, right-wing attacks energized supporters of social justice and stimulated new scientific perspectives, including arguments that gender identities and sexual orientation assume many, even fluid forms, none more normal than the others.[123]

The tumult of recent decades strengthened the resolve of many physical educators and coaches. Some took tentative steps toward breaking their field's silence and rectifying discrimination. More courageously, others pushed for frank discussion and fundamental reform. Thanks to the perseverance of committed leaders and researchers, professional conferences and journals now cover topics of sexuality and homophobia more often than before. Progressive schools have created affirmative environments and implemented nondiscrimination policies. Advocacy groups, such as the Women's Sports Foundation, have aided the cause through websites, reports, and workshops.

At same time, social conditions have reinforced HPER's wariness about gay issues. Because the profession's reputation and roles are tenuous, its official stance on sexual orientation remains cautious. Since America depends on exercise and sports to embody normative gender and sexuality, physical educators face constant scrutiny as members of a body-centered profession. Consequently, lesbian teachers, coaches, and administrators must still negotiate significant risks while doing their jobs and living their lives.

"It's just the gym"

In many respects, physical education and sports after mid-century simply replicated America's general pattern of sex discrimination. As HPER sought a niche within educational institutions and health-related professions, it often marginalized female personnel. As physical education requirements steadily declined, women staff either shouldered other responsibilities or disappeared. As competitive sports for girls and women gained importance, female coaches and administrators were relegated to the periphery. The largest inequities occurred at the top and bottom of the occupational ladder—the very jobs where status and authority were either concentrated or denied. Overall, power gravitated to male personnel and resources flowed primarily to programs for boys and men. These gender disparities were interlocked with race and sexual orientation. A predominantly white profession discriminated against black personnel; likewise, the heterosexist ethos of physical education and sports stigmatized and often silenced lesbian teachers and coaches. In sum, the profession reproduced familiar hierarchies of difference; being female, black, and/or gay disqualified individuals from full membership and leadership positions in a field that trained bodies and developed athleticism.

The centrality of active bodies, though, underscores the field's unique features. Being a gym teacher or coach downgraded women's status compared to their counterparts in more prestigious professions. Conversely, being female was disadvantageous in a field so intent on privileging men and male physicality. The devaluation of most female experts not only solidified men's institutional power, but also represented physical aptitude as a masculine trait. Similarly, discrimination based on race and sexual orientation insulated the profession from common stereotypes about "dumb jocks" and "butch women" in the gym. Although Americans are now accustomed to watching black athletes, male and female, perform, they still see relatively few African Americans in leadership positions in interscholastic and intercollegiate sports. Likewise, the preponderance of men coaches for both male and female athletes sends a clear message about gender and sexuality; men are deemed qualified and trustworthy regardless of whom they train, whereas women's professional abilities and interactions with other females are universally suspect. This system preserves the masculinist, heterosexist profile of sports and oppresses all women, whatever their sexual orientation.

Although inequities pervade American society, the interconnected hierarchies of gender, race, and sexual orientation have special salience in physical education and sports. They constitute difference in both symbolic and material terms: Who supposedly understands the world of physicality and athleticism, and who does not? Who wields power and makes decisions in the realm of active bodies, and who may not? The gym is far more than "just the gym."

{8}

Physical Fairness

SCIENCE, FEMINISM, AND SEX DIFFERENCES, 1950–2005

> When we had tennis class [in the late 1920s], the men would come and
> hang on the fences, and [shout] "haw, haw, look at them try to play."
> That did things to the girls. They didn't want to be laughed at, so they
> didn't play. And if they played, they didn't want to be so good that they
> might be noticed. That's why to me the progress that's been made has
> been like a revolution. Now men invite women to play tennis.
>
> —Professor Laura J. Huelster, *University of Illinois, 1974*

Even as the status of teachers changed after mid-century, a corresponding revolution swept up their students. The expansion of women's sports and exercise in schools and throughout society encouraged new ideas about active female bodies. Americans increasingly acknowledged women's physical capacity and athletic talent. This cultural reassessment of sex differences prompted gym teachers to reconsider their concepts of equity: Whether activities were coed or single-sex, what did "physical fairness" now mean?[1] Although this question had puzzled physical educators for decades, developments in American law, politics, and science stimulated new perspectives during the second half of the twentieth century.

Court rulings and federal legislation stipulated that activity programs include individuals once regarded as different. In 1954 *Brown v. Board of Education of Topeka* directed dual school systems to desegregate, and this included the schools' programs of athletics and physical education. Title IX of the 1972 Educational Amendments Act opened numerous academic and non-academic opportunities to girls and women; in the name of gender equity, many high schools expanded girls' sports and replaced sex-segregated gym class with coed instruction. In 1973, Section 504 of the Rehabilitation Act banned recipients of federal money from discriminating against individuals with disabilities; specifically, school-based physical education and sports programs had to "provide equal opportunities for comparable participation" to qualified handicapped students.[2] The new legal standards of the 1970s coincided with a revitalized women's movement.

Along with other campaigns for social justice, second- and then third-wave feminism influenced public policy, daily life, and popular attitudes by asking whether men and women were alike or dissimilar, and if biology or culture made them so. By century's end, traditional boundaries between masculinity and femininity no longer seemed absolute or even sensible to some Americans. Similar disagreements arose among biological and social scientists. Research on sex differences reinvigorated debates over women's "nature": Did femaleness (one complementary state in the presumed dualism of sex) determine behavior or did socialization create womanliness (one position in the supposed binary of gender)?

These developments permeated American physical education, especially the work of female teachers and coaches. Because many still dealt primarily with adolescents and young women, female professionals reevaluated their students and programs: What did a fair chance for the "fair sex" now mean? Just as their predecessors had in the early 1900s, female physical educators after mid-century used their remarks on difference and fairness to articulate broad philosophies and exert professional power. This chapter examines how women physical educators, coaches, and administrators—predominantly middle-class whites—conceptualized difference and equity between 1950 and 2005. Although consensus was rare, majority opinions in each decade tended to agree with mainstream feminism, science, and culture. While most white female teachers played it safe, however, a few mavericks envisioned more radical forms of justice in the gym.

Democratic Fitness in the 1950s

During the late 1940s and 1950s, strength and security became national watchwords. Preoccupied with the Cold War, political leaders declared that the country's domestic interests and global power were interdependent; to ensure vitality here and abroad, they proclaimed, American education, capitalism, technology, and defense must be augmented through heavy investments in scientific research, military readiness, and economic growth. President Dwight D. Eisenhower insisted that physical fitness was equally important. His concern was both personal and strategic; advised after a heart attack in 1955 to exercise more, Eisenhower also worried about national weakness, since American youngsters seemed less fit than European children. Several highly publicized studies, particularly by Hans Kraus and Ruth Hirschland, indicated that a majority of the country's children "failed to meet even a minimum standard [of strength and flexibility] required for health."[3] At a special White House Conference on Fitness of American Youth in 1956, delegates concluded that giving physical education the same weight as other school subjects would elevate fitness as a national priority. Eisenhower immediately created a cabinet-level body, the President's Council on Youth Fitness (PCYF), and doctors, educators, and sports experts hailed the new emphasis on exercise and health. Labor unions, the Girl Scouts and Boy Scouts, and other private groups sponsored recreational and outdoor activities. Whether seeking fitness or fun, more citizens participated in bowling, bicycling, golf, tennis, boating, and swimming.[4] In word and deed, the country seemed committed to fitness.

Behind the scenes, though, health experts and government officials argued over how to define and measure fitness, as well as who should lead the nation's campaign. Despite this in-fighting, most professionals believed that exercise was a critical component, as long as people's activities suited their physical and personal makeup. Sex differences figured prominently in a 1958 statement by the American Medical Association and the American Association for Health, Physical Education, and Recreation (AAHPER).[5] "There are measurable differences between the sexes in heart capacity, muscular strength, and skeletal proportions," the two groups declared, that "set certain limitations for women in activities of strength, speed, and endurance." Nevertheless, the report concluded, "social custom" also strongly influenced female activity and the "range of physical capacities in individuals of both sexes is great." In short, nature and nurture together produced both differences and similarities among active males and females. At mid-century, however, claims about exercise rested on meager research. Although the principles of physical activity, especially "how the body responded to exercise, how to assess physical fitness, and how to increase fitness in youth and adults," intrigued many scientists, their data were sketchy and theories quite speculative—leaving doctors and other professionals unsure how to apply the information.[6] These problems led diverse researchers and practitioners to band together in such organizations as the American College of Sports Medicine, founded in 1954.

Physical educators were ambivalent about the fitness crusade. On the one hand, it could enhance their professional stature while improving the public's health. On the other hand, dismal reports about unfit youth and sedentary adults cast doubt on the field's effectiveness: Why were Americans so out-of-shape despite decades of mandatory gym class? Eager to seize the moment without accepting blame, physical educators mobilized. They conducted studies on the value of instructional exercise, lobbied for stronger requirements in public schools, and developed an independent battery of fitness tests and standards.[7] These initiatives raised questions about sex differences. Since physical and psychosocial health varied by age and sex, gym teachers wondered how to characterize female fitness. Which activities—conditioning exercise, recreational games, or competitive sports—would best promote girls' vigor? Given that boys outperformed girls on most motor ability tests, did biology or culture limit female development? Only a few women physical educators regarded males and females as completely dissimilar due solely to biology or as socially and physically identical, other than reproduction. Instead, white female teachers usually asserted that biology and socialization made the two sexes both alike and different, rendering females at once admirable and deficient.

Starting with the body, teachers catalogued the physical traits that active males and females shared. Regardless of sex, they believed, motor skills typically improved as one's body matured; conversely, activity fostered strength, endurance, and other aspects of fitness. Some anatomical features, though, disadvantaged girls and women. According to one high school instructor, the female's "wider hips" and "broader pelvis with shorter oblique legs" precluded efficient running and jumping. By contrast, the "male physique—broader shoulders, narrow hips, the bones of the upper leg nearly parallel and perpendicular to the floor"—aided performance.[8] Physical activity, teachers reasoned, must take such differences into account.[9] Volleyball nets should be lowered to match average female height. Softball catchers ought to learn a special crouch to accommodate their broad hips. Although many aspects of basketball seemed sex-neutral, rules about guarding and physical contact must be modified to respect girls' limited stamina and skill. Some experts opposed allowing the "ball to be tied or taken from an opponent" because girls' arms were too short and their body control too tenuous to "execute this technique without contact."[10] Absent such adaptations, teachers warned, physical education would be counterproductive, even harmful.

They wondered, however, if biology acted alone. Without doubt, a respected researcher acknowledged, average body composition produces stark disparities in power. "In every sport where strength and/or speed is important, men have (and will always have!) a tremendous advantage." But, Anna S. Espenschade continued, performance gaps also arise from interest, experience, and other psychosocial factors.[11] This argument implied that novelty, not anatomy, caused girls' awkwardness when they first played field hockey or tried track and field. Every novice feels clumsy and self-conscious, teachers observed, whether executing basic skills or a technical sport. Many girls, one high school teacher reported, "push [a] ball instead of throwing it" and "close their eyes and shy away" when catching. The remedy, Amy Brown proposed, is instruction and practice. "Correct body training" is precisely what a shy, inept beginner needs to "build [her] confidence and physical fitness."[12] If softball players seem timid, then train them how to slide, swing a bat, and field a ground ball. If you spot an adolescent or undergraduate running with "side flings of the legs" and "'flapping' her arms," then teach proper technique at a young age.[13] Experience develops new skills and, conversely, "ability encourages participation."[14]

Because activity depended as much on interest as skill, teachers next described the personal attributes that the two sexes brought to the gym.[15] As do boys, many girls "have a desire to run, jump and throw, to indulge in self-testing skills, and to compete against themselves and with others." In fact, the "will to win and competitive spirit" were an integral "part of human nature." Moreover, recreation and sports could teach everyone—young and old, male or female—basic lessons in democratic conduct. General traits aside, though, teachers regarded females as unique, individually and collectively. Although each girl and woman follows her own path, they explained, some roles and behaviors seemed to be universal among females. Similarly, each girl learns skills in the gym her own way, but girls' and boys' preferences rarely coincide.[16]

Consequently, co-recreation was the biggest obstacle to physical fairness. By the 1950s virtually all physical educators advocated mixed activities of some kind for every age group. Interaction with the opposite sex, they reasoned, matched "real life situations," promoted "mutual respect and understanding," and prepared for "a sound, happy marital and family life."[17] When sex differences in body and character were negligible or irrelevant, as in social dance, the path to fairness was straightforward. Certain coeducational sports also seemed feasible. In track and field "events requiring speed, agility, and coordination, such as the running events, the high jump, and the throw for accuracy," two teachers argued in 1958, "girls and boys compete with equal chances of success. They may therefore be scheduled either together or separately."[18] By contrast, if one sex held a significant advantage, then an activity's rules, objectives, or team composition should be modified to neutralize the disparity. Coed volleyball could require that "a boy plays the ball once," whereas girls are permitted to "set it up to themselves or someone else." Coed games could reward skill, rather than strength, and emphasize "social development" and cooperation, rather than competition. Coed softball might use "a girl battery for the boys team and a boy battery for the girls team."[19] One teacher even puzzled over pin setting in coed bowling:

> Girls should not set pins for boys because boys roll such a fast ball that there is danger from flying pins. Several solutions are possible. One method is to have boys and girls on each alley, but have only boys set pins. This has two disadvantages: (1) boys have less bowling time; and (2) girls are deprived of the valuable experience of pin setting. Another, and better, method is to assign boys and girls on alternate alleys. Thus, only boys set pins for the male bowlers, yet opportunity is provided for all to benefit from the advantages of a coeducational class.[20]

This scenario suggested another approach to fair play: If biological or cultural differences were insurmountable, then the two sexes should play separately. Some sex-segregated schemes in the 1950s retained the illusion of co-recreation. Two high school teachers proposed a version of three-on-three basketball in which six boys (three guards and three forwards) played against each other at one end of the court and six girls played at the opposite end; "the boy guards pass [the ball] to girl forwards and vice versa." More commonly, teachers simply ran different activities; boys wrestled and played football, while girls participated in tumbling and other activities requiring "grace and flexibility."[21] Whether de facto or de jure, sex-segregated activities were intended to give boys and girls comparable opportunities to succeed (the standard of equality) by respecting their differences (the foundation of equity).

Despite hints of gender consciousness, teachers' views largely agreed with scientific interpretations at mid-century.[22] Few biological or social scientists were strict biodeterminists, attributing every aspect of human life to raw material forces; such reductive views were unpopular, at least temporarily, following the excesses of the eugenics movement and the Nazis' "final solution." Likewise, although psychologists, sociologists, and anthropologists favored cultural explanations of behavior, they rarely discounted the role of biology. Amid these balanced perspectives, some rigid views also gained favor; increasingly, many disciplines posited a sharp distinction between sex and gender—between the immutable bedrock of male versus female and the fluid effects of culture on masculine and feminine identity. Most white physical educators found middle ground on these issues: Sex formed a clear binary, they said, but some attributes and rights were not gendered. Anatomy *was* destiny in the gym, but socialization also affected motor skill and interests.

Teachers' complex perspective suited the political environment. In the 1950s mainstream culture and political discourse celebrated prosperity, consumerism, family, and motherhood as the markers of white, middle-class women's lives. Cold War ideology praised American individualism; unlike conformity and oppression under totalitarian regimes, the argument ran, the United States was egalitarian, with every man, woman, and child enjoying freedom of choice. In the gym, therefore, everyone deserved a chance to participate and learn. This represented the principle of similarity and equality. But the gym must be fair as well; every participant was entitled to be treated as an individual or group member with distinctive biological and psychosocial traits. This upheld the principle of difference and equity. Confident that human beings were similar and equal, white physical educators nonetheless perceived basic divisions by sex, race, and class. White teachers' allegiance to traditional norms of gender and sexuality, and a sharp divergence between men's and women's lives, reflected their status as white, middle-class Americans. Recognizing that broader opportunities for girls and women were approaching, perhaps inexorably, physical educators' nuanced model of active womanhood opened some doors but kept others closed. White female instructors accepted feminine skill but not unfettered athleticism. They envisioned a gymnasium full of white, middle-class, heterosexual girls and boys who were capable and cooperative. As did their profession at large, white female teachers remained oblivious to, at least silent about, inequities related to race, class, and sexuality.

The Turbulent 1960s

Holding the middle ground proved difficult in the 1960s as intellectual and social tremors shook the field. Biomedical experts reworked the meaning of personal and public health. Natural and social scientists pushed more reductive biological interpretations of human development. With the Vietnam War raising critical issues of political authority and social engagement, activists called upon the United States to honor its democratic ideals. Although this tug-of-war over justice and power drew many Americans into the public arena, the "silent majority" simply warned of moral collapse or retreated into their private lives. These broad developments complicated gym teachers' customary judgments about active womanhood.

During the 1960s and 1970s, the prevalence of cancer, heart disease, and other chronic illnesses drew experts' attention to the social, behavioral, and environmental factors that might render individuals more vulnerable to these disorders. The role of personal habits, acquired and practiced throughout one's life, seemed especially important in managing risk.[23] While scientists sought to connect specific behaviors and ailments, public health officials preached about the dangers of smoking, alcohol, and physical inactivity. Despite inconclusive research on the physiological and medical benefits of exercise, the renamed President's Council on Physical Fitness (PCPF) and related groups championed physical activity by conducting surveys, issuing how-to booklets, promoting standardized fitness tests, evaluating school programs, and advocating more opportunities for girls and women.[24] Health-centered exercise, though, drew a lukewarm response from physical educators. Despite revisions, AAHPER's Youth Fitness Test still involved sports-related skills differentiated by sex.[25] Instructional programs also continued to emphasize team sports. Although some postsecondary curricula introduced more recreational games and exercise, these health-related activities seemed secondary given America's obsession with athletics.[26]

Research on human behavior and sex differences proliferated in the 1960s, with a decided tilt toward biological interpretations.[27] At the forefront were scientists who argued that brain development in males and females was mediated by prenatal hormones in sex-specific ways—a process culminating in permanent, gendered character. Two classes of chemicals supposedly made two types of brains resulting in two patterns of behavior. Highly reductive and dualistic, the "organization theory" quickly permeated physiology and neuro-endocrinology in the 1960s, and other disciplines followed suit. Since sexual development had two natural paths leading to two distinct identities, some psychologists claimed, biology intended intersexuals to be either a man or woman, regardless of ambiguous genitalia. Similarly, anthropologists and sociologists applied simple binaries of sex and gender to explain diverse human experiences, past and present. Although some researchers dissented, biodeterminism and dualisms dominated the natural and social sciences in the 1960s.

Beyond the laboratory, sex and gender seemed less clear-cut. A resurgent women's movement raised critical questions about difference, equality, and social change.[28] Mainstream white feminists tended to accept liberal Western ideals of human equality, rationality, and agency. Because Nature endowed the two sexes with comparable rights and abilities, they said, women were entitled to the same opportunities as men; any disparities were the result of societal attitudes and institutions. To ensure gender neutrality in employment, education, and other domains, liberals concluded, antidiscrimination laws were necessary. Although this analysis of similarity and equality interrupted the simple mapping of sex onto gender, it naturalized the male/female binary and protected America's investment in marriage and heterosexuality. By contrast, radical feminists associated with civil rights, gay rights, the New Left, and the antiwar movement considered the two sexes to be fundamentally different; a significant number valorized women's innate values as superior to men's. Whether biological essentialists or not, many radicals held patriarchy responsible for women's social subordination and deemed separation from men the only route to liberation. Despite these internal conflicts, the women's movement secured vital legislative reforms and, along with other activists, made the tidy categories of sex and gender seem less obvious and absolute.

These intellectual and political currents swept through American physical education in the 1960s. Given its preoccupation with sex differences, the field had to reassess active womanhood and the nature/nurture relationship. White female teachers wondered how research on bodies and difference, and the new politics of gender and fairness, might reshape American life. "The topic of 'male and female' pervades our society today as never before," one teacher exclaimed. "Changing and challenging views of masculine and feminine roles are evidenced. . . . Artificial differences between the sexes—hairstyles, clothing, professional pursuits—are particularly under fire. 'Unisex' has become a meaningful term."[29] Other teachers, however, celebrated their "dynamic, mobile society," anticipating that the "liberating movements for women" would broaden female interests and roles.[30] Whether uneasy or enthusiastic, white female teachers reconsidered the meaning of difference and fairness in the gym. The unresolved issue of competitive sports illustrates how divisive their discussions became.

As social sanction for women's athletics increased, physical educators faced difficult decisions about supporting certain team sports. In the mid-1960s, their primary national organization revisited the "perennial problem" of football for girls and women.[31] Having previously vetoed the game as too rough, professional leaders again concentrated on safety. Opponents considered risk an empirical question to be settled by experts' "accurate information," not teachers' "personal bias."[32] While acknowledging gaps in the scientific evidence, football's detractors cited doctors' opinion that the game was "not an appropriate physical education activity for girls." Of greatest concern was the possibility that sudden or repeated trauma to the breasts contributed to cancer.[33] Since biology constituted human beings, they elaborated, the body automatically set females apart from males, and because sex made gender, protecting female anatomy was comparable to defending womanhood. As one football critic exclaimed in

1967, "Let's keep our young girls as ladies not tomboys!!!"[34] This declaration was antifeminist code for conventional femininity and compulsory heterosexuality. Opponents' only concession came in the late 1960s when they approved a "non-contact football-type" game whose rules would "prohibit roughness and dangerous play."[35]

Behind the scenes, some leaders suspected that a cultural bias against contact sports for women, rather than established facts, influenced football's detractors.[36] This argument rang true for the game's supporters. As "experience and knowledge gained from the past" demonstrated, advocates said, well-trained girls and women could play basketball and other vigorous sports "without ill-effect." Whereas society once condemned such activities as dangerous and "not ladylike," changes in "customs and attitudes" were opening new options. Specifically, football's rising popularity signified America's less "static or rigid" values as well as girls' "motivation and incentive" for physical challenges.[37] Without denying a sexual duality, proponents regarded gender as so fluid that womanhood could encompass any interest or talent females exhibited. Instead of trying to explain current enthusiasm for football, they maintained, people should simply accept girls' "demands . . . for more active sports and better competition."[38] The football controversy illustrated the polarization between conservative physical educators who placed restrictions on female athleticism and their more liberal colleagues who defended women's right to equal opportunity. As this rift widened in the 1960s, most female teachers sought safe, intermediate positions on difference/similarity, sex/gender, and biology/culture.

THE MIDDLE GROUND

In 1965 physical educators and other experts gathered in Lansing, Michigan, for the Second National Institute on Girls Sports. Sponsored by the U.S. Olympic Development Committee and AAHPER's Division for Girls and Women's Sports (DGWS), the conference allowed participants to exchange scientific and practical information as well as discuss broad philosophical issues. Laura J. Huelster, a prominent teacher and administrator at the University of Illinois, spoke on "The Role of Sports in the Culture of Girls."[39] Viewing athletic motions as "learned acts," Huelster was confident that girls could "learn the designed precision and control of these neuromuscular sport skills as well as boys" and, with training, would develop sufficient "cardiovascular efficiency" for sustained activity. Physical differences, though, seemed just as obvious; boys naturally exerted "great muscle force and power," whereas girls exhibited "flexibility, agility, and enough strength to propel the body and objects in beautifully coordinated skill patterns." Personality differences also were self-evident; boys displayed an "aggressive drive," while girls had an aesthetic sensibility. Reinforcing these innate styles, society "does not expect and certainly does not demand that women compete in sports." At the same time, because the "cultural environment is increasingly favorable to women's self-assertion," female lives and aspirations were changing. Since both sexes need physical activity for "self-hood" and "self-mastery," Huelster explained, girls and women are entitled to "equal sports rights" through fair (even extra) activities, facilities, and leadership. But to guarantee equity, the two sexes should not compete with or against each other, unless coed teams were "organized in a comparable manner" and "physical contact" was not involved.

The majority of Huelster's peers concurred. Many physical attributes, they agreed, are universal: All bodies need activity for proper development and function; females and males alike enjoy running, jumping, and other basic activities; the mechanics of skilled movement are generic, as are the physiological benefits of exercise.[40] Lest the point be lost, one college teacher simplified the principles of structure and performance. "Isn't the female body composed of the same nine basic body systems as that of the male?" Eleanor Rynda asked. Regardless of one's sex, "it is muscles, nerves, lungs, heart, and blood vessels, etc. that must function at maximum level when training and competing."[41] This reality, asserted Virginia Crafts of the Ohio State University, demolished the "false premise" that women were "incapable of handling the physiological and psychological stresses inherent in vigorous activity and sports competition." Her colleague Phebe Scott went further; women are not merely sturdy but exceptional, she declared, as evidenced by their early maturation, resistance to illness, and longevity compared to men.[42] Citing current research, including studies sponsored by their professional organizations, most white female teachers affirmed women's physical potential.[43]

Nevertheless, "Eve just is not the same as Adam."[44] Despite the two sexes' similar design, no one would confuse them. The average male is bigger, taller, and more muscular than the typical female. His shoulders are broader, his femur less oblique, his lung capacity greater, even his thumbs are longer. Teachers attributed these differences to puberty, when natural processes took young male and female bodies down divergent paths. The implications for the gym seemed undeniable. Men's physique conferred speed, strength, and endurance; when boys throw "an object for distance," their "larger forearm length and girth" give them a "mechanical and strength advantage" and more mature technique.[45] Despite being agile and flexible, the female body seemed handicapped; small hands, for example, made hook passes in basketball difficult and accurate long-distance shots virtually impossible.[46] Overall, teachers' analysis sent mixed messages. By calling attention to physical similarities, they lessened the ostensible gap between male and female bodies. On the other hand, they regarded most differences as innate and asymmetric; accepting male performance as the standard, few doubted that nature played favorites in the gym or that women's deficiencies barred them from participating, much less excelling in certain activities.

Conversely, though, might experience foster skill? Explaining how nurture sits on top of nature, a 1967 textbook declared that a "human being starts life as a biological organism and at what we may call cultural zero." The organism develops and learns according to natural law, but "cultural factors have a determining role in shaping the individual."[47] Applying this biosocial paradigm to physical activity, white gym teachers argued that nature set upper limits on motor skill, but nurture controlled the ways and extent to which an active female realized her potential. Compared to the applause showered on male athletes, "social attitudes and customs" had stifled female sports and "choked out any natural motivation [women] might have had" to be competitive.[48] A vicious cycle ensued. If America tells girls that a "lady does not strike things," then softball players "tend to recoil as contact is made in hitting the ball"—which supposedly proves they cannot hit.[49] Similarly, the stereotype that muscles are unfeminine deters women from building strength and learning to throw; weak arms contribute to poor technique, which reinforces the myth that females cannot throw and discourages further activity.[50] Learned incompetence could be dangerous as well as self-perpetuating. If no one teaches a girl how to catch a ball, her bruised fingers prevent further practice and her skills erode; the misperception that girls cannot catch makes them unwilling to try again.[51] Instruction interrupted this cycle by building skill and confidence, which, in turn, fostered more participation and proficiency.

These interactions between nature and nurture drew teachers' attention to psychosocial factors. Given a fair chance to practice "cooperation, loyalty, and emotional control," one teacher declared, women "will develop them in the same degree as men."[52] Behavioral differences, though, also were apparent. By ages ten to twelve, girls and boys preferred different activities, had unique styles of play, and gained physical confidence in distinct ways. Being "aggressive and individualistic," boys liked sports that featured muscular strength; by contrast, girls' enthusiasm for competition waned during puberty, whereas their body awareness and interest in graceful activities grew.[53] Few teachers, however, regarded these preferences as innate. Instead, boys liked building muscle because society equated masculinity and strength; a sixth grader will try bulking up by practicing the climbing bar over and over again "with the hope of achieving this mark of masculinity. He will work until he is exhausted to chin himself more times than he did yesterday."[54] Compared to the "culturally approving environment" in which boys exercise, two researchers concluded, America's indifference, even hostility, to female performance helps explain girls' halfhearted effort during fitness tests.[55]

Having addressed body and behavior, similarities and differences, biology and culture, physical educators were ready to define "fairness." They opted for equality *and* equity. On the one hand, they argued, girls and women have the same right as boys and men to develop their full potential. Instead of teaching girls to be prissy, inept, and timid, America should prepare them to be skilled, confident young women. On the other hand, teachers must not treat the two sexes as interchangeable. Special equipment was required to help girls succeed:

Light archery bows, low-compression golf balls, and light, three-fingered bowling balls to accommodate girls' lack of strength, small basketballs to fit their small hands, and chest protectors in fencing to shield their developing breasts.[56] Likewise, sports rules should not undercut safety or proficiency; well into the 1960s, many white female teachers opposed full-court girls' basketball with body contact as too vigorous.[57] Finally, changes during puberty raised the issue of coed versus segregated activity. "As boys are stronger and more intensely interested in activity than girls are," Evelyn Schurr reasoned, "it is important that the teacher not use an organization that permits boys to dominate game play and exclude girls. There are many activities in which boys and girls can play together harmoniously and on even terms, but boys and girls should be separated for some sports activities because of the differences in their interests in vigorous participation."[58]

Although teachers' compromise between equality and equity seems vague, their separation of sex and gender was unambiguous. White instructors depicted bodies as material systems that followed natural laws of organization and function. Despite regarding female bodies as more competent and resilient than their predecessors had, many teachers still saw the sexual binary as asymmetric and slanted toward male norms. While regarding human behavior as bimodal, physical educators called American norms of femininity too restrictive. Gender's plasticity gave them hope that society would approve a wider range of womanly roles and attributes. This was not a call for revolution—Eve was entitled to new opportunities, but her world would not and should not merge with Adam's. For most white female teachers, Eve was white, middle-class, and heterosexual. They understood that the rhythms of infancy, adolescence, and adulthood would change Eve's physical needs. Besides age, however, only gender seemed relevant. Yet again, white teachers typically overlooked how race, ethnicity, class, and sexual orientation affected physical experience.

QUESTIONING THE DUALITIES

Despite teachers' insistence that sex and gender were all-encompassing, even these analytical categories proved unstable in the 1960s. According to some scientists and feminists, sex did not produce gender and the border between masculinity and femininity was not rigid. Encountering these ideas while debating women's athletics, a small cohort of physical educators, white and black, explored alternate models of active womanhood by challenging traditional dualities. Gender proved an easy target. Mavericks began by noting Americans' inclination to classify everything as "masculine" or "feminine"—associating, for example, team sports with boys and dancing and rope jumping with girls. Far from being intrinsic, renegades countered, these connotations were assigned by culture. Social expectations were so powerful that young boys, for example, are "reluctant to be observed publicly jumping rope." An activity's valence, however, could change, as happened when boys and men began to rope-jump as a "training and conditioning device."[59] By implying that girls jumped for fun, whereas boys did so to be more athletic, this example unintentionally reinforced gender norms. Other physical educators and coaches were less obliging. For Patsy Neal and like-minded critics, gender conventions were harmful "myths and superstitions" that intimidated active girls and women. Afraid their image would be "mangled by a narrow-minded public" through epithets of "masculine, unladylike, or low-class," athletic females often surrendered by adopting the "protective coloration society demands: marrying, raising a family, and being a good homemaker." Neal hoped the turbulent 1960s would enable American females to explore their physical potential as fully as women in other countries did.[60]

Nonconformist teachers next disputed the link between physical activity and the sex binary, despite its presumed biological basis. Beginning with the simple observation that individuals vary, they pointed to large differences in body type, ability, and interests among active females and males.[61] Women's physicality is so diverse, they continued, that it overlaps with male bodies and aptitude, especially before puberty.[62] If no typical female exists and aptitude does not divide neatly by sex, then being male or female cannot predict an individual's motor performance.

Mavericks therefore considered other biological variables. Chronological age and physical size seemed uninformative; after all, even small girls could learn difficult activities, such as putting the shot. Perhaps developmental stage was the key, since girls' technique often improved as they matured, regardless of rate or age. Yet, talent and training could compensate for physical immaturity. Maybe physique determined skill? On the contrary, argued Nell Jackson, the black Olympic runner and college coach, "every girl regardless of her size, shape, or age can find herself a place" in track and field programs, because events involve agility, coordination, and other skills unrelated to build. "Runners come in all shapes and sizes—some are tall, some are of medium height and some are even short." Similarly, "throwers ... are not necessarily the heaviest girls."[63] In sum, sex, age, physique, and other biological factors failed to predict motor ability.

This insight was transformative. Instead of looking for the correlates of skill, some teachers dismantled "skill" itself. Each sport, they explained, involves distinct skills requiring specific techniques. Patsy Neal, a champion basketball player who taught at North Carolina's Brevard College in the late 1960s, gave an example from her favorite sport. "To shoot a jump shot in basketball means that a person has to be able to jump high into the air, bring the ball above his or her head, and release it with a flip of the wrist and an extension of the arm at the height of the jump."[64] Success, Neal continued, depends on technique:

This is why good women athletes perform in a way that is basically similar to that of men. At the same time, it is why good men athletes perform in a way basically similar to that of women. Women, like men, wish to execute movements in the most efficient way, to get the most out of the ability they have, and to use scientific techniques. Because of the human body's limitations, anatomy, and physiological workings, certain movements must be made in a specific pattern, whether they are done by a man or a woman.[65]

The point was not that a skillful girl "'plays like a boy'" but that "her movements are such that they produce the greatest efficiency." This logic refuted the old premise that "male" techniques were consummate and unique.

Such critiques were too extreme for most white female teachers in the 1960s. Despite welcoming women's broader aspirations, the majority shunned the radical streams of American feminism and politics; to protect their work and reputations, they talked as if everyone in the gym were white, middle-class, and heterosexual. Only dissidents shattered the accustomed binaries of gender and sex. Their views so blurred the gender line that androgyny seem plausible, although they never quite said so. They argued, furthermore, that the existence of two sexes did not mean that males alone were physically gifted, much less normative. By taking traditional discourses of difference apart, progressive physical educators exposed their field's timidity. Notably, their insights also had no clear parallel among contemporary researchers of human development or champions of women's rights.

The 1970s and 1980s

During the next two decades, powerful forces disrupted American physical education. Health-related exercise gained ground in popular and scientific circles. Determined to jog and bike their way to health and happiness, active citizens helped spark a fitness boom. Meanwhile, public health officials, biomedical scientists, and behavioral epidemiologists expanded their proposition that regular exercise and other healthy habits reduced the risk of chronic disease. Despite tenuous data about the benefits of "lifestyle management," experts prescribed regular "doses" of vigorous aerobic activity for all Americans. Physical educators, though, were wary of the ascendant ideology (and business) of health-based exercise; its effectiveness in motivating disinterested, inactive girls and women seemed especially doubtful.[66]

Title IX also raised tough questions. Although the new law did not explicitly mandate coed gym class, this arrangement seemed a logical way to equalize opportunities for older pupils. Teachers wondered, however, if mixed instruction could accommodate boys' and girls' varied interests and abilities. In athletics, concern over disparities in size and strength usually quashed coed competition; most institutions pursued gender equity by adding girls' and women's teams.

Meanwhile, disturbing reports surfaced of musculoskeletal injuries and reproductive problems among female athletes. At the very time when competitive opportunities finally increased, high school and college coaches now had to worry about pushing participants too far.

These developments thrust physical educators into broader scientific and political controversies. New research on sex differences intensified old debates over the roots of human behavior.[67] Between 1967 and 1985 the number of biomedical publications on behavioral sex differences quadrupled. Many scientists, especially experts on brain development, still advanced biological explanations of sex and gender. Increasingly, however, reductive models of supposedly dimorphic phenomena came under fire, with women researchers leading the critique. Bitter disputes arose among natural and social scientists over binary models of human anatomy, behavior, and sexuality, and the relative weight of biology and culture. Amid the turmoil, many researchers agreed to separate sex and gender, that is, biological infrastructure and social character. By depicting socialization as a cloth draped over the body, the "coatrack" model of human identity and experience created, in effect, yet another duality.[68]

While scientists investigated sex and gender in the lab, social conditions brought women's daily lives into the public spotlight. The second-wave women's movement became more assertive and diverse. Although schisms persisted across race, class, and sexual orientation, the liberal and radical camps remained dominant.[69] Adhering to the principle of equality, mainstream liberals, especially white middle-class women, argued for parity in education, employment, legal rights, and health. This approach, objected radical feminists, would merely assimilate women into a male-dominated system; true liberation required valuing sex differences and foregrounding women's unique qualities. Despite these disagreements, both groups accepted the basic distinction between sex and gender, while remaining uncertain about biology's impact on behavior. Likewise, both camps were slow to recognize that female experience in the United States and across the globe was far from uniform—a blind spot that alienated many women of color and the working class. Nonetheless, the feminist movement stimulated political participation and defended education initiatives, affirmative action mandates, and reproductive rights, while its central themes gradually seeped into American culture.

A NEW DAY

"The 1970's and 1980's," declared Dorothy V. Harris, "will surely be known as the decades of women in sport." Harris, a prominent sport psychologist at Penn State University, was excited: "Females from age six to sixty and beyond are running, jumping, swimming, and hitting and kicking balls as never before. Sweat is no longer a stigma; society has moved beyond the notion that 'horses sweat, men perspire and ladies glow.'" Nevertheless, Harris was disappointed that "the world of competitive sport is still the male's domain in which females are the intruders, not rightful heirs."[70] Welcoming America's more liberal view of active womanhood, many female physical educators wanted to open the door even wider. New legal and political concepts of equality, however, left them uncertain what the revolution in exercise and sports should entail. Whether we identify with "Women's Lib" or not, one leader observed in 1972, current trends were forcing physical educators to "examine the position we take on issues regarding discrimination, liberation, and assimilation."[71]

Although legislative signposts were helpful, most teachers regarded scientific knowledge as fundamental to decisions about female exercise. They sought information about how a woman's aerobic capacity, performance potential, and risk of injury compared to those of a man. They wondered if sex differences in motor skill were irrelevant or so pronounced as to preclude elite female competition, especially against males. They discussed whether sex differences were built into nature or represented a legacy of history and culture. At present, Dorothy Harris lamented, most answers are based on "misconceptions, hearsay, chauvinism, old wives tales, and genuine sparseness" of good data.[72] Replacing assumptions with facts required new research on female physicality. Professional leaders—especially those with scientific backgrounds—insisted that investigators follow standard protocol in experimental design and data analysis.[73] Another source of information was even closer at hand; given the surge in female exercise and sports, Barbara Drinkwater observed, the "entire country has become a laboratory" for testing the impact of biology and society on women's physical capacity.[74] In effect, cultural changes were as vital to scientific discovery as research was to social progress.

Female teachers reached some basic agreements about difference and physicality. Most joined America's scientists and feminists in adopting the new "coatrack" distinction between sex and gender. As Dorothy Harris observed, "Individuals are born either male or female; they must learn to be masculine or feminine."[75] Addressing the male/female duality first, most teachers accepted scientists' conclusion that physical sex differences among children were minor. During puberty, though, hormonal changes produced absolute disparities in average height and weight, body composition, metabolic rate, hemoglobin level, and maximum oxygen uptake—with a male advantage in each case. These differences, teachers continued, affected motor performance; endowed with bigger hearts and more muscle, males typically had greater strength, speed, and aerobic capacity. No amount of instruction or practice, they believed, could overcome the biological cap on female potential, including that of athletes. Well-trained women, one teacher conceded, were "still smaller, slower, less strong, and less powerful than their male counterparts." Even the "hormonal manipulation" of female athletes in socialist countries had not enabled them to match men's performances.[76]

Lest these examples exaggerate the male/female divide, physical educators cited uniformity as well. Nature does not discriminate by sex, they asserted, in biomechanics, physiological responses to exercise, or activity-related improvements in health.[77] Furthermore, any review of physique and skill by sex shows more overlap than separation. The "short boy and the tall girl also exist," just as the "wide hips-narrow shoulder shape" occurs among both sexes; similarly, performance measures—such as "strength, speed, and power"—vary considerably "'both *within and between* [the] sexes.'"[78] To a greater extent than their predecessors had, teachers rehabilitated the female body by representing physical sex differences as matters of degree, not kind.

This revision owed much to women researchers. As did their counterparts in other disciplines, female scientists in physical education debunked popular stereotypes about sex differences. They argued that women's oxygen uptake readily supported aerobic exercise, female pelvic structure did not impede running, and active women did not wilt in hot weather.[79] Far from being inevitable, the relative weakness of women's bones probably stemmed from inactivity, that is, "lesser muscle forces acting on the bones to stimulate the bone-cell response system." This problem may disappear, one researcher speculated, once women experience "more sports competition, better conditioning programs, and a more equitable sociological life."[80]

The indirect effect of social status on bone density illustrated teachers' belief that America stifled women's recreation and sports. Every cultural barrier, they argued, added to the cycle of female inactivity and apparent incompetence. Consider physical aptitude after age fourteen; girls' "performance curves tend to level off or even drop," whereas boys' fitness scores "continue to rise for some time." This pattern, explained Bonnie J. Purdy from the University of Washington, "appears to reflect cultural influences more than an actual change in ability to learn or perform. In our society, physical ineptness is accepted and perhaps even expected of women after puberty."[81] Purdy's distinction between bodies and society was appealing because it justified additional exercise and sports. Gym teachers disagreed, however, about the direction and pace of such growth. Paralleling the two main strands of American feminism, some physical educators pursued equity by leveraging sex differences, while others promoted equality by demanding gender-neutral opportunities. Though not mutually exclusive, these two positions represented well-defined strategies in the acrimonious politics of women's athletics during the 1970s and 1980s.

DIFFERENCE AND EQUITY

In 1973 a Vermont physical educator sought advice from national leaders about the "problem of ice hockey for girls." Many schoolgirls in the state, she reported, "have a great desire to play" the game; one even insisted on "trying out for our Boys Varsity Team as a goalie." The response from the Research Committee

of the Division for Girls and Women's Sports (DGWS) typified the difference-
and-equity position.[82] Although there was no physiological or biomechanical
reason to prohibit girls' ice hockey, the chair observed, allowing girls and boys
to try out for the same team would be unfair because "lesser skilled girls" would
be "eliminated from play" due to boys' greater muscle mass, bulk, and ability
"to withstand the blows of body impact during a contact sport." Since the aim
was to keep youngsters' opportunities "on an even keel," sex-segregated competition was the best arrangement. The DGWS official recommended that Vermont teachers develop a modified version of ice hockey in which girls played
against "girls of their own size and with rules" that limited "body contact."

    Many white leaders and rank-and-file teachers endorsed this view. Fair-
ness meant providing diverse opportunities for girls and women to learn, play,
compete, and excel, just as active boys and men were accustomed to being
challenged. Such opportunities, however, must respect the "sex-determined
physiological disadvantages of females" in strength, speed, and aerobic capacity.[83] If teachers and coaches overlooked these innate deficits, the argument
ran, they would scuttle any prospect of equity.

    Mixed activities posed the biggest challenge. Equity supporters feared that
boys would dominate coed gym class by virtue of their superior motor performance. Although teachers could imagine ways of neutralizing this advantage during instructional activities, coed sports seemed inherently unwise and
unfair; after puberty, boys' skillfulness would either preclude girls from making
a team or subject female participants to physical harm.[84] At the very time when
"opportunity is knocking [for women] on gymnasium doors," teachers warned,
their participation could actually decline; institutions might use open eligibility
for coed teams "as an alibi . . . to avoid hiring staff, allocation of facilities, and
funds for an adequate girls program."[85] To guarantee fairness, the logic ran,
most sports should be sex-segregated. "Teams for girls and women," a panel of
experts declared in 1971, "should be provided for all girls and women who desire
competitive athletic experiences." Chaired by Dorothy Harris, the DGWS Special Committee on Women on Men's Teams concluded that female participation on male teams should be "rare and should be judged acceptable only as an
interim procedure for use until women's programs can be initiated."[86] By 1973
the DGWS resolved that "mixed teams" were appropriate only "in such activities as volleyball, tennis, badminton, and golf when there are equal numbers
of participants of both sexes."[87] Fairness also required professional autonomy;
sports for girls and women, equity supporters declared, must epitomize female-
guided education and development, not male-driven commercialism.

    This version of equity reflected recent developments in American science,
law, and feminism. First, teachers' perspective coincided with the dominant
threads of contemporary research, namely, the male/female duality and the
primacy of biological difference. Teachers also found support in Title IX,
which approved (but did not require) sex segregation when gym class involved

contact sports; likewise, it permitted separate male and female teams in intramural, interscholastic, and intercollegiate programs when the "activity is a
contact sport" or "when competitive skill determines membership."[88] Finally,
teachers' position drew strength from the radical strand of second-wave feminism. Although physical educators rarely identified themselves as essentialists,
their emphasis on woman-centered values and self-governance corresponded to
the politics of difference that attracted many feminist activists and academics
during the 1970s and 1980s.

Despite its female-friendly agenda, the difference-and-equity position had
serious shortcomings. The most glaring was physical educators' naïve expectation that sex segregation could be fair, that an "equal, but different system"
would produce "equal opportunity through programs for women supported
and conducted on an equal basis with men's athletic programs."[89] Across the
decades, female teachers had learned firsthand that men's monopoly on institutional resources rendered separate as inherently unequal. Equity proponents
exacerbated the situation by practicing discrimination, as illustrated by the
AIAW's initial opposition to college scholarships. Designed to preserve the educational integrity of women's programs, the policy denied female athletes opportunities equal to those afforded male athletes.[90] Such practices also stemmed
from teachers' formulation of difference. By deeming male ability superior and
female bodies deficient, they inevitably shackled the pursuit of equity; underestimating how much culture, rather than biology, set the parameters of active
womanhood, physical educators misjudged the extent of women's marginalization in a society that equated manhood with power.

Despite their sincere belief in female potential and education-centered
sports, difference-and-equity proponents were unwilling to flout tradition at
a time when their authority over women's sports was so contested and consequential. Instead, they accepted America's asymmetric dualism of sex and,
with it, conventional views of gender and sexuality. This cautious stance not
only denied athletic opportunities to girls and women but also weakened physical educators' objectives and clout. Locked into the hierarchical binary of sex,
they pursued equity, but sacrificed equality.

SIMILARITY AND EQUALITY

The second position that appealed to female physical educators during the
1970s and 1980s was similarity and equality. If someone asked them why softball players rarely threw overarm, or females reacted more slowly than males
during motor tasks, or adolescent girls looked uncoordinated, or female pole
vaulting was uncommon, equality supporters would focus on gender norms
rather than biological dictates.[91] Convinced that femininity was malleable, they
hailed modern America's acceptance of more diverse roles for women as another step toward the democratic ideal of individualism. "Our culture values

equality and the right for each person to become the best that they are capable of becoming," applauded a college instructor in 1987. In gym class and athletics, equality "means having opportunities to develop skill, and to test that skill against others of equal or better ability."[92] Accordingly, a female should "be encouraged and directed to develop her potential strength, endurance, and sport skills in the same way that males are."[93]

In grades K–12, two approaches seemed especially promising. First and foremost, physical education must become gender neutral; all activities should be open to every individual based on interest, not a game's supposedly masculine or feminine valence. At recess, do not automatically "hand jump ropes to the girls and balls to the boys."[94] During class, let girls play football and rugby, and teach field hockey and synchronized swimming to boys.[95] For androgynous curricula to succeed, teachers must also eliminate gendered language and assumptions.[96] Creating a gender-free gym was more likely, teachers continued, if classes were coed. For advocates of similarity-and-equality, physical education's long-standing practice of sex segregation seemed "unnecessary and unfounded" on several grounds.[97] First, as a matter of principle, boys and girls should "learn and enjoy sport together without regard for the artificial expectations and limitations imposed by sex segregation and stereotyping."[98] Second, science had undercut many "assumptions regarding bio-physiological and social-psychological sex differences," including a host of "unexamined beliefs regarding what feminine and masculine roles are thought to be."[99] Third, Title IX honored the concept of universal needs and rights by prohibiting sex discrimination in education. Physical education, equality advocates concluded, should finally join the modern school curriculum by transmitting common material to coed groups—just as English, mathematics, and other subjects did. Teachers understood, however, that gender neutrality did not guarantee gender equality. For example, scoring children's fitness tests by a single standard or running coed activities irrespective of skill could disadvantage girls.[100] Achieving parity in athletics looked even more difficult; simply adding sports for girls would not rectify the "very real day-to-day instances of [sex] discrimination in getting gymnasium and field space, equal time, equal pay for coaches, equal numbers of teams, [or] equal numbers of games."[101]

Despite these challenges, many teachers sided with liberal feminism and legal precedent by declaring that everyone in the "land of opportunity" deserved a fair chance to be active and skilled. This allegiance to basic American principles inoculated women physical educators against any doubts that school officials or the public harbored about their political leanings or sexual orientation. Teachers also embraced new psychosocial interpretations of human behavior by uncoupling sex and gender, and regarding masculinity and femininity as social constructs separated by artificial boundaries.

One tough question remained: Could the two sexes be equal without being identical? "Women do not want to become men," insisted Pamela Peridier, a junior high school teacher, "but surely they have the same right as men to live to the fullest of their capacities."[102] Exercising this right in gym class and sports, a "predominantly male-oriented activity," though, might be difficult. Her students, Peridier hoped, would "be aggressive and assertive in play. In coeducational classes, we wish the girls to play well, not be 'meekly feminine.'" Peridier probably did not recognize the levy she had placed on equality; instead of being active on their own (meek) terms, girls and women would be competent and competitive—qualities that society usually ascribed to boys and men. By viewing gender similarity as women's capacity to express "male" traits, physical educators construed equality as the opportunity to enter an androcentric system of performance and competition. Apparently, assimilation was the price of admission to the "male-oriented" world of physical activity.

Teachers' predicament was not unique. Many liberal reformers in the 1970s and 1980s also chose access over contestation. By seeking full entry to American society without seriously challenging gender constructs or male privilege, mainstream white feminists opened doors but left patriarchy intact. Liberalism's shortcomings extended beyond issues of sex and gender. Looking at society through white middle-class eyes, conventional feminists often failed to oppose racism, classism, and heterosexism.[103] Many physical educators were equally tone-deaf. Middle-class whites still dominated the profession's leadership and agenda; instead of confronting racism and heterosexism in the gym, they favored middle-of-the-road reforms. In the end, the similarity-and-equality position was neither gender-blind nor democratic. Preoccupied with gender disparities, advocates pursued fair opportunities without questioning androcentric norms or social hierarchies. They sought equality, but sacrificed equity.

OUTSIDE THE BINARY BOX

Other teachers argued that liberating the gym required thinking well outside the boxes of male/female and man/woman. Among the most visible innovators were university teachers and researchers, including Susan Birrell, Alyce Cheska, Mary E. Duquin, Jan Felshin, Susan Greendorfer, Pat Griffin, Dorothy V. Harris, Carole Oglesby, and Christine L. Wells. They drew inspiration from progressive feminists and radical theorists who were questioning long-standing assumptions about human bodies, identity, dualities, and difference—portraying each as fluid, constructed, relational, and contested.[104] These critics judged the established philosophies of the women's movement as being "too singular an account of power relations and too monolithic an account of gender."[105] Accordingly, black activists, lesbian feminists, and progressive intellectuals disputed popular interpretations of sex and gender, while placing racism and heterosexism on the political agenda as well. These breakthroughs also encouraged a feminist interrogation of science that challenged many disciplines' binary approaches to sex difference research.[106]

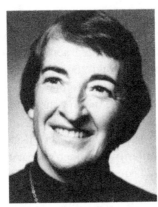

FIGURE 8.1 *Dorothy V. Harris (1931–91). Courtesy of Penn State University Archives, Eberly Special Collections Library, The Pennsylvania State University.*

To introduce these issues to physical educators, innovative teachers began, as their field often did, with the body. While stressing individual variations, they accepted that males and females were physically alike and dissimilar. The next step usually was to evaluate the effect of sex differences on physical activity. Instead of quarreling over the answer, however, progressive teachers disputed the question itself; they dismantled the sex binary and destabilized the male standard of skill. The male/female duality, they maintained, does not shed much light on active bodies or aptitude. "Male and female basketball players," one researcher explained, "are more alike than male gymnasts and male football linemen."[107] One's sex did not dictate build or choice of activity; instead, individual physique—regardless of sex—predicted a person's preferred sport. Nevertheless, it seemed that males usually outperformed females; if Americans compared male and female basketball players of similar physique, would not most assert that men were naturally more gifted? This belief, progressive teachers quickly countered, owes more to social expectation than biological fact.

Dorothy Harris outlined the cultural invention and spurious logic of male skill: America favors activities requiring strength, power, and speed; it equates these qualities with skill; males are deemed physically superior because many have these traits; females are considered incompetent precisely because they are not males; the only skilled female is one who, contrary to her nature, "'plays like a man.'"[108] This fraudulent reasoning, Harris pointed out, overlooks the many boys and men who fall short of male performance norms. People often asked her, Harris reported, if a "female will ever break the four-minute-mile barrier. My answer has always been that there are a lot of males that will never break that barrier either. There might be a female one day who will."[109] If sex did not correlate with performance, then the fabled "typical male" was a bogus standard in the gym.

Perhaps a woman could take his place. Consider the observation that active females usually sweat less than active males do. Instead of asking why women's response to heat stress was defective, Christine Wells inverted both the question and frame-of-reference. The issue, she declared in 1977, is not "which sex performs best in the heat. Instead, it is a matter of which thermoregulatory mechanisms are used by each sex and to what extent." Further research, she conjectured, may show that "women are more efficient regulators of their body temperatures" although they sweat less than men.[110] By "having to sweat sooner in order to cool his body," Dorothy Harris shrewdly suggested, the average male "compensates because he differs from the female."[111] Having dislodged the male norm, Wells, Harris, and like-minded colleagues sometimes retreated to the difference-and-equity position, arguing that women's bodies should be judged by female-specific criteria. Nevertheless, their insights stood: The male/female binary does not elucidate performance, and the cultural association of maleness and skill misrepresents reality at women's expense.

Having deconstructed sex, progressive physical educators set their sights on gender. According to Dorothy Harris, the well-documented overlap between men's and women's behavior proved that gender was not a clean binary. The diverse traits that different societies throughout history had associated with men and women also showed that "human personality is highly malleable."[112] For example, although people considered aggression a universal male attribute, it was a multifaceted behavior that both men and women expressed, depending on culture and circumstance.[113] Since the masculine/feminine divide made no sense, in theory or practice, Harris and like-minded teachers sought alternate formulations. One option was simply to declare that "what a *woman* does *is* feminine."[114] Other proposals were more radical; dispensing with gender altogether, perhaps teachers and researchers should think about "HUMAN behavior ... along a continuum," with no trace of "polarized masculine-feminine stereotypes."[115]

Although androgyny probably seemed far-fetched, most women physical educators understood that gender was more than a behavior manual; it also regulated access to roles and activities, including sports. For progressive teachers, the most salient issue was *why* American society deployed its gender schema in particular ways. Masculinity and femininity, Alyce Cheska asserted in 1981, constitute hierarchical relationships through which men maintain social power and physical control. Competitive activities replicate this larger system; sports symbolically display male prowess and literally exclude women as "inappropriate and ineffective game contenders."[116] Although Cheska's critique probably struck many gym teachers as too radical, it would have resonated with feminist activists and scholars.[117] Many academicians argued that gender and difference were relational, not simply classificatory, and constitutive, not just ideological. Because mainstream reforms preserved traditional gender schema, women's liberation required more emancipatory strategies.

Progressive physical educators agreed. Social justice, they said, required a different "cultural reality" that replaced oppressive gender dualities with an ethos of self-determination. Similarly, the "social power hierarchy" and its "male-defined sport system" must give way to practices that democratized activity and empowered girls and women.[118] This agenda entailed both access and fairness; everyone had a right to activity and competition but in a context that supported individual development and success. Balancing equality and equity "requires nothing less," one teacher declared in 1988, "than a complete reconstruction of the content and process of physical education" and sports.[119] To eliminate "sex stereotyping and discrimination" in gym class, schools could not simply put boys and girls together; instead, physical educators had to undo gender expectations and interrupt "stereotyped interaction and participation patterns." For the sake of equity, teachers must treat boys and girls as individuals whose participation styles and skill levels varied widely.[120]

Gender, however, was not the only axis of injustice. For decades, black physical educators had called attention to their field's racial inequities. A growing number of white colleagues, too, acknowledged that racism operated alongside sexism in the gym. Some perceived how gender norms sustained heterosexism. As Dorothy Harris contended in 1981, a female "is socialised to use her body to attract and please the male while the male learns to use his body to please himself, to develop social and behavioural skills, and to gain recognitions for his abilities."[121] By contrast, when a girl or woman "displays physical prowess and skill in sports," her supposed masculinity calls her sexual orientation into question. The stigma of lesbianism, Harris observed, is an "'old male tactic' to curtail support [for] women in sport," and physical education was complicit through its silence.[122] Although Harris and other progressive teachers were unsure how to eradicate heterosexism, their impatience with homophobia was manifest. As the twentieth century closed, pressure mounted for all physical educators to pay more attention to sexual orientation and other axes of difference.

Diversity in the Gym, 1990–2005

At the turn of the twenty-first century, physical education returned to the public spotlight as scholars, citizens, and policymakers alike focused on the body and health.[123] Some Americans tried achieving physical "perfection" through extreme and costly measures, goaded on by the mass media and makeover hucksters. For girls and women seeking balanced fitness, not simply ideal figures, the country's "'body-centric' attitude" inspired regular exercise and competitive athletics.[124] As the "body craze" spread through popular culture, government officials, exercise scientists, and health professionals named physical activity a vital public health priority. In his landmark report of 1996, the U.S. Surgeon General declared that the United States "must accord [physical activity] the same level of attention that we give other important public health practices that affect the entire nation."[125] The Department of Health and Human Services' Healthy People 2010 initiative ranked physical activity and fitness a critical "focus area" and first among its top ten "leading health indicators." In 2005 the Department of Agriculture's revised Food Pyramid featured an energetic stick figure climbing toward health—reminding Americans that good nutrition and regular exercise were equally important "steps to a healthier you."[126]

This intentional play on words represented a new interpretation of the relationship between physical activity and health. Moving away from the clinical standard of cardiovascular fitness, exercise scientists and public health officials recommended that people of all ages and abilities participate in a "broader range of health-enhancing physical activities."[127] The list comprised not only leisure-time choices but also domestic chores, work-related exertion, and active transportation, including walking and bicycling. Bouts of healthy activity could be moderate in intensity and of medium duration; even several small doses accumulated during the day seemed beneficial.[128] To popularize this kinder, gentler paradigm, experts envisioned partnerships between families, communities, schools, voluntary organizations, and government agencies. Heading virtually everyone's agenda was quality school-based physical education; gym class represented a safe, supervised setting in which millions of young Americans could "develop the knowledge, attitudes, skills, behaviors, and confidence needed to be physically active for life."[129] Creating an active citizenry, though, looked daunting. According to Healthy People 2010, the "proportion of the population reporting no leisure-time physical activity is higher among women than men, higher among African Americans and Hispanics than whites, higher among older adults than younger adults, and higher among the less affluent than the more affluent. Participation in all types of physical activity declines strikingly as age or grade in school increases." For health policies to succeed, the project advised, experts must "identify barriers to physical activity faced by particular population groups and develop interventions that address these barriers."[130] Public health had discovered "diversity."

Experts began analyzing physical activity's connection to age, sex, ethnicity, religion, and the built environment (the physical spaces in which people live, work, and play). Although age stood out as the most critical factor, sex was a close second.[131] The consensus that females were less active than males prompted exercise scientists, sociologists, women's health advocates, and public health experts to examine women's lives more closely.[132] Researchers interested in psychosocial patterns studied how age, income, education, race, and region affected female activity rates and confidence levels, as well as which interventions might increase girls' and women's willingness and ability to be active. Other scientists focused on physical sex differences by comparing male and female adaptations to exercise and training. Of particular concern was whether inactive girls and women incurred special burdens, while active ones acquired unique benefits or hazards, such as torn knee ligaments and menstrual disorders.

Investigations of physical activity followed general trends in research on human development and behavior. Biomedical science became increasingly reductive; most notably, genetic paradigms asserted that virtually every aspect of life was hardwired at the molecular level, forming a material base for all observed differences. Rejecting this new version of biodeterminism, other researchers explored the impact of social systems and life experience on identity and behavior. Mediating between these two extremes were models that depicted humans as both similar and diverse, and biosocial interactions as complex. The nature/nurture debate was by no means over.

A "NEW PE" FOR ONE AND ALL

Developments in public health and exercise science intersected with school activity programs in critical ways. Potentially, gym teachers and coaches could be vital partners in the campaign to get Americans moving. Physical activity rates, though, represented a challenge—some might say a disgrace—for the profession. Despite decades of physical education, most Americans seemed averse to being active. Along with fast food and electronic entertainment, two teachers grumbled, gym class had "produced . . . unmotivated, overweight, inactive, technological couch potatoes."[133] The situation among girls and women was especially disheartening. Although athletes usually remained active throughout their lives, physical educators lamented that the sports revolution following Title IX had not created a broader ethos of female exercise and recreation.[134]

Maybe gym class needed a radical overhaul. Instead of concentrating on sports-related skills, some leaders urged, programs should embrace the new paradigm of lifetime activity by fostering "the physical competence, health-related fitness, self-responsibility, and enjoyment of physical activity for all [youngsters] so that they can establish physical activity as a natural part of everyday life."[135] Advocates devised new health-related curricula, from outdoor adventures to high-tech workouts resembling those at an upscale health club. For other teachers, however, the so-called "new PE" seemed unproven; innovative activities might not engage girls and boys equally nor change youngsters' basic attitudes and habits. Concerned about sex differences in motor skill and participation styles, some critics suggested that re-segregating gym class might particularly benefit girls.[136] Physical educators faced a tough predicament; they wanted to encourage regular activity, even high-level sports, among girls and women but without compromising female health or gender equity.

Sex and gender, though, were not the only relevant variables. Much as "diversity" arrived as a catchphrase in American education and public health, physical educators became increasingly aware that their students varied by race, ethnicity, culture, and religion. Whereas some politicians and health experts trumpeted pluralism in the abstract, gym teachers and coaches encountered it "in the flesh" every day. Although physical disparities still mattered to instructors, students' complex backgrounds seemed to present a more acute challenge; which culturally sensitive activities would promote physical fairness for everyone in an inclusive environment? Despite Title IX and other initiatives, one teacher observed, gender equity remained elusive as did the broader goal of ensuring that "all students, regardless of gender, race, social class or motor ability have the opportunity to maximize their participation, enjoyment and achievement."[137] This project took center stage as the 1990s began.

Two approaches emerged and, in many respects, still dominate. The first can be called diversity-and-equity; it represents a "culturally responsive pedagogy" that values and adapts to students' diversity.[138] The second is social justice; it contests the wide-ranging inequities that physical education has replicated so quietly for so long. Both philosophies owed a debt to feminism. During the 1990s feminist scholars and activists in the United States and other countries articulated new concepts of body, gender, difference, and equity. While some intellectuals intensified their critique of the male/female duality in Western science, postmodern feminists, queer theorists, and women of color scrutinized other standard binaries.[139] Did "masculinity" and "femininity" represent cohesive oppositional states or universalizing categories that obscured the "multiplicities of sameness and difference among women and among men and within individuals as well"? Similarly, is sexuality a continuum of expression and self-perception, rather than a neat dyad of heterosexuality and homosexuality? Is "race" the product of biological nature or do "white" and "black," for example, signify historically specific political relationships?

Together, the collapse of old dualisms and the emphasis on diversity prompted "a reformulation of the difference perspective (focusing on differences among women rather than differences between women and men)" as well as a reexamination of the apparent paradox between equality and difference. More than any other problem, states the political theorist Judith Squires, the latter debate "clearly and decisively shaped feminist theorizing during the 1980s and 1990s."[140] While some theorists sought to reconcile equality and difference, others discarded this stubborn dichotomy by testing entirely new perspectives.[141]

These developments affected HPER professionals as new exchanges opened between academic feminists, advocacy groups, sports scholars, and physical educators.[142] Although older views of difference and fairness lingered, most gym teachers and coaches became frustrated with similarity-and-equality and other mainstream positions. The majority adopted the diversity-and-equity perspective, while a smaller group endorsed social justice.

DIVERSITY AND EQUITY

The diversity-and-equity philosophy has dominated curricular literature, research studies, and professional commentaries over the past twenty years.[143] Gym class and sports, it posits, should afford every participant a fair chance to learn and succeed in a "supportive atmosphere" that affirms multiple differences.[144] Whereas earlier paradigms stressed physical disparities, "diversity" focuses on cultural attitudes and backgrounds. For example, a "gender-fair environment" would empower girls and boys to be physically active and confident by recognizing youngsters' "schemas about gender-appropriate physical activities" as well as their gendered beliefs, experiences, interests, and problems.[145] To create a girl-friendly gym, curriculum planners have proposed task-oriented activities and fitness units, because "structured physical activity environments" and health goals supposedly appeal to girls more than free play and sports competition do. In addition, since girls "are often more cooperative, social, creative, and mature than" boys, instructors should engage small single-sex groups in student-centered projects. Finally, to build girls' interest and self-esteem, teachers might offer aerobics and other "'feminine'-typed activity."[146]

Though necessary, teachers continue, gender-based strategies are insufficient. A truly equitable gym must ensure "opportunity for successful participation and exposure to instruction regardless of gender, race, ethnicity, religion, sexual orientation, social class, or motor ability."[147] To promote inclusiveness, teachers should model behaviors and introduce activities that enable every student to feel "accepted and appreciated," irrespective of religion, language, clothing, or play style.[148] To internationalize the curriculum, instructors could incorporate games and dances from other cultures. To work more effectively with minority athletes, a coach should recognize their unique backgrounds, while avoiding racial and class stereotypes. Overall, inclusiveness "reflects and embraces the diversity of the world in which we live," and teaches everyone "that 'different' is okay."[149]

As some supporters understand, however, valuing diversity can degenerate into old-fashioned stereotyping. Girl-friendly pedagogies might reproduce and essentialize the very differences that teachers regard as social constructs. For example, modifying the rules of a coed game to ensure girls' interest and participation "sends the message that girls need special treatment, which only serves to reinforce the stereotype that girls are not as competent as boys."[150] Culturally responsive curricula can also mask variety within groups. A physical educator might assemble a "Latino-specific bag of tricks" for working with all Hispanic youngsters—when "no such bag" exists.[151] Instead of validating diversity and advancing equity, some teachers realize, multicultural adaptations often homogenize and stigmatize "special" groups. Despite these inherent contradictions, the diversity-and-equity approach remains popular in physical education, thereby keeping the profession in line with mainstream feminism, education, and public health.

SOCIAL JUSTICE IN THE GYM

For progressive teachers, however, "happy pluralism" is unacceptable.[152] Besides solidifying stereotypes, they maintain, theories of diversity naturalize "difference" by concealing socio-historical context and compartmentalize it by obscuring the interplay of gender, race, ethnicity, and sexuality. Despite sounding egalitarian, they argue, the pledge to tolerate, even affirm diversity simply protects the privileges of dominant groups; an inclusive gym allows teachers to be sensitive and fair, without challenging systemic inequities among their pupils. "Noticeably absent from the diversity discourse," several teachers conclude, "is a strong commitment to social/institutional change."[153]

Emancipating gym class for everyone, progressives believe, requires a new set of objectives and approaches. Discrimination should be confronted directly, customary power relationships must be scrambled, all pupils must be valued and empowered, and a sense of "community and connection" should be fostered.[154] To bridge theory and practice, advocates have undertaken various pilot projects, focusing particularly on gender. One experiment featured classroom activities that divided pupils according to skill, not sex, emphasized "the process of playing rather than the outcome of winning," and offered pupils regular opportunities to share their opinions. These changes "began to reconstruct the gendered relationships . . . and helped the children to see themselves and each other as capable and valuable."[155] Another innovative curriculum, called "Sport for Peace," sought to transform traditional sport-based physical education in ways that "enhance[d] students' opportunities to participate within an equitably structured environment."[156] Teams comprised members of "relatively equal skill and playing ability" who were required "to participate in a number of roles and assume a variety of community-oriented responsibilities." While teaching physical skills through multiple "second chances," the curriculum also emphasized student ownership of class sessions, "conflict negotiation, care and concern for others, and self and social responsibility." These approaches helped low-skilled girls and boys feel less alienated and more competent, while enabling higher-skilled pupils to interact more positively with their classmates. Other projects have attempted to connect gym class to the real world by focusing on self-defense and other "life skills" and involving "students, their families, and friends in all kinds of physical activities and community events."[157]

Progressive reformers have also addressed race, ethnicity, and class, especially in urban schools where African American or Hispanic pupils from low- and middle-income families often predominate. One program deliberately retained basketball because of the game's centrality to black youngsters' identity and experience; at the same time, teachers redirected boys' "free-play" style toward more collaboration, while helping lesser-skilled boys and girls become more proficient and engaged.[158] By highlighting the "core values of care, compassion, and interdependence," the Sport for Peace curriculum tried to encourage African American pupils "to reconnect with a sense of family and kinship that is consistent with their culture and sense of self."[159] Whatever their successes and disappointments to date, progressive teachers remain committed to confronting and reordering every social hierarchy in the gym.[160]

Physical Education and Binary Boxes

Physical educators' ideas about difference and fairness changed significantly during the second half of the twentieth century. Nevertheless, several constants remained. Most white female teachers retained familiar dualisms of male/female, man/woman, sex/gender, and biology/culture. Few resolved the apparent dichotomy between equality and equity. Women physical educators thought about these issues using the terms that American culture, science, and feminism made available to them. As researchers, academics, and political activists grappled with questions of difference and fairness in the late twentieth century, binary thinking and the seemingly irreconcilable strategies of equity/equality persisted in popular culture and expert domains.

Physical educators faced unique pressures as well. Their basic conservatism suited a beleaguered profession handling high expectations about its social role but saddled with low prestige and uncertain resources. The rising popularity of sports and the emergence of physical activity as a public health priority did not improve the field's shaky position. The women represented in this chapter had even more reason to be cautious. Most were white, middle-class professionals working as teachers, coaches, or administrators in grades K–12 or at the collegiate level. Structural changes and marginal status after mid-century undercut their authority; power struggles over programs and governance were demoralizing; the field's intransigent racism and homophobia hung over white and black women, gay and straight alike. As the century closed, many white teachers welcomed the diversity paradigm because they could revitalize the gym without forcefully confronting contentious issues. In many respects, a racialized model of athletic Eve—white, feminine, and heterosexual—remained, even as physical educators' white-dominated profession and the country as a whole came to appreciate multiculturalism.

Despite their deep-rooted caution, female teachers and coaches advanced fairness for the "fair sex." Progress toward gender parity in physical education and sports would have been slower during the second half of the twentieth century had women professionals not pressed the issue. On the other hand, each leading interpretation of difference and fairness exacted a high price. The argument that women and men are similar accepted women's assimilation into an androcentric world. The argument that anatomy is destiny invoked a "biological justification for a sociological restriction."[161] The argument that socialization made women "special" perpetuated gender stereotypes and inequities. Instead of securing fairness, these three viewpoints constrained active girls and women. In each case, the flaw was teachers' expectation that dualistic thinking could deliver justice in a non-egalitarian society. In the United States, one physical educator realized, "differences [are] directives for disadvantage."[162]

These conditions made alternate paradigms unlikely but not impossible. Energized by feminist theory and politics, some maverick physical educators proposed unconventional ideas about difference, gender, and fairness. This eclectic group included research scientists, educators with advanced training in the social sciences, coaches who supported elite competition, and progressives who broke their field's silence about racism and heterosexism. In various ways, the renegades politicized the central tenets of physical education and American society, aiming to enact in the gym a form of social justice that contested the status quo while democratizing physical activity and sports.

Exercising Caution

PHYSICAL ACTIVITY AND REPRODUCTIVE HEALTH,
1940–2005

In 1912 *Harper's Bazaar*, a popular women's magazine, posed an ominous question: "Are athletics a menace to motherhood?" Nearly seventy-five years later, the periodical sounded the same alarm by asking "Can Sports Make You Sterile?"[1] In 1915 a letter to the *Journal of the American Medical Association* described the "effects of athletic competition on childbirth." Eight decades later, *JAMA* reviewed the "evaluation and management of menstrual dysfunction in athletes."[2] In 1925 an article in the country's leading physical education journal considered the "conflicting medical and lay opinion as to the effect of exercise on the reproductive functions of women." As the century closed, the same journal analyzed the "Female Athlete Triad"—the "collective syndrome" of amenorrhea, disordered eating, and premature osteoporosis among highly trained girls and young women.[3]

Despite their longevity, discussions about exercise and reproductive health, especially menstruation, were far from uniform. From the 1940s through 1960s, most experts concluded that physical activity was not likely to disrupt monthly cycles, even among elite athletes. Beginning in the 1970s, however, apprehension grew with reports of "athletic amenorrhea" in young competitors. During the 1980s and 1990s, concern spiked; experts warned that vigorous training, even routine exercise, could produce both clinical and asymptomatic reproductive disorders along with other health problems in the near and long term. As researchers probed various causes and solutions, many lay and professional groups joined the conversation. By the turn of the twenty-first century, specialized journals and the mass media alike featured commentaries by gynecologists, pediatricians, family physicians, endocrinologists, exercise physiologists, sports medicine experts, athletic trainers, dieticians, school health leaders, physical educators, women's health advocates, and fitness entrepreneurs. In discussions ranging from levelheaded to hyperbolic, both scientific and professional issues hung in the balance. Many experts vied to control if, when, how much, and in what way girls and women would exercise—in short, to claim ownership over the active female body.

To stake their claim, specialists deployed one or more of the paradigms that developed in reproductive biology between the mid-nineteenth and late twentieth centuries.[4] The oldest was the economic or mechanical metaphor—it likened the human body to a small business balancing revenue and expenses or a "living machine" whose smooth operation depended on steady intake and output. A second option appeared in the early 1900s—the engineering metaphor represented the body as a self-regulating system trying to maintain equilibrium. By the late 1940s a third view emerged—the cybernetic model described the body as a complex "communications network" that transmitted and processed information through feedback loops connected to some master control. Scientists, doctors, and other experts selected the model that best suited their distinctive perspective and purpose, be it to study, treat, or educate the populace, and that justified their field's intervention in women's lives.[5]

In the early 1900s no single group dominated the interpretation of exercise and reproductive health. By mid-century, biomedical theories and practices were steadily overtaking physical education and other applied fields. Despite losing stature, female gym teachers and coaches retained the critical responsibility of supervising active girls and women. This chapter explores the controversy over physical activity and menstrual health during the second half of the twentieth century, focusing on women physical educators' ideas and adaptations as the gymnasium lost ground to the laboratory and clinic.

The Calm before the Storm: 1940s–1960s

Between the 1940s and 1960s, physically active women became more visible in the United States. Belying the postwar "return to domesticity," they continued to hold demanding jobs and participated in diverse sports and recreation. Although the physical challenges that females routinely met as mothers, homemakers, paid workers, and athletes were undeniable, Americans worried about the impact of exercise on reproductive health. Family physicians offered reassurance. Except for "activities involving greater increased intra-abdominal pressure," the American Medical Association and National Education Association stated in 1943, women "will profit from most forms of exercise." Individual circumstances might require some females to reduce, even stop physical activity during their periods, but many do "not need to modify their exercise at all."[6] Two decades later, general practitioners still endorsed regular exercise during menses "if it is well tolerated." As the AMA and AAHPER declared in 1964, "No harm to normal menstrual function has been shown to result from vigorous exercise. In fact, exercise can be beneficial in relieving certain types of menstrual pain."[7] Opinions among medical specialists were less consistent. In 1948 a leading gynecologist observed that "reasonable activities, such as golf or even a leisurely game of tennis should not be harmful to the normally menstruating girl," but "violent exercise" posed risks.[8] The American Academy of Pediatrics' 1956 policy statement on competitive athletics for prepubescent children raised concern about injuries, fatigue, and emotional strain but did not mention delayed menarche.[9]

Doctors' cautious optimism stemmed partly from contemporary data. During the 1950s and 1960s American and European scientists conducted numerous surveys among elite female athletes, such as participants in the Olympic Games. Despite uncovering some menstrual irregularities, researchers concluded that physical activity, even high-level competition, usually was not detrimental to monthly periods, fertility, or childbirth.[10] As an eminent exercise physiologist exclaimed in 1956, "Millions of girls have indulged in sports, gymnastics and games; competed in swimming, on track and field and on horseback; women have climbed some of the highest mountains and swum through a thousand rivers and lakes" without summoning the "evil ghosts" of masculinization and reproductive damage. Railing against "millennia of prejudice and ignorance," some scientists championed physical activity as a woman's right.[11]

With moderate exercise exonerated, the cause of delayed menarche, irregular periods, and secondary amenorrhea (the cessation of periods after menarche) remained unsolved. Gynecology textbooks cited anatomical abnormalities, constitutional diseases, environmental conditions, and developmental instability, along with emotional trauma and improper hygiene.[12] Whatever the specific trigger, the underlying mechanism of menstrual problems, experts hypothesized in the 1940s, was "endocrinopathic."[13] Between the 1920s and 1940s scientists had isolated several reproductive hormones, including estrogen, progesterone, follicle stimulating hormone, and lutenizing hormone.[14] Investigating the interactions between the hypothalamus and various endocrine glands, especially the pituitary and ovaries, researchers proposed that chemical miscommunication disrupted critical hormone levels, resulting in amenorrhea. By the late 1940s endocrinologists likened this mechanism to cybernetics, from a Greek word meaning "helmsman"; perhaps the "engineer's concept of feedback control [could] be applied to biologic systems."[15] Extending the analogy, gynecologists depicted the female body as a sensitive network that relied on the endocrine system to mediate complications; monitoring this chemical feedback, the hypothalamus, as the master control, regulated the body's efforts to restore equilibrium.[16] Before doctors assisted this internal process with drugs or other therapies, they were advised to ascertain a patient's specific problem. In most cases, experts stated, physical activity would not be the leading suspect.

PHYSICAL EDUCATION, 1940s–1950s

While researchers unraveled the science of menstruation, physical educators managed its implications in the gym. During the 1940s women's professional organizations usually adopted a "policy of caution" about vigorous activity during menses.[17] The official aquatics guide for 1941 recommended that pool swimming be off-limits during a girl's period; similarly, the 1946 basketball manual advised against participation in "strenuous" games "during the first day or so" of menstrual flow.[18] At the same time, many instructors and administrators believed that specific exercises relieved dysmenorrhea, that is, painful periods.[19] Other teachers took bolder steps. A girls' boarding school recounted in 1943 its successful experiment with swimming during menstruation, and a key organization declared that girls and young women could swim and play certain sports during menses with their supervisor's approval and, if necessary, a medical consultation.[20]

Surveys in the 1950s indicated growing confidence among some parents, teachers, administrators, and athletes that vigorous activity did not compromise menstruation or general health. Sports advocates were especially encouraged by data compiled by the Amateur Athletic Union (AAU), which sponsored competitive events for males and females.[21] When nurses and health educators visited schools, girls expressed uneasiness by asking "Is exercise harmful during the menstrual period?" and "Is it all right to swim during the menstrual period?" Underlying their confusion was a clear desire for more opportunities to play, train, and compete.[22]

Many professional leaders, rank-and-file gym teachers, and recreation workers also endorsed more diverse activities. To make the case they had to overcome the menstrual barrier, the very beliefs and practices they once used to limit exercise and sports. Teachers turned to science for help. Whereas previous generations had justified prudence by citing biomedical uncertainty, physical educators at mid-century enlisted the emerging scientific consensus to dismiss restrictions as old-fashioned and unnecessary.[23] Their effort to liberalize policy was conscious and public. The National Section on Women's Athletics (NSWA) and it successors (NSGWS and DGWS) built a scientific case and packaged it for "'popular' consumption."[24] In the late 1950s, the group decided to update *The Doctor Answers Some Practical Questions on Menstruation*, a booklet for girls and young women written by Margaret Bell in 1937 and revised in 1952. The pamphlet, leaders insisted, "'should adopt a more modern concept and application to sports participation.'"[25] The organization also asked its Research Committee to undertake a study that "might aid in increasing participation in sports activities during menstruation."[26] After several false starts, this charge evolved into a survey of medical opinion about "physical activity, sports competition, and swimming during the menstrual period." Based on responses from seventeen physicians and gynecologists, the committee concluded that the "large majority of doctors place no restrictions" on activity "during any phase of the menstrual period for girls and women who are free from menstrual disturbances."[27] The report thereby met the sponsors' goal of marshaling "sufficient scientific evidence to back up our beliefs" for more liberal standards in women's athletics.[28]

Other stakeholders were equally upbeat. Manufacturers of hygiene products assured girls and young women that they could remain quite active during their periods. Although companies' advertisements, brochures, and educational films carried many negative messages about adolescent bodies and sexuality, these materials declared that, with common sense and the right napkin or tampon, females could swim, bathe, exercise, and play sports, in moderation, throughout their monthly cycles.[29] Since hygiene companies regularly advertised in physical education journals and provided classroom films, pamphlets, and product samples, gym teachers had ready access to commercial resources.

Old practices, though, were hard to break. During the 1950s the profession's general guidelines about activity and menstruation remained conservative, while recommendations for specific sports eased up—a discrepancy that confused many teachers. Institutions also sent mixed messages; although Smith College expected students to participate in gym class during their periods, those with severe cramps were excused, and swimmers attended class in street clothes.[30] Elsewhere, policies were more relaxed. High schools in Mississippi permitted basketball players to compete during their periods, while Stanford University directed female students "to participate in physical education unless there is an abnormality existing where activity should be limited."[31]

PHYSICAL EDUCATION, 1960s

During the 1960s some veteran teachers still worried that vigorous activity jeopardized menstruation, pregnancy, and childbirth. Increasingly, however, professional articles, textbooks, and research studies argued that exercise, sports, and menstruation were compatible. This outlook fit physical educators' general goal of rehabilitating the female body by debunking popular beliefs and normalizing women's "peculiarities." Menstruation, one health educator stated in 1965, is a "normal female bodily function, which every girl should proudly, easily, normally, regularly, and not uncomfortably, accept."[32] The monthly cycle also seemed resilient enough to handle regular exercise, even sports. As a physical educator at the University of Oregon explained in 1969:

> We now know that, unless pathological or structural defects are present, the female benefits from mild to moderate exercise during menstruation. . . . Only jumping, which results in hard vertical landings, and heavy lifting are to be avoided during the menstrual period, for these activities can place increased pressure on the pelvic floor of the abdominal area.[33]

During menses, Betty McCue continued, an individual may follow her regular pattern of exercise, "even if this activity is highly competitive," as long as her cycle "'does not show unfavorable change'" and her athletic performance does not suffer.[34] Moreover, other teachers noted, a history of activity aided pregnancy and childbirth because "strong abdominal muscles are a decided asset during the second stage of labor."[35] Finally, hygiene did not preclude swimming during menses; "normal menstrual fluid," a high school instructor stated, "is virtually 'clean' when compared with the normal bacteria on the skin or in the nose, mouth, and anal areas."[36]

Research by colleagues and outside experts buttressed these claims. By the mid-1960s gym teachers could draw upon numerous scientific studies and informal surveys, especially the work of P.-O. Åstrand, Gyula J. Erdelyi, Ernst Jokl, and the AAU as well as Anna Espenschade and other physical educators. These investigations demonstrate, several teachers confidently declared in 1964, that "vigorous exercise will not harm reproductive functions."[37] Common sense and experience also proved that active girls and women usually experienced trouble-free cycles. Sports "matches, meets, [and] tournaments," one instructor noted, "are never changed, never cancelled, never forfeited because of menstrual problems."[38] After ten years of "everyday experience coaching a university women's swimming team," a Michigan State staff member reported that her athletes' "health was not impaired" nor did their grades or social life suffer; "all are married now and have from two to six youngsters."[39] Elite champions also had "pretty well settled" the question of competition during menses; "they all do it," Anna Espenschade proclaimed in 1965.[40]

Nevertheless, policies and practices lagged behind. The DGWS gradually deemed "play during the menstrual period" as "permissible" in basketball, softball, track and field, and other sports, "with referral to a physician in case of uncertainty."[41] For nearly a decade, however, the group's general statement of philosophy and standards failed to address menstruation. Reinstated in 1969, the revised guideline declared:

> Participation in sports during the menstrual period should be guided by knowledge of the demands of the activity, the physical condition of the girl, and her health history record. It is the opinion of many doctors and physiologists that the menses should not inhibit motor performance; however, premenstrual fluid retention may cause temporary anxiety and fatigue. In the absence of knowledge of the individual's physical reaction to vigorous activity, or if the participant has a history of menstrual disorders, procedure should be reasonably conservative.[42]

This timid conclusion contradicted the organization's up-to-date information.[43] Because its Research Committee wondered if the DGWS "standard in regard to menstruation [is] reasonable," members regularly summarized current scientific studies for the group's officers.[44] Using gentle prose, the committee's abstract of Erdelyi's 1962 report on "highly trained female athletes" observed that "it would appear that the participation of girls and women in normal physical education activities would result in very few unfavorable changes in the menstrual cycle," and even elite competition did not jeopardize pregnancy "in later years."[45] Erdelyi's work and similar projects appeared in DGWS bibliographies, but not in its policies. Torn by controversies over competition in the 1960s, the national organization deferred to its conservative and moderate wings, while hiding other members' more progressive attitudes. Science was useful, but less compelling than internal politics.

THE ENGINEERING METAPHOR

Between the 1940s and 1960s many female teachers and coaches gradually accepted more liberal views of menstruation and physical activity, including competitive sports. Borrowing biomedicine's paradigm, teachers described the reproductive cycle as a sensitive chemical system. "The menstrual cycle," observed a Smith College instructor, "is a continuous process governed by rhythmical hormonal changes" responding to numerous factors.[46] As staff members at Kent State University elaborated, "Changes in living arrangements, climate, or emotional upsets are sufficient to alter endocrine secretions. As a result the variations that occur when coming to college often cause fluctuation in one's 'normal' cycle."[47] This perspective portrayed the female body as both vulnerable and resilient; the ups-and-downs of daily life could upset women's reproductive system, but strenuous activity did not seem intrinsically harmful.

To overcome traditional beliefs about physical activity and reproductive health, reform-minded teachers had to normalize menstruation and destigmatize exercise. The engineering metaphor served both purposes; positing that systems were designed for stability, the model judged some disturbances to be more calamitous than others. All else being equal, sports advocates insisted, the load imposed by moderate exercise, even competitive activities, was less than a woman's body faced in many everyday situations. Why that was true did not interest most physical educators. Setting aside the complexities of reproductive endocrinology, they focused instead on real people, daily experience, and practical solutions: Which girls need exercises to relieve dysmenorrhea? How can girls and women manage life's ordinary stresses that disrupt their cycles? How might colleagues be persuaded that females can exercise, swim, and compete with little immediate or delayed risk? This real-world perspective set physical education apart from biomedicine. Working on the front lines of physical activity and female health, teachers and coaches focused on actual bodies and regular lives. Determined to expand women's opportunities, some female physical educators reformulated the engineering model of reproductive physiology to liberalize their field's perspective on exercise, sports, and menstruation.

The Storm, 1970–95

During the 1970s reports surfaced of delayed menarche and secondary amenor-rhea among young athletes. A furious debate ensued about prevalence, causes, solutions, and long-term effects. Specialists in gynecology, exercise physiology, sports medicine, and reproductive endocrinology produced conflicting data and hypotheses about the relationship between vigorous exercise and the onset and regularity of menstruation. Clinicians discussed whether "athletic amen-orrhea" was a distinct entity and which diagnostic and treatment protocols were effective. Sports governance groups revised their policies regarding ado-lescent training and competition. Professional organizations sponsored work-shops and developed position papers. Among the most influential was a report issued by the American College of Sports Medicine after its 1992 conference on amenorrhea, osteoporosis, and eating disorders—three conditions the group designated the Female Athlete Triad.[48] The ACSM subsequently cautioned that these problems could arise, together or separately, in any active female.[49] In 1995 one physician declared the Triad a national "epidemic."[50] Accounts in the popular media were even more sensational; as one magazine warned in 1988, "Babies or Barbells: Make Your Choice."[51] The controversy had two phases: a short downpour in the 1970s, followed by a full-blown storm between 1980 and 1995. During both stages, physical educators had to reconsider their standpoint and role as biomedicine steadily gained the upper hand.

In the 1970s researchers observed delayed menarche and secondary amenor-rhea among some athletes.[52] To explain these phenomena, many experts seized upon the work of Rose Frisch, a population specialist at Harvard University. Noting a correlation between height, weight, and various markers of puberty, Frisch hypothesized that a minimum body weight "may trigger" menarche and other "adolescent events" through changes in metabolism, growth hormones, and the "ovarian-hypothalamus feedback" system.[53] Her later iteration focused on critical body fat; as the experiences of anorectics and other undernour-ished females suggest, a "minimum level of stored, easily mobilized energy is necessary for ovulation and menstrual cycles."[54] Perhaps, other experts rea-soned, lean athletes also have insufficient body fat to initiate and maintain men-ses. Popular media immediately publicized these speculations, complete with photos and grim stories of skinny runners.

The storm then subsided. While some specialists challenged Frisch's statis-tical analysis, others cited counterevidence, such as slender athletes with reg-ular periods and large active women with menstrual disorders. Gynecologists and pediatricians pointed out that life crises and crash diets also altered hy-pothalamic function; regardless of cause, however, they were confident that hormone therapy could "reawaken" normal communication between the hypothalamus, pituitary gland, and ovaries, commonly known as the HPO axis.[55] Convinced that the benefits of exercise far outweighed the risks, medical organizations asserted that secondary amenorrhea probably was benign, reversible, and uncommon—a phenomenon limited to long-distance runners and other special groups.[56] Biomedical reviews also concluded that most girls and women could be active, even competitive, without reproductive harm.[57] Finally, popular media lowered the decibel level with more balanced accounts of contradictory scientific data.[58]

Reactions among physical educators varied widely in the 1970s. Although general textbooks and journals paid scant attention to the controversy, sports advocates could not ignore it. Hoping that Title IX would expand competition, some teachers and coaches cited outdated studies of healthy active females, while overlooking recent reports of reproductive problems.[59] By contrast, physical educators with research backgrounds challenged the new empirical data directly. "Strenuous activity" does not cause "uterine damage," exercise physiologist Christine Wells maintained in 1978.[60] "There is no experimental or clinical evidence to suggest that women, who have participated frequently in vigorous athletic activities with high level training programs and regular competition, have experienced any gynecological or obstetrical abnormalities because of that participation." Wells's message about monthly periods was equally encouraging: Since activity generally need not "be adjusted or modified during any phase of the menstrual cycle for the normally functioning female athlete," an individual's "freedom of choice" should be paramount.

This focus on personal circumstances was critical to Dorothy V. Harris, a leading sports psychologist. Any discussion of sports and reproductive health, she insisted, must take into account wide variations in women's cycles as well as highly individual responses to exercise and other stresses. Every active female, Harris recommended, should find her "pattern of training and performance that is compatible for her menstrual cycle" along with solutions she deemed acceptable for any problems.[61] By inviting athletes to trust their own bodies and judgments, Harris challenged the medicalization of menstruation. Why should we regard secondary amenorrhea as pathological, she asked, when most cases are short-term and reversible? Why prescribe hormones when simple adjustments in training probably will suffice? Harris's argument was shrewd; marshaling science to defuse the exercise-menstruation controversy, she nonetheless deemed active women the real experts.

Scary forecasts of amenorrhea, though, might dissuade girls and women from being active. As Harris and like-minded colleagues understood, this was simply the latest flare-up in the politics of sex differences. If the "'effects of heavy exercise on the body'" were the main issue, remarked Barbara Drinkwater, a prominent physical education-based researcher, then scientists would study both males and females; instead, they focused on menstrual disturbances, the "'more visible'" response unique to girls and women.[62] For Dorothy Harris as well, the social impetus behind demonizing exercise and pathologizing women's bodies was clear. "Females have been restricted in their pursuit of vigorous and competitive sport down through the ages," she explained, "because of misconceptions, old wives' tales, ignorance, and male chauvinism." Classifying menstrual changes as problems and attributing them to exercise perpetuated long-standing myths about female frailty.[63] This analysis struck a chord with doctors who were athletes. Why all the fuss about sports? asked Tenley Albright, a surgeon and the 1956 Olympic gold medalist in figure skating. It seemed "amusing" that people "worry about how much physical activity girls have, when no one has ever worried about how hard a woman has to work keeping house, helping to run a farm, beating laundry in a cold stream, carrying water, protecting her children, [or] pioneering across this country hundreds of years ago." Apparently, a woman who expends energy on "her role in the family" is "all right," whereas a "stigma" is attached to "those who participate in sports."[64]

Such critiques did not reject science. Research-based physical educators and women doctors accepted the endocrinologic paradigm of female physiology and valued biomedical studies as an antidote to conventional wisdom about women's "peculiar" bodies. As the storm over sports and reproductive health brewed in the 1970s, they employed science to reassure colleagues and the lay public that the menstrual cycle was resilient and exercise was safe. They also understood, however, that hormones were a pawn in gender politics: the real issue was not the status of the HPO axis but the future of women's sports. Against the backdrop of Title IX and second-wave feminism, some female experts insisted that imperfect science should not override the testimony of healthy athletes or scuttle their ambitions.

SCIENTIFIC DISPUTES, 1980–95

During the 1980s and early 1990s, the storm intensified again. Investigators reported a wider array of serious disorders among more diverse cohorts of active girls and women. Reproductive endocrinologists, sports medicine experts, and exercise physiologists argued about risk factors, mechanisms, and therapeutic strategies. Doctors, nurses, and health advocates joined the debate, and popular media eagerly covered it. Fueled by widespread alarm and technical disputes, the storm lasted about fifteen years, with three scientific issues at the forefront: the range of health problems, risk factors and causes, and possible solutions.[65] The first seemed clear-cut and empirical. Although concern about delayed menarche and secondary amenorrhea continued, experts turned their attention to less noticeable conditions. Since the late 1970s, researchers had described anovulatory cycles among athletes, which exposed them to excess estrogen; other women had a shortened luteal phase between ovulation and bleeding, which rendered them infertile.[66] Because cycles might seem normal, specialists warned, these two phenomena probably were more common than athletes or their doctors realized. To organize their findings, experts proposed a continuum of "exercise-induced perturbations" from amenorrhea and other "obvious clinical presentations" to the "less obvious subclinical presentations" of anovulation and luteal inadequacy.[67] Such constructs suggested an ominous, perhaps inevitable progression from subtle events to chronic dysfunction.

In the mid-1980s evidence appeared of nonreproductive problems including electrolyte imbalances and heightened risk of heart disease and breast cancer. Experts also described a propensity for skeletal injuries among young amenorrheic runners and dancers, whose bone mineral density resembled that of postmenopausal women. Although subsequent work revealed partial remineralization once training tapered off and menses resumed, the alarm bell had sounded and research accelerated.[68] Between 1984 and 1987, the number of studies on "athletic amenorrhea" was "more than four times that of all previously published papers."[69] With premature bone loss looming as the "black cloud overshadowing women's athletics," one insider recalled, scientists' "complacency" gave way to apprehension.[70] In the late 1980s and early 1990s, the ante rose even higher when researchers suspected that reproductive, skeletal, dietary, and psychological problems occurred in clusters—an idea reified in 1992 as the Female Athlete Triad. On its own, one doctor warned, athletic amenorrhea signified a "system edging toward collapse." "At the extreme," another declared, the Triad's three conditions together could "affect every organ system and even lead to premature death."[71]

As the inventory of problems grew, so did the list of predisposing factors. A "complex interplay of physical, hormonal, nutritional, psychological, and environmental factors" seemed likely, one doctor observed. Examples included body composition, dietary and caloric deficits, menstrual and obstetric history, physical and psychological stress, intensity of training, hormone profiles, and the catchall category of "other factors."[72] Further research yielded the consensus that no single variable independently produced menstrual dysfunction. In fact, known risk factors and their combinations probably accounted for only 30 percent "of menstrual status variability" among athletes.[73] Nevertheless, common terminology, such as "exercise-induced amenorrhea," cast physical activity and sports as the chief suspect, with other factors being mere accomplices.

Still undetermined was how exercise and its partners triggered physiological problems. During the 1980s and early 1990s, simple hypotheses, such as low body fat, gave way to complex explanations involving the HPO axis.[74] Cybernetic metaphors ruled. Regardless of specialty, experts viewed reproductive functions as part of a communications network through which chemicals transmitted information under the direction of the "pacemaker" hypothalamus and some "master switch" in the central nervous system. Extending the electrical imagery, they speculated about the transduction of neuronal signals into endocrine messages, the modulation of the frequency and amplitude of chemical pulses, and the rhythmic movement of inputs through feedback channels that needed fine-tuning. Several gynecologists even likened the HPO axis to the "multiple components of a modern hi-fi stereo system with tuners, tape decks, preamplifiers, amplifiers, and speakers" whose complicated connections and "switch stations" sometimes required the services of a "radio repair expert." With the information-processing paradigm firmly in place, scientists disagreed primarily over why certain messages became erratic or inappropriately loud or soft.[75]

Finally, experts asked which girls and women were vulnerable and what could be done for them. International studies described reproductive complications among skiers, rowers, speed skaters, swimmers, volleyball players, and fencers. Some scientists warned that menstrual disturbances "may be the rule rather than the exception in a high proportion of exercising women," including recreational joggers and other moderately active females.[76] Nonreproductive problems seemed likely as well. "Potentially all physically active girls and women," an ACSM panel asserted, "could be at risk for developing one or more components of the [Female Athlete] Triad."[77] As methods of restoring menses, bone, and nutrients multiplied, leading experts cautioned against radical approaches. "'If we don't know precisely what mechanism turns off the menstrual cycle,'" one researcher observed, "'we can't say what turns it on.'"[78]

Although questions remained, the science of exercise and menstruation had been transformed. In the 1970s researchers had regarded secondary amenorrhea a benign condition limited to elite young athletes in particular sports; by the early 1990s they envisioned a spectrum of clinical and subclinical disorders produced by multiple factors that, through complex mechanisms, could affect all females over various age groups and activity levels. "It used to be simple," sighed a Canadian endocrinologist in 1985. "Exercise had no effect on reproduction. Then came a letter reporting amenorrhea in intercollegiate track women. . . . It is no longer simple."[79]

This revolution captured wide attention. Clinical guides alerted gynecologists and pediatricians to the role of exercise in reproductive disorders, while assuring them that such cases were manageable.[80] Family physicians, orthopedic surgeons, reproductive endocrinologists, physical therapists, nurses, and sports doctors pondered their involvement in this complicated area of practice. If specialized literature was sober, more public discourse seemed quite agitated. Professional organizations revised their guidelines about female exercise.[81] Sports governance groups modified their policies on training and competition to protect young participants.[82] In the 1980s New York State prohibited girls who had not yet menstruated from competing in interscholastic events.[83] The federal Women's Health Equity Act of 1993 identified education about eating disorders a top priority.[84] Many lay health guides offered sensible, but somber advice about exercise and menstruation, expressing particular concern about weakened bones.[85] Other sources simply fanned the flames. A health book by several gynecologists warned that women suffering bone loss due to low estrogen—even young athletes with otherwise "excellent exercise and diet"—might "face serious illness and deformity from the fragile bones of osteoporosis within just a few years."[86] Equally certain about the line between health and hazard, another specialist advised "any woman who trains to the point where she stops menstruating" to "seriously reevaluate her priorities."[87] Articles in general magazines also fell into hyperbole: "Should Women Stop Jogging?" and "How Exercise Can K-O Your Period."[88] The implications were unsettling: Maybe menstrual irregularities were serious and widespread. Perhaps active girls and women should eat more, exercise less, see a doctor, and take hormones.

As clinicians and scientists interpreted these matters for lay and professional audiences, two perspectives emerged. Although some experts straddled the line, the majority tended to distrust female bodies and exercise, while a small group challenged orthodoxy and its gender politics. For mainstream experts, menstrual changes generally signified pathology. Although some variations, even interruptions, were natural, "exercise-induced amenorrhea" violated biology's plan and female identity. To avoid implicating *all* forms of physical activity, orthodox specialists clarified the difference between fitness and catastrophe; the boundary stood wherever nature, not personal ambition or cultural fads, set it. As one self-confessed old fogey declared in 1985, "There are unique aspects of female biology that impose definite constraints on women's athletic achievements and expose them to special hazards."[89] Another commentator put the issue more starkly: "Does high-level competition take a woman's body on a journey it was never meant to take?"[90] Accordingly, one doctor's algorithm for curing "athletic amenorrhea" focused on reducing women's "training to the point at which seemingly normal menstrual cycling begins." As long as she bled, a female was normal and well.[91]

By blaming exercise for producing unnatural bodies, orthodox experts helped "secure the border of the sexualized self."[92] A slender, amenorrheic, undernourished female body suffering infertility and brittle bones fell outside the male/female duality. A natural female was well-fed, moderately fit, fertile, and eumenorrheic (normal cycles). A natural male—the "default norm of the public person"—was solid, steady, athletic, and nonmenstrual; his reproductive system easily withstood physical activity and competition. Occupying neither of these two states, the disordered female athlete was caught in limbo. To obey the "telos of reproductive biology," the athlete must yield to the female; as ovulation and menses returned, she properly ceded the world of sports to boys and men.

Not every active female mattered, however.[93] Initial research emphasized young long-distance runners, whose slender, athletic bodies seemed almost "masculine." Next came gymnasts, ballet dancers, and other lean performers; perhaps even socially sanctioned pursuits could render women "unsexed" and infertile. Subsequent studies examined physiques carrying disparate gender images, from figure skating to body building. Despite the apparent range of research subjects, each of these sports was restricted chiefly to participants with ample resources and opportunities. By focusing on exclusive sports, establishment scientists betrayed a class and racial bias. Virtually no mainstream expert analyzed physical activities that attracted a broad range of girls and women; almost no one asked if race, ethnicity, and class were relevant in the epidemiology of delayed menarche and athletic amenorrhea. Instead, conventional researchers wondered if the reproductive status of privileged white females was in jeopardy. Might *these* high-value bodies, they asked, become too active, hungry, infertile, lean, brittle, or "male"?

The majority's perspective drew criticism from some doctors, scientists, and women's health advocates. While agreeing that bone loss in amenorrheic athletes was serious, they doubted that subclinical menstrual changes or the Female Athlete Triad were common.[94] Moreover, prevalence would not necessarily signify importance. As one health educator explained, many active females noticed variations in their periods and lab tests could detect their hormonal fluctuations, but the real issue "is how significant from physiological or clinical perspectives are these changes?"[95] Even this question sounded too orthodox for some critics. Rejecting the disease model altogether, they asked why twelve cycles per year—what "most Western-trained doctors" expected for the "sedentary, overfat female of mid-twentieth-century America"—were considered the norm, when menstrual patterns around the world are so diverse.[96] Rather than being medical crises, endocrine responses to exercise were normal, even desirable adaptations. Just as physical activity affected a woman's cardiovascular, musculoskeletal, and metabolic systems, athletic training stimulated a gradual, functional "process of 'hypothalamic conditioning.'"[97] Across the centuries "Mother Nature" had reduced the likelihood of pregnancy "when there [were] other physical or psychological demands upon the reproductive system." Females in nomadic hunter-gatherer tribes, for example, are "extremely active, nurse their children for several years and average only one to two periods a year."[98]

This argument inverted mainstream perspectives: The female body is resilient, not fragile; menstrual variations are normal, not pathological; athletes fall within, not outside femaleness; and biological processes are wise, not punitive. Mother Nature is not a tyrant who penalizes athletes but is a "gentle hand" helping humans "maintain a hardy species."[99] Following nature's counsel, a young woman with no interest in conceiving might accept anovulatory cycles. A competitive athlete might welcome breaks from her periods or conclude that intensive training lowered her cancer risk by reducing lifetime exposure to estrogen. Women are self-determining agents, critics insisted, with the right and capacity to assess their own reproductive health.[100]

Moreover, most cases of infertility and menstrual irregularity occurred among non-athletes.[101] To skeptics, this suggested that majority views were not "concepts based on thorough evaluation of prospective studies," but "medical expressions of cultural attitudes towards women and sport."[102] Popular anxiety about female competition, critics explained, had pulled scientific research toward the experiences of high-level athletes. Because the real crisis was too little physical activity among women, rather than too much, the broad population of average, sedentary females should be investigators' primary focus. Overall, skeptics rehabilitated the female body, defused concern about women's sports, and exposed the gender politics underlying disputes over exercise and menstruation. At the same time, they rarely challenged the standard image of active females as white, middle-class, and heterosexual or asked whether the dynamics of exercise and reproductive health varied by race, class, or sexual orientation.

PHYSICAL EDUCATION, 1980–95

The storm over exercise and menstruation posed a dilemma for female teachers and coaches. Despite feeling obliged to join the debate, they also recognized how the controversy could impede women's sports. Most decided to keep a low profile. In the early 1980s physical education journals and textbooks paid scant attention to athletic amenorrhea, with medical specialists and research-based teachers providing only occasional commentaries.[103] Subsequent reports of eating disorders and osteoporosis, though, prompted gym teachers to ask "Can an athlete be too thin? Yes, yes, yes!"[104] Leaving the details of endocrinology to other experts, physical educators and coaches seized on nutrition and skeletal health as practical matters they could address with young students and competitors. By taking the onus off sports, teachers' emphasis on weight, diet, and bones enabled them to promote health and physical activity without undercutting women's athletics.[105]

By contrast, research-based colleagues marched directly into the storm. Building on their physical education backgrounds, Barbara Drinkwater, Dorothy V. Harris, Sharon A. Plowman, Charlotte Feicht Sanborn, and Christine Wells became leading specialists in sport science. Determined to influence scientific knowledge, public opinion, and sports policy, they engaged the controversy over exercise and menstruation in both professional and popular settings. At first glance, their views seem orthodox. They worried about secondary amenorrhea as well as nutritional and skeletal problems among active females. Adopting cybernetic metaphors, they likened reproductive processes to an "intricate negative and positive feedback system" and visualized physiological changes as communication disturbances and "inappropriate feedback."[106] Criticizing the sloppy methods and analyses plaguing the science of exercise, they contributed seminal studies, including a 1978 report by Charlotte Feicht (Sanborn) on the menstrual status of collegiate athletes and Barbara Drinkwater's work in the 1980s on bone loss and remineralization.[107]

Women scientists, however, also sided with the debate's skeptics. Warning against facile generalizations, they noted that the prevalence of menstrual problems among athletes compared to the general population was unknown. In fact, was "problems" even the correct term? If the "'only regular aspect of the menstrual cycle is that it is irregular,'" one exercise scientist observed, then calling any period normal or aberrant was questionable.[108] By corollary, if a particular change was common, perhaps it should be considered normal. Maybe secondary amenorrhea and the subsequent resumption of menses, Dorothy Harris suggested, were "indicative of the body's ability to respond and adapt to stress." If menstrual variability is frequent and reversible, Harris mused, "perhaps we've been using [the] wrong standard for 'normal.' Maybe women don't need to menstruate every month?"[109] This logic overturned conventional assumptions: Menstrual irregularities became common variations, abnormalities became natural adaptations, and monthly periods were no longer the litmus test of female health.

Having deconstructed menstrual "disorders," women researchers moved on to the supposed cause, namely, exercise. Beginning with a familiar admonition against jumping to conclusions, they maintained that physiological changes in active females did not mean exercise was responsible; diet, emotional stress, and numerous other factors might be involved, and their interactions were complex and individual. Researchers' commitment to credible data and comprehensive theories was political as well as intellectual; they understood the power of science to shape popular attitudes, women's lives, and sports policy. "'The potential benefits of exercise are just so great,'" Barbara Drinkwater remarked in 1986, "'that it would be devastating to think that women are being frightened away from activity'" by scientific reports and "'media misrepresentation.'"[110] For decades, Christine Wells concurred, society's quarrels over menstruation had been a "major stumbling block" to women's participation "in strenuous physical activity."[111]

As Wells perceived, the science of sex differences and the politics of active bodies were inseparable. The debate over exercise and menstruation was intertwined with arguments about gender equity and women's rights. Physical education researchers and other skeptics lent support to feminist causes by normalizing reproduction, redefining female "nature," and shattering the sexual dualism that privileged men's physical activities. By contrast, opponents of women's rights could enlist orthodox science to recommend shutting the gymnasium door; for conservatives, menstrual disorders among active females signaled the primacy of reproductive imperatives and the unquestioned prerogative of active males.

Boys and men, though, were conspicuous by their absence. Between 1980 and 1995 researchers rarely examined reproductive health in active males.[112] Instead of studying "the sexual maturation of the young male athlete," scientists simply assumed that boys were innately robust and their athleticism improved during

puberty—although males probably are "more sensitive to environmental influences than females during growth and development."[113] Likewise, most scientists believed that hormonal responses among active adult men were minor,
while the "absence of a clear indicator" comparable to menstrual variations
made male reproductive distress too hard to study.[114] Neither assumption was
valid; physical training can disturb men's reproductive status and the effects are
detectable. Nevertheless, scientists' emphasis on girls and women implied that
they alone must exercise caution in the gym. Equally hidden were variations
in reproductive "disorders" among active Americans across race, class, and
other social variables. Most experts, orthodox and renegade alike, envisioned
the ideal female as a white, middle-class heterosexual with moderate fitness,
regular menses, and the prospect of pregnancy.

New Storm Surge, 1995–2005

In recent years biomedical experts converged on a single hypothesis about
physical activity and reproductive processes. Most now attribute menstrual
disturbances in active females to a chronic imbalance between energy intake
and expenditure. Researchers first proposed a link between energy shortage and
athletic amenorrhea in the 1980s. Noting the connection between "undernutrition and altered reproductive function" in anorexia nervosa, they speculated
that high energy use during physical activity also produced a "relative metabolic deficit."[115] Although the "energy drain" theory acquired various names
and meanings during the 1980s and 1990s, each version emphasized the role
of intensive exercise in energy debt and subsequent menstrual changes. Over
the past decade the energy paradigm came to dominate scientific thinking.[116]
All mammals, including humans, the argument runs, "partition dietary energy
among five major metabolic activities (cellular maintenance, thermoregula-
tion, locomotion, growth, and reproduction)."[117] If the body detects a short-
fall between intake and expenditure, it enters survival mode by concentrating
energy on "life-sustaining metabolic functions," while suppressing high-cost,
noncritical processes such as reproduction.[118]

Applying this idea to physical activity, many specialists use the concept of
energy availability, that is, the energy remaining "to support all other physiological processes" once "exercise energy expenditure" has been subtracted
from "dietary energy intake."[119] Among active girls and women, especially
competitive athletes, this balance can be quite small because, deliberately or
inadvertently, their caloric intake might not cover their high activity level.
Facing "an energy-deficient diet," the active female body shuts down reproductive functions as "an energy-conserving adaptation."[120] How this adjustment
occurs is unclear. Employing the cybernetic metaphor, researchers speculate
that "energy deficit elicits a cascade of endocrine-metabolic aberrations that

are interrelated in terms of their regulation and magnitude."[121] They disagree, however, over which specific chemicals transmit information about energy reserves to the brain.

Real-world questions also persist. Scientists do not know why problems are more common among adolescents than mature females or why larger, well-nourished athletes, such as swimmers, also experience reproductive irregular-ities.[122] Nor can the energy paradigm account for the distribution of the Female Athlete Triad's three components, either separately or concurrently; to date, "only three studies of female athletes have investigated the simultaneous occur-rence of disordered eating, menstrual disorders, and low [bone mineral density]" using established definitions and measurements. Without accurate prevalence data, a causal model cannot be confirmed.[123] Moreover, doctors and other pro-fessionals are divided over how to screen for and treat the Triad because few prospective studies of different interventions have been undertaken.[124]

Despite these critical gaps, the energy availability hypothesis has consoli-dated the analysis of exercise and reproductive health. The theory enjoys almost universal support in North American biomedicine, including obste-tricians and gynecologists, pediatricians, general practitioners, physical thera-pists, and reproductive endocrinologists. Numerous professional organizations have adopted the paradigm, as has the Female Athlete Triad Coalition, spear-headed by the American College of Sports Medicine (ACSM).[125] The Women's Sports Foundation and other advocacy groups have signed on, as have sports governance organizations, including the NCAA.[126] Books and articles for pop-ular audiences also refer to the energy model.[127] Despite this broad consensus, the emergence of two interpretations of the energy paradigm in the mid-1990s fueled a new storm surge.

The dominant version cloaked old suspicions about active female bodies in modern scientific language. According to the biomedical establishment, the Female Athlete Triad is a collection of severe pathologies. The absence of men-ses raises a "red flag," signaling internal disturbances that are "never healthy, desirable or acceptable."[128] Premature bone loss is said to occur throughout an athlete's body, including sites where exercise loads normally boost skeletal health.[129] However dire the Triad's components seem individually, specialists regard their simultaneity as "even more serious, and often life-threatening."[130] Eventually, an ACSM panel recently concluded, "sustained low energy avail-ability" can compromise every aspect of mental and physical health.[131] A prac-tical guide for athletes and coaches asserts that the Triad could "decimate the lives of the best and brightest women." Nothing less than a "hidden epidemic," the authors conclude, the Triad "is silently affecting [athletes'] health and per-formance now, and it could erupt like a time bomb in the future."[132]

Whereas the Triad originally entailed three specific problems (clinical eating disorders, amenorrhea, and osteoporosis), recent formulations recognize the more general phenomena of "disordered eating, menstrual dysfunction, and altered bone mineral density."[133] Each category occurs along a continuum from mild to severe states, with intermediate points being a precursor to the next more serious condition.[134] This construct implies that *all* female athletes, "training in all sports and activities, from aerobics and badminton to softball and tennis," live on a slippery slope of pathology.[135] Lacking sufficient fuel, *any* physically active female of *any* age—the exercise addict, recreational jogger, or average health club member—may experience one or more parts of the Triad, thereby extending its reach to the "entire population."[136]

To some extent, clinicians and researchers blame contemporary cultural norms of slender, fit womanhood. Athletes, they acknowledge, face the extra burden of resolving "conflicting requirements for aggressiveness and sweetness, strength and daintiness, and optimal weight for performance and desired thinness for look."[137] Many experts, though, believe that biology also places girls and women at risk, because the threshold between exercise's benefits and costs supposedly is lower in females than in males.[138] Whether society or nature rules, both explanations suggest that women, especially athletes, mismanage their energy accounts. Living in denial, the argument runs, athletes are reluctant, even hostile patients who prioritize sports over health and resist sensible advice.[139] Despite valuing regular physical activity, the orthodox version of the energy paradigm perpetuates negative judgments. By asserting that all girls and women are at risk, the mainstream view indicts exercise and sports as singular hazards, and medicalizes the experiences of athletes—the very girls and women whose active, disciplined bodies seem closest to cultural standards.

Recast, however, the energy theory can break each link in the causal chain that once explained athletes' situation. First, if reproductive and skeletal problems arise from overall energy imbalances, not specific expenditures, then the model exonerates physical activity per se. Second, some specialists no longer attribute low bone mineral density solely to the suppression of estrogen accompanying so-called athletic amenorrhea; instead, many believe that osteopenia and osteoporosis in active women may be related primarily to "undernutrition and its metabolic consequences."[140] If exercise itself does not interrupt menstruation and "athletic amenorrhea" does not weaken bones directly, then old constructs fall apart and alternate views of the female body become possible.

By allowing one to see monthly cycles as smart and resilient, the energy paradigm redefines secondary amenorrhea as a normal adaptation to intensive exercise and other costly functions. "This protective system," two experts observe, "has been in place in our bodies for millions of years to protect women from getting pregnant during starvation or energy deficiency." Even though we are not prehistoric women, they continue, "our reproductive systems are still programmed to stop or slow down if there is an energy imbalance."[141] Accordingly, amenorrheic athletes are not uncooperative patients with defective bodies but are self-determining individuals endowed with physiological wisdom. Moreover, by portraying nature's laws as universal and energy arithmetic as sex-neutral, the energy theory overturns the old supposition that female bodies operate by strange rules and suffer unique breakdowns.[142] In sum, the alternate version of the energy paradigm could vindicate exercise and sports, normalize reproductive changes, displace menstruation as the core of women's physical identity, and destabilize the sex binary.

PHYSICAL EDUCATORS AND COACHES

Whether orthodoxy or dissent prevails, science now stands as the undisputed authority on exercise and reproductive health. The less prestigious job of applying biomedical knowledge falls to physical education and other practical fields. To prepare teachers and coaches for this role, recent literature by and for HPER professionals has covered exercise science and reproductive health, including both mainstream and revisionist analyses of the Female Athlete Triad.[143] As do biomedical experts, physical educators perceive many risk factors among virtually all active females and arrange each potential outcome along a continuum from mild to severe. Insisting that amenorrhea is neither normal nor desirable, they also express concern for women's skeletal health and warn that disordered eating may foreshadow life-threatening problems.[144] Using mainstream logic, teachers and coaches maintain that physical activities, especially competitive sports, can be dangerous, energy deficits might spiral into medical crises, and girls and women are uniquely vulnerable, due to biology and culture.[145]

At the same time, physical educators and coaches have distinguished themselves from other professions by highlighting their close relationships with students and athletes. Our field is positioned, leaders observe, to do either the most harm or the most good for young women. Coaches can "treat . . . athletes as machines," driving them to physical and emotional breakdowns for the sake of championships, or help "young, active females consume a healthy diet and maintain the energy needed in order to maintain a regular menstrual cycle for optimal health and performance."[146] As mentors at the gym, training room, and athletic field, physical educators can detect problems and intervene sooner than a friend, parent, or doctor might. Accordingly, the profession has focused on converting scientific information into practical action: What do young athletes need to know about menstruation, bone health, nutrition, and training? How can teachers refute competitors' belief that amenorrhea is normal, strict diets are necessary, and osteoporosis is a distant threat?[147] Stopping short of orthodox judgments, most physical educators and coaches attribute the Triad and other problems to general energy deficits, not physical activity per se. Moreover, by emphasizing how amenorrhea impairs health and athletic performance, they have humanized science's arcane theories, and depicted exercise and menstruation in more female-positive, sports-friendly terms.

These convoluted views stemmed from social conditions and professional concerns. Between 1995 and 2005 exercise scientists and public health leaders stressed the role of physical activity in health, weight control, and disease prevention, especially for girls and women. Meanwhile, American support for women's sports, both amateur and professional, continued to grow, bringing with it higher expectations, more money, and media attention, along with renewed battles over Title IX. In this environment, physical educators carefully defended physical activity and sports; without ignoring potential problems, they impugned neither exercise nor female physiology. As diverse specialists asserted control over active female bodies and appropriated the Triad as an area of expertise, gym teachers and coaches cast themselves as intermediaries between science and practice, between research and the real world. By virtue of working closely with active girls and women every day, physical educators laid claim to actual female bodies, both in motion and distress.

{Conclusion}

Justice in the Gym

Throughout the twentieth century, women physical educators influenced American views and experiences of the body-in-motion. They taught exercise and games to innumerable children and adults, supervised activity programs in diverse institutions, and interpreted female fitness for professional peers and popular audiences. Their work with girls and women was a critical site where the scientific and social meanings of gender, race, and sexuality were debated, presumed differences between people were embodied and resisted, professional authority was asserted or lost, and physical fairness was advanced or thwarted. A review of the past one hundred years offers both hope and doubt about the prospects for justice in the gym.

Today, being female no longer disqualifies one from becoming skilled and athletic or from being recognized as such. Fewer Americans assume that all female bodies are unstable or that physical activity invariably compromises women's identity and reproductive health. Girls and women of more diverse backgrounds have greater opportunities for recreation and competition than did their counterparts a century ago. This progress was associated with broad historical developments. Movements for social justice toppled familiar norms of womanhood and catalyzed fundamental (albeit incomplete) reforms in American laws. Although the science of exercise often upheld tradition, many researchers refuted long-standing ideas about sex differences and biodeterminism. In the gym and on the athletic field, active girls and women demolished old beliefs about their supposed shortcomings. Some female physical educators, white and black, championed more enlightened perspectives and equitable programs, with lasting effects. Compared to their predecessors, current teachers and coaches are more optimistic about women's physical potential, more enthusiastic about high-level fitness and competition, and more committed to broad-based equity in the gym.

Conceptualizing justice, much less achieving it, proved difficult. Because white and black women worked at their profession's margins with people deemed second class, they deliberated at length over fairness for the "fair sex." The majority viewed parity in exercise and sports through the lens of sex differences. Even at the turn of the twenty-first century, most aspects of the field—from pedagogical strategies and fitness tests to research studies and teacher training—still revolved around the axes of male/female and man/woman.[1] Tackling a project that most whites avoided, black female teachers questioned mainstream assumptions about race, femininity, and physicality. Until the 1980s, though, a conspiracy of silence, among black and white professionals alike, hindered examining justice in relation to sexual orientation.

Far from reaching consensus during the twentieth century, disagreements over difference and fairness escalated as physical educators addressed complex issues, from reproductive health and competitive sports to departmental structure and professional autonomy. Each approach—including similarity and equality, difference and equity, difference and equality, diversity and equity, and social justice—had merit and drew fervent support. Whether flattening or accentuating difference, however, these philosophies usually judged every individual by masculine standards of skill and behavior. Strategies of equality applied male-based criteria to girls and women by treating everyone "the same." Schemes that emphasized difference tended to marginalize females; whether girls were relegated to a separate gym or accommodated in mixed classes, their bodies and activities were devalued. Concepts of similarity and difference both held reproductive processes sacrosanct; gym teachers worried that exercise threatened menstruation and fertility but rarely asked if monthly cycles impinged on physical ability. Nor did most white teachers challenge dominant depictions of athletic black women as mannish, sexualized oddities. Although the diversity perspective of the 1990s expanded the categories of difference and inclusion—from race and ethnicity to religion and cultural background—it did not necessarily reduce the stigma of otherness or rectify inequities between privileged and subordinate groups.

The blind spots in physical education exemplified American and, more generally, Western concepts of difference. Asserting that maleness or femaleness permeated every aspect of a person's body, the modern sexual binary seemed free of any overlap or uncertainty.[2] As the physical and social signature of womanhood, a female's reproductive system delineated her basic roles and behavior. By connecting sex directly to gender, standard theories represented women as if they were (or should be) identical based solely on common anatomy and physiology. By limiting human identities, homogenization condemned anyone who fell outside the norm, while masking people's variability, ambiguities, and remarkable individuality. The claim that human character and the social order stemmed from biology, not culture, reified and naturalized various hierarchies of "difference."

Barriers to justice are especially high when difference is located in the body. Regardless of time or place, the body "plays a pivotal role [in] the formation and maintenance of self-identity, in our understanding of who we are and of our location or positioning in social life."[3] In the modern era, Westerners came to regard the physical self as the primary expression of a person's identity and worth.[4] Twentieth-century Americans learned to rehearse difference and regulate their bodies in routine ways in ordinary places, both public and private.[5] Venues for physical activity gained special meaning; in the gymnasium, sports arena, and health club, the body seemed to confirm, in stark ways, that differences not only existed but that they indeed mattered. Recreation and athletics have long served to constitute the self and social relationships, and the twentieth century's preoccupation with the body made the embodiment of identity and inequity through physical activity even more significant.

Because physical education is intrinsically body-centered, its ideas and curricula connect average Americans to modern discourses of the body and difference. The process is subtle but compelling; in the gym, social rules and relationships are quietly integrated into people's everyday practices and sense of self.[6] Ascertaining physical education's power requires "bringing bodies back in."[7] By examining the scientific infrastructure of gym class—that is, teachers' theories of anatomy and physiology, analyses of physical and psychosocial difference, and debates over the relative impact of biology and culture on women's exercise, one can perceive how instructional physical education strengthened its social impact by affiliating with the natural and social sciences.[8]

Given the burdens of "difference," it is tempting to conclude that physical education should abandon this core concept. Although paradigms of difference have serious intellectual flaws, their underlying problem is political: How does a given society deploy and embody difference? Do its schemes denigrate and disadvantage certain people or affirm and empower everyone? Being classified as male or female, white or black, straight or gay, able or disabled in the gym and American society has very real consequences. Denouncing these categories is a necessary but insufficient step so long as the contexts in which they operate remain unjust.

Throughout the nineteenth and twentieth centuries, Americans devised ideas and actions that subverted "difference" and promoted justice. Political activists mobilized for human rights. Social reformers tried to alleviate poverty, illiteracy, and disease. Working-class and professional women of all races challenged discrimination on the job. Girls and women invaded the gym, competed on the field, and took to the road. In 1893, when Frances E. Willard was fifty-three years old, she learned how to ride a bicycle. Despite poor health and time-consuming obligations, the noted suffragist and temperance reformer was determined to give the novel contraption a try. As Willard became comfortable on "Gladys," her new set of wheels, she learned as much about women's rights as the laws of physics. Just as steady riding depended on good instruction, balance, and persistence, so too, she believed, social progress required cooperative efforts, strong wills, and an abiding faith that women would overcome the "bluff, the swagger, the bravado of young men" who deemed them inferior.[9]

Willard understood that the female body could serve both prejudice and liberation. On the one hand, she observed, "old fables, myths, and follies" about women's physical "incompetence" abounded. On the other hand, these barriers to equality would crumble once women displayed their ability to "handle bat and oar, bridle and rein, and at last the cross-bar of the bicycle" with "nimbleness, agility, and skill." Willard recognized that the confidence women gained through physical activity would enable them to master their "wobbling will" and turn the wheels of social reform "at the right moment on the right angle."[10] As Willard discovered, exercise can be a potent engine of change. Physical activity inspires what anthropologist Emily Martin has called the "embodiment of oppositions"—a process of "questioning, opposing, resisting, rejecting, and reformulating the ways in which [we] live and the ways in which the society might work."[11] In the gym, so-called dubs discover power and agency. On the playground and athletic field, disadvantaged groups challenge discrimination. Exercise and sports are especially empowering for girls and women, both physically and personally. Active females develop strength and skill, thereby dispelling myths of women's frailty and men's superiority. Some physiques and movements are visibly transgressive. Female athletes who are large and graceful, small and tough, or talented "despite" being blind, disabled, injured, or elderly disrupt conventions of femininity. Female bodies that flaunt muscle, look androgynous, "kick butt," or say "No" threaten "to dismantle the heterosexualized femininity in which women's bodies are cast."[12] Instead of being fragile and sexually vulnerable, an active woman learns to own her body, not only in the gym but in other contexts as well. Teenage girls who participate in sports improve their health, body image, and academic performance, while reducing their risk of substance abuse or an unwanted pregnancy. Through recreation, individuals can re-create themselves, in literal and symbolic ways.[13]

The playing field, however, is not yet level. The chance to participate and excel in diverse physical activities is still limited by social address—not only gender but also age, race, ethnicity, class, sexuality, religion, and locality. Institutional barriers and resource disparities remain in physical education and recreation, as do deep-rooted prejudices about race and sexual orientation in relation to sports. Inequality also persists in the profession. As various sectors of Health, Physical Education, and Recreation (HPER) have waxed and waned in recent decades, many female teachers, coaches, and administrators have faced old and new disadvantages relative to their male counterparts.

Perhaps physical education can serve justice more fully and consistently in the twenty-first century. After all, Frances Willard did not learn to ride a bicycle by herself. More than a dozen people helped her during a visit to England in the early 1890s and back in the United States, before her death in 1898. Her early teachers included "three young Englishmen, all strong-armed and accomplished bicyclers, [who] held the machine in place while [she] climbed timidly into the saddle." Increasingly, however, she relied on female acquaintances. Unfortunately, one lady "had not a scintilla of knowledge concerning the machine." Another was so "timorous" that the whole bicycle (and Willard's nerve) quaked when the assistant held it. A third woman "was a fine, brave character" who cheered Willard on, but "never relinquished her strong grasp on the cross-bar," lest the novice rider falter. Her best instructor, Willard decided, was the person whose approach was to "'Let go, but stand by.'" This motto represented the "only rule that at once respects the individuality of another and yet adds one's own, so far as may be, to another's momentum in the struggle of life." The philosophy suits physical educators as well: Teach *and* liberate, guide *and* affirm.[14]

Judging from the historical record, physical education's willingness and capacity to accept this role seem mixed. As members of a young, insecure profession in the twentieth century, male and female instructors favored security over confrontation. They built connections with natural and social science, reflected mainstream ideologies of citizenship and individualism, and absorbed each new definition of fitness that arose through the decades. This conservatism certainly benefited the field's white male leaders. Many women, too, believed that discretion was the better part of valor. White and black female teachers alike often invoked traditional paradigms of difference to validate their work, assert professional authority, and restrict female sports. Weighed down by intellectual, social, and professional burdens, few sought true justice for their programs or themselves.

In each generation, however, some female teachers, administrators, and researchers opposed the status quo. Between the 1920s and 1950s, African American physical educators in the public schools of Washington, D.C., demanded equity for their segregated programs and fostered racial pride through innovative curricula. During the last quarter of the twentieth century, some teachers and researchers successfully challenged oppressive and inflexible labels of sex, gender, and sexual orientation. Since the 1990s, advocates of social justice have exposed the ways in which gender-friendly, multicultural instruction can perpetuate prejudice and injustice. Reexamining gym class through a feminist lens, some teachers and coaches have proposed remedies for gender inequities.[15] As critiques of American physical education and athletics multiply, scholars in sports studies have developed alternate theories of difference and fairness.[16]

These examples, past and present, have several things in common. Escaping binary thinking, they usually accept human identity as malleable. Most attach "difference" to history and culture, rather than to biology alone. Some even reinterpret women's reproductive health, arguably the most stubborn sexual duality. Above all, progressive physical educators have politicized "difference" by exposing the deep relationships between physical activity, racism and heterosexism, male privilege, women's autonomy, and social progress. They embrace opposition and justice in the gym, as a principle and practice. To be fully realized, this goal requires a new paradigm in which difference becomes a creative force, not an obstacle to be ignored or overcome.[17] Reform, of course, necessitates actions as well as ideas. Can American physical education deploy "difference" in ways that contest, rather than embody inequity? Following the lead of its progressive wing, perhaps the field will create a gym that affirms each individual and empowers every active body.

{ ENDNOTE ABBREVIATIONS }

AAHPER	American Association for Health, Physical Education, and Recreation
AAHPERD	American Alliance for Health, Physical Education, Recreation and Dance
ACOG	American College of Obstetricians and Gynecologists
APEA	American Physical Education Association
APER	*American Physical Education Review*
APNEA	*Addresses and Proceedings of the National Education Association*
BHL-UM	Bentley Historical Library, University of Michigan
BL-UCB	Bancroft Library, University of California at Berkeley
BMC	Archives, Bryn Mawr College
BNSG	Boston Normal School of Gymnastics
CA-RI	College Archives, Radcliffe Institute, Harvard University
CSSMA	Charles Sumner School Museum and Archives, Washington, D.C.
DGWS	Division of Girls and Women's Sports
ESDPECW	Eastern Society of Directors of Physical Education for College Women
ESSR	*Exercise and Sport Sciences Reviews*
GPO	Government Printing Office
HG-UCB	Hearst Gymnasium Historical Collections, University of California at Berkeley
HUA	Hampton University Archives, Hampton University
JAMA	*Journal of the American Medical Association*
JNE	*Journal of Negro Education*
JOAAHPER	*Journal of the American Association for Health, Physical Education, and Recreation*
JOHPE	*Journal of Health and Physical Education*
JOHPER	*Journal of Health, Physical Education, and Recreation*
JOPER	*Journal of Physical Education and Recreation*
JOPERD	*Journal of Physical Education, Recreation, and Dance*
JSH	*Journal of Sport History*
JTPE	*Journal of Teaching in Physical Education*
MBB	*Memories Beyond Bloomers (1924–1954)*, by Mabel Lee
MBG	*Memories of a Bloomer Girl (1894–1924)*, by Mabel Lee
MDA-LU	Milwaukee-Downer College, Archives, at Lawrence University
MHAAB	*Mary Hemenway Alumnae Association Bulletin*
MSRC	Moorland-Spingarn Research Center, Howard University

MSS	*Medicine and Science in Sports*
MSSE	*Medicine and Science in Sports and Exercise*
NAPECW	National Association of Physical Education for College Women
NASPE	National Association for Sport and Physical Education
NEA	National Education Association
NEJM	*New England Journal of Medicine*
NSGWS	National Section for Girls and Women's Sports
NSWA	National Section on Women's Athletics
OCA	Oberlin College Archives, Oberlin College
PCPFS	President's Council on Physical Fitness and Sports
PCPFS Research Digest	*President's Council on Physical Fitness and Sports Research Digest*
PE	*The Physical Educator*
Proc. AAAPE	*Proceedings of the American Association for the Advancement of Physical Education*
PSM	*The Physician and Sportsmedicine*
PSU	Special Collections and University Archives, Penn State University
RQ	*Research Quarterly*
RQES	*Research Quarterly for Exercise and Sport*
SA-UW	Steenbock Archives, Steenbock Memorial Library, University of Wisconsin at Madison
SC-Duke	Special Collections, William R. Perkins Library, Duke University
SC-SU	Department of Special Collections, Green Library, Stanford University
SC-UNCG	Special Collections, Walter Clinton Jackson Library, University of North Carolina at Greensboro
SCA	Spelman College Archives, Spelman College
SCA-SC	Smith College Archives, Smith College
SSC-SC	Sophia Smith Collection, Smith College
UA-Duke	University Archives, William R. Perkins Library, Duke University
UA-OSU	University Archives, Ohio State University
UA-TU	University Archives, Tuskegee University
UA-UI	University Archives, University of Illinois at Urbana-Champaign
UA-UMN	University Archives, University of Minnesota
UA-UNCG	University Archives, University of North Carolina at Greensboro
UA-UNL	University Archives, University of Nebraska at Lincoln.
UA-UW	University Archives, University of Wisconsin at Madison
WAS	Women's Athletic Section
WCA	Wellesley College Archives, Wellesley College
WD-NAAF	Women's Division of the National Amateur Athletic Federation
WSPAJ	*Women in Sport and Physical Activity Journal*

{ NOTES }

Introduction

1. Marie M. Ready, *Physical Education in City Public Schools*, Bureau of Education Physical Education Series, no. 10 (Washington, D.C.: GPO, 1929); James Frederick Rogers, *State-Wide Trends in School Hygiene and Physical Education*, Office of Education Pamphlet no. 5, rev. (Washington, D.C.: GPO, 1934), 4–10, 13; and Thomas A. Storey, Willard S. Small, and Elon G. Salisbury, *Recent State Legislation for Physical Education*, Bureau of Education Bulletin, 1922, no. 1 (Washington, D.C.: GPO, 1922).

2. Galen Cranz, "Women in Urban Parks," *Signs* 5, no. 3 suppl. (1980): S79–S95.

3. Linda J. Borish, "'An Interest in Physical Well-Being Among the Feminine Membership': Sporting Activities for Women at Young Men's and Young Women's Hebrew Associations," *American Jewish History* 87 (1999): 61–93; and Martha H. Verbrugge, "Recreation and Racial Politics in the Young Women's Christian Association of the United States, 1920s–1950s," *International Journal of the History of Sport* 27 (2010): 1191–1218.

4. Linda Jean Carpenter and R. Vivian Acosta, *Title IX* (Champaign, Ill.: Human Kinetics, 2005), 35–63.

5. Ron French et al., "Revisiting Section 504, Physical Education, and Sport," *JOPERD* 69 (September 1998): 58.

6. Karen L. Butt and Markella L. Pahnos, "Why We Need a Multicultural Focus in Our Schools," *JOPERD* 66 (January 1995): 48.

7. Data from Centers for Disease Control and Prevention, "National Youth Risk Behavior Survey, 1991–2005: Trends in the Prevalence of Physical Activity," http://www.cdc.gov/HealthyYouth/YRBS/pdf/trends/2005_YRBS_Physical_Activity.pdf (accessed February 15, 2008); and National Association for Sport and Physical Education and American Heart Association, *2006 Shape of the Nation Report: Status of Physical Education in the USA*, http://www.aahperd.org/naspe/ShapeOfTheNation/ (accessed February 15, 2008).

8. Sarah G. McCallister, Elaine M. Blinde, and Jessie M. Phillips, "Prospects for Change in a New Millennium: Gender Beliefs of Young Girls in Sport and Physical Activity," *WSPAJ* 12 (2003): 94, 96.

9. My students provided the example. For analysis, see Susan Wilkinson, Kay M. Williamson, and Ruth Rozdilsky, "Gender and Fitness Standards," *WSPAJ* 5 (1996): 1–25.

10. Deborah Tannehill and Dorothy Zakrajsek, "Student Attitudes Towards Physical Education: A Multicultural Study," *JTPE* 13 (1993): 80.

11. Lynn E. Couturier, Steveda Chepko, and Mary Ann Coughlin, "Student Voices—What Middle and High School Students Have to Say about Physical Education," *PE* 62 (Early Winter 2005): 172.

12. Ronald G. Morrow and Diane L. Gill, "Perceptions of Homophobia and Heterosexism in Physical Education," *RQES* 74 (2003): 205–14.

13. Scott Mccredie, "Unicycles in the Gym Class?" *Daily Item (Sunbury, Pa.)*, September 10, 2002, sec. E4.

14. Julie Bosman, "Putting the Gym Back in Gym Class," *New York Times*, October 13, 2005, G10. An informative website is http://www.pe4life.org.

15. Sam Dillon, "Online Classes Offer Virtual Dissection, but Gym Still Takes Sweat," *New York Times*, August 2, 2005, A14. For a critique, see Craig Buschner, "Online Physical Education: Wires and Lights in a Box," *JOPERD* 77 (February 2006): 3–5, 8.

16. Jan Hoffman, "Crunching Fitness into Phys Ed at School," *New York Times*, November 24, 2004, B2; and Susan Saulny, "Schools Pushing for Exercise, Even Without a Place to Play," *New York Times*, November 11, 2004, A1.

17. Based on U. S. Census Bureau, *Statistical Abstract of the United States, 1951*, 124 (Table 149), http://www2.census.gov/prod2/statcomp/documents/1951-01.pdf; U. S. Census Bureau, *Statistical Abstract of the United States, 1976*, 147 (Table 247), http://www2.census.gov/prod2/statcomp/documents/1976-02.pdf; and National Center for Education Statistics, "Bachelor's, master's, and doctor's degrees conferred by degree-granting institutions, by sex of student and field of study: 1997–98," Table 257, in *Digest of Education Statistics: Tables and Figures, 2000*, http://nces.ed.gov/programs/digest/d00. All items accessed March 19, 2006.

18. Darrell Crase and Hollie Walker Jr., "The Black Physical Educator: An Endangered Species," *JOPERD* 59 (October 1988): 65–69.

19. Melvin I. Evans, "The Vanishing Americans," *JOHPER* 44 (October 1973): 55–57.

20. Bonnie J. Hultstrand, "Women in High School PE Teaching Positions—Diminishing Numbers," *JOPERD* 61 (November–December 1990): 19–21; and Lynda E. Randall, "Employment Statistics: A National Survey in Public School Physical Education," *JOPERD* 57 (January 1986): 23. On 1966–2001, see National Center for Education Statistics, *Digest of Education Statistics: Tables and Figures, 2004*, Table 70, http://nces.ed.gov/programs/digest/d04/tables/dt04_070.asp (accessed March 19, 2006).

21. Mary C. Lydon, "Secondary School Programs: Diversity in Practice," in *Women in Sport: Issues and Controversies*, ed. Greta L. Cohen (Thousand Oaks, Calif.: Sage, 1993), 95–103; and Becky L. Sisley and Susan A. Capel, "High School Coaching Filled With Gender Differences," *JOPERD* 57 (March 1986): 39–43.

22. R. Vivian Acosta and Linda Jean Carpenter, "Women in Intercollegiate Sport: A Longitudinal, National Study—Twenty Seven Year Update: 1977–2004," *WSPAJ* 13 (Spring 2004): 62–89; and Richard Lapchick, with Jenny Brenden, "The 2005 Racial and Gender Report Card: College Sports," http://www.bus.ucf.edu/sport/public/downloads/2005_Racial_Gender_Report_Card_Colleges.pdf (accessed January 11, 2007).

23. See Pat Griffin, *Strong Women, Deep Closets: Lesbians and Homophobia in Sport* (Champaign, Ill.: Human Kinetics, 1998), 27–49, 78–89, 133–56; and Sherry E. Woods and Karen M. Harbeck, "Living in Two Worlds: The Identity Management Strategies Used by Lesbian Physical Educators," in *Coming Out of the Classroom Closet: Gay and Lesbian Students, Teachers, and Curricula*, ed. Karen M. Harbeck (New York: Haworth Press, 1992), 141–66.

24. Jepkorir Rose Chepyator-Thomson, JeongAe You, and Brent Hardin, "Issues and Perspectives on Gender in Physical Education," *WSPAJ* 9 (Fall 2000): 99–121; and Patricia A. Vertinsky, "Reclaiming Space, Revisioning the Body: The Quest for Gender-Sensitive Physical Education," *Quest* 44 (1992): 373–76.

25. Pat Griffin, "Homophobia in Physical Education," *CAHPER Journal* 55 (March–April 1989): 27–31; and Morrow and Gill, "Perceptions."

26. Patricia Vertinsky and Gwendolyn Captain, "More Myth than History: American Culture and the Representation of the Black Female's Athletic Ability," *JSH* 25 (1998): 549–52.

27. Barbara A. Barnes, Susan G. Zieff, and David I. Anderson, "Racial Difference and Social Meanings: Research on 'Black' and 'White' Infants' Motor Development, c. 1931–1992," *Quest* 51 (1999): 328–45; and Patrick B. Miller, "The Anatomy of Scientific Racism: Racialist Responses to Black Athletic Achievement," *JSH* 25 (1998): 119–51.

28. Critiques of "biological foundationalism" include Elizabeth Grosz, "Notes Towards a Corporeal Feminism," *Australian Feminist Studies* 5 (1987): 1–16; and Linda Nicholson, "Interpreting Gender," *Signs* 20 (1994): 79–105. Lynda Birke, Anne Fausto-Sterling, Thomas Laqueur, Nelly Oudshoorn, Cynthia Eagle Russett, Londa Schiebinger, and Marianne van den Wijngaard have explored specific historical examples.

29. See Evelynn M. Hammonds and Rebecca M. Herzig, eds., *The Nature of Difference: Sciences of Race in the United States from Jefferson to Genomics* (Cambridge, Mass.: MIT Press, 2009); and Jennifer Terry, *An American Obsession: Science, Medicine, and Homosexuality in Modern Society* (Chicago: University of Chicago Press, 1999).

30. General critiques include works by Linda L. Bain, David Kirk, and Nancy Theberge. Many scholars, notably M. Ann Hall, Jennifer Hargreaves, Michael A. Messner, and Sheila Scraton, have spearheaded gender analysis. Susan Birrell, Sheila Scraton, and Yevonne R. Smith have brought questions of race to the forefront.

31. Morrow and Gill, "Perceptions."

32. Quoted phrase from Peter McLaren, "Schooling the Postmodern Body: Critical Pedagogy and the Politics of Enfleshment," in *Postmodernism, Feminism, and Cultural Politics: Redrawing Educational Boundaries*, ed. Henry A. Giroux (Albany: State University of New York Press, 1991), 154.

33. Alyce T. Cheska, "Women's Sports—The Unlikely Myth of Equality," in *The Female Athlete: A Socio-Psychological and Kinanthropometric Approach*, ed. Jan Borms, Marcel Hebbelinck, and Antonio Venerando, Medicine and Sport Series, vol. 15 (Basel: Karger, 1981), 9.

34. Theoretical perspectives on the body in modern society, especially the work of Sandra Lee Bartky, Susan R. Bordo, and Kathy Davis, informed my analysis of physical education.

35. See Roberta J. Park, "The Emergence of the Academic Discipline of Physical Education in the United States," in *Perspectives on the Academic Discipline of Physical Education*, ed. George A. Brooks (Champaign, Ill.: Human Kinetics, 1981), 20–45; and Patricia Vertinsky, "Science, Social Science, and the 'Hunger for Wonders' in Physical Education: Moving Toward a Future Healthy Society," in *New Possibilities, New Paradigms?*, American Academy of Physical Education Papers, no. 24 (Champaign, Ill.: Human Kinetics, 1991), 70–88.

36. Paula Rogers Lupcho, "The Professionalization of American Physical Education, 1885–1930" (Ph.D. diss., University of California, Berkeley, 1986), 15–21; and Magali Sarfatti Larson, *The Rise of Professionalism: A Sociological Analysis* (Berkeley: University of California Press, 1977), x–xviii.

37. Shirl J. Hoffman, "In My View: Therapy for an Ailing Profession," *JOPERD* 56 (November–December 1985): 17.

38. See Roberta J. Park, "Physiologists, Physicians, and Physical Educators: Nineteenth-Century Biology and Exercise, *Hygienic* and *Educative*," *JSH* 14 (1987): 28–60; and Patricia A. Vertinsky, "Embodying Normalcy: Anthropometry and the Long Arm of William H. Sheldon's Somatotyping Project," *JSH* 29 (2002): 95–133.

39. A classic statement is Jesse F. Williams, "Education Through the Physical," *Journal of Higher Education* 1 (May 1930): 279–82.

40. By contrast, critiques of physical education in other Western countries often reflect a clear historical and theoretical sensibility. Good examples include works by Jennifer Hargreaves, David Kirk, and Gertrud Pfister. Likewise, historians such as Susan Cahn, Mark Dyreson, Pamela Grundy, Patrick Miller, and David K. Wiggins have contextualized twentieth-century American sports.

41. Besides its differentiation from sports, physical education is distinct from (albeit related to) several other fields. On dance, see Linda J. Tomko, *Dancing Class: Gender, Ethnicity, and Social Divides in American Dance, 1890–1920* (Bloomington: Indiana University Press, 1999). On health education, see Susan G. Zieff, "The American 'Alliance' of Health and Physical Education: Scholastic Programs and Professional Organizations, 1920–1950," *RQES* 77 (2006): 437–50. On health services, see Heather Munro Prescott, *Student Bodies: The Influence of Student Health Services in American Society and Medicine* (Ann Arbor: University of Michigan Press, 2007).

42. Studying white and black female physical educators also allows similarities and contrasts—both within and between—the two cohorts to become apparent, thereby correcting misleading generalizations in extant scholarship.

Chapter 1

1. Quoted in Hazel M. Gross, "Recognition for Outstanding Service," 3, typescript, CAHPER banquet, March 20, 1947, Folder: Biography, Papers of Winifred Van Hagen, Hearst Gymnasium Historical Collections, University of California at Berkeley, Berkeley, Calif. A published tribute is "Winifred Van Hagen, 1881–1968," *JOHPER* 40 (May 1969): 89.

2. Paula Rogers Lupcho, "The Professionalization of American Physical Education, 1885–1930" (Ph.D. diss., University of California, Berkeley, 1986), 15–21; and Magali Sarfatti Larson, *The Rise of Professionalism: A Sociological Analysis* (Berkeley: University of California Press, 1977), x–xviii.

3. James C. Boykin, "Physical Training," in *Report of the [U.S.] Commissioner of Education for the Year 1891–92* (Washington, D.C.: GPO, 1894), 1:580–94.

4. Angela Lumpkin and Jane Jenkins, "Basic Instruction Programs: A Brief History," *JOPERD* 64 (August 1993): 33–36; and Joseph B. Oxendine, "100 Years of Basic Instruction," *JOPERD* 56 (September 1985): 32–36.

5. On curricula, see Roberta J. Park, "1989 C. H. McCloy Research Lecture: Health, Exercise, and the Biomedical Impulse, 1870–1914," *RQES* 61 (1990): 133. On students and graduates by sex, see Delphine Hanna, "Present Status of Physical Training in Normal Schools," *APER* 8 (1903): 296–97.

6. Isabel C. Barrows, ed., *Physical Training. A Full Report of the Papers and Discussions of the Conference Held in Boston in November, 1889* (Boston: George H. Ellis, 1890).

7. Arthur Weston, *The Making of American Physical Education* (New York: Appleton-Century-Crofts, 1962), 40–41. In 1937 the APEA merged with NEA's division of School Health and Physical Education. In 1969 it became a national affiliate of NEA.

8. "Our Official Publications," *JOHPER* 31 (April 1960): 74–75.

9. Lupcho, "Professionalization," 250–96.

10. Mabel Lee, *A History of Physical Education and Sports in the U.S.A.* (New York: John Wiley and Sons, 1983), 166–68; and Lupcho, "Professionalization," 256–62.

11. Roberta J. Park, *Measurement of Physical Fitness: A Historical Perspective*, ODPHP Monograph Series (Washington, D.C.: U.S. Department of Health and Human Services, Public Health Service, 1989), 8.

12. Helen McKinstry, "Organization of Work for Women, with Special Consideration of the Type of Work for Which Colleges Might Reasonably Be Expected to Give Credit," *APER* 22 (1917): 344.

13. Generalizations are based on diverse archival and published materials. For a profile of the first 212 female graduates of the BNSG, see Martha H. Verbrugge, *Able-Bodied Womanhood: Personal Health and Social Change in Nineteenth-Century Boston* (New York: Oxford University Press, 1988), 162–91, 258–66.

14. See Regina Markell Morantz-Sanchez, *Sympathy and Science: Women Physicians in American Medicine* (New York: Oxford University Press, 1985); and Margaret W. Rossiter, *Women Scientists in America: Struggles and Strategies to 1940* (Baltimore, Md.: Johns Hopkins University Press, 1982).

15. "Personal Recollections of Our Family Life in the Early 1900s," 5, 7, Box: Correspondence, Writings, Addresses, Folder: Addresses and Writings, 1937–1982, Grout Family Papers, Special Collections Department, William R. Perkins Library, Duke University, Durham, N.C.

16. "The Sportswoman Prior to 1920," 1, speech for NAPECW, December 1963, Box 6, Folder: Speeches, 1928–1963, Dorothy S. Ainsworth Papers, Smith College Archives, Smith College, Northampton, Mass. (Hereafter, depository cited as SCA-SC.)

17. See ibid., 1–3; and Ainsworth's letters to her family, Box 1: Ainsworth A-N, Folder: Correspondence, 1912–1913, Faculty Papers: Individuals (Coll. 42), SCA-SC.

18. Ethel Perrin, "Ethel Perrin—An Autobiography," *RQ* 12, suppl. (October 1941): 682. Perrin's administrative positions with the Detroit public schools and the American Child Health Association highlighted a distinguished career of nearly four decades.

19. Transcript of "Groundbreakers Interview [1979]," 12, in Diaries, Box 3, Papers of Mabel Lee, Archives, American Alliance for Health, Physical Education, Recreation and Dance. (Hereafter, depository cited as AAHPERD.)

20. Mabel Lee, *Memories of a Bloomer Girl (1894–1924)* (Washington, D.C.: AAHPERD, 1977), 38.

21. Ibid., 26.

22. Ibid., 49–79; and "Groundbreakers," 18–20, Lee Papers.

23. Information from Betty Spears, "Success, Women, and Physical Education," in *Women as Leaders in Physical Education and Sports*, eds. M. Gladys Scott and Mary J. Hoferek (Iowa City: University of Iowa Press, 1979), 9; Mabel Lee, "A Tribute to J. Anna Norris," speech, Middle West Association of Physical Education for College Women, October 20, 1979, typescript from University Archives, University of Minnesota; and Gertrude Baker, oral history, tape recording, May 24, 1968, in Baker Papers, University Archives, University of Minnesota, Minneapolis, Minn. (Hereafter, depository cited as UA-UMN.)

24. "In Memoriam," *JOHPER* 35 (October 1964): 87; and Marianna Trekell, "Gertrude Evelyn Moulton, M.D.: Her Life and Professional Career in Health and Physical Education" (Ph.D. diss., Ohio State University, 1962).

25. Trekell, "Moulton," 27–30, 57–59, 67–68, 105.

26. Debora Lynn Cottrell, "Women's Minds, Women's Bodies: The Influence of the Sargent School for Physical Education" (Ph.D. diss., University of Texas at Austin, 1993), 445–48. Anna Hiss's career at the University of Texas spanned nearly forty years. One of her brothers was Alger Hiss, the lawyer and diplomat accused of espionage in the late 1940s.

27. "Brief Outline of the Life and Work of Dr. Delphine Hanna," *RQ* 12, suppl. (October 1941): 646–52; and Cottrell, "Women's Minds, Women's Bodies," 245–303.

28. Elizabeth Claire Umstead, "Mary Channing Coleman: Her Life and Contributions to Health, Physical Education and Recreation, 1883–1947" (Ed.D. diss., University of North Carolina at Chapel Hill, 1967).

29. Elizabeth B. Griego, "The Making of a 'Misfit': Clelia Duel Mosher, 1863–1940," in *Lone Voyagers: Academic Women in Coeducational Universities, 1870–1937*, ed. Geraldine Jonçich Clifford (New York: Feminist Press, 1989), 147–82; and Martha H. Verbrugge, "Clelia Duel Mosher," in *American National Biography*, ed. John A. Garraty and Mark C. Carnes (New York: Oxford University Press, 1999), 15:976–78.

30. See Alison M. Wrynn, "A Fine Balance: Margaret Bell, Physician and Physical Educator," *RQES* 76 (2005): 149–65.

31. Cottrell, "Women's Minds, Women's Bodies," 393–443; and Marilyn B. Weissman, "Elizabeth Burchenal," in *Notable American Women: The Modern Period*, eds. Barbara Sicherman and Carol Hurd Green (Cambridge, Mass.: Belknap Press of Harvard University Press, 1980), 121–22. After training at the Sargent School, Burchenal directed girls' physical activity in New York City's public schools (1906–16) and spearheaded America's folk dance movement.

32. Information from "In Memoriam," *JOHPER* 36 (February 1965): 78; and documents in Box 14, Folders I-5 and I-9, Papers of School of Education: Department of Women's Physical Education—Blanche Trilling Files (Acc. 82/50), Archives, Steenbock Memorial Library, University of Wisconsin, Madison, Wisc. Hereafter, collection cited as Trilling Files, SA-UW (82/50). I-# refers to folder number as listed on printed inventory.

33. Edwin B. Henderson, *The Negro in Sports*, rev. ed. (Washington, D.C.: Associated Publishers, 1949), 237–39; Nina Jo Wooley Smith, "'Out of Adversity We Survived': Oral Histories of Seven Black Women Physical Educators" (master's thesis, San Francisco State University, 1992), 77–78; and Janell Walden, "Sports," in *Contributions of Black Women to America*, ed. Marianna W. Davis (Columbia, S.C.: Kenday, 1982), 1:572–73.

34. "Jessie Harriet (Scott) Abbott," in *Black Women Oral History Project*, ed. Ruth Edmonds Hill (Westport, Conn.: Meckler, 1990), 1:1–38.

35. Information from *Biographical Directory of the Public Schools of the District of Columbia*, rev. ed. (Washington, D.C.: Office of the Statistician, 1953), 83–85; obituary in *Washington Tribune*, February 15, 1941; and Leon N. Coursey, "Anita J. Turner: Early Black Female Physical Educator," *JOHPER* 45 (March 1974): 71–72.

36. Information gleaned from Thomas's forms in the student records of the Papers of the Department of Hygiene and Physical Education, and in Biographical Data: Classes 1891–1900, Records of the Alumnae Association: Hygiene and Physical Education, Wellesley College Archives, Wellesley College, Wellesley, Mass. (Hereafter, depository cited as WCA.)

37. Papers of Maryrose Reeves Allen, Manuscript Division, Moorland-Spingarn Research Center (MSRC), Howard University, Washington, D.C.

38. Joseph A. Hill, *Women in Gainful Occupations, 1870 to 1920*, Census Monographs 9 (Washington, D.C.: GPO, 1929; repr. ed., New York: Johnson Reprint, 1972), 32–45; and Janet M. Hooks, *Women's Occupations Through Seven Decades*, Women's Bureau Bulletin, no. 218 (Washington, D.C.: GPO, 1947), 52, 59, 157–61.

39. John L. Rury, "Who Became Teachers? The Social Characteristics of Teachers in American History," in *American Teachers: Histories of a Profession at Work*, ed. Donald Warren (New York: Macmillan, 1989), 9–11, 23–33.

40. Darlene Clark Hine and Kathleen Thompson, *A Shining Thread of Hope: The History of Black Women in America* (New York: Broadway Books, 1998), 247.

41. Paula Giddings, *When and Where I Enter: The Impact of Black Women on Race and Sex in America*, 2nd ed. (New York: William Morrow, 1996), 58–64, 95–102, 108–17, 184–97.

42. Elizabeth Higginbotham, "Employment for Professional Black Women in the Twentieth Century," in *Ingredients for Women's Employment Policy*, ed. Christine Bose and Glenna Spitze (Albany: State University of New York Press, 1987), 73–83; and Marion Kilson, "Black Women in the Professions, 1890–1970," *Monthly Labor Review* 100 (May 1977): 38–41.

43. Hine and Thompson, *Shining Thread of Hope*, 222–28.

44. Katherine M. Cook, *State Laws and Regulations Governing Teachers' Certificates*, Bureau of Education Bulletin, 1927, no. 19 (Washington, D.C.: GPO, 1928), 21–22, 268–74, 278–79; *Biennial Survey of Education, 1928–1930*, Office of Education Bulletin, 1931, no. 20 (Washington, D.C.: GPO, 1932), 373; and Lupcho, "Professionalization," 281–83.

45. On white women, see Dorothy S. Ainsworth, *The History of Physical Education in Colleges for Women* (New York: A. S. Barnes, 1930), 52–55; and Miriam Gray, ed., *A Century of Growth: The Historical Development of Physical Education for Women in Selected Colleges of Six Midwestern States* (Ann Arbor: Edwards Brothers, 1951), 30–32. On black teachers, see Pat A. Brandford, "Training and Opportunities for Negro Women in Physical Education" (master's thesis, State University of Iowa, 1939), 11; and John Harold Burr, "A Survey of Physical Education in Negro Colleges and Universities" (master's [Ed.] thesis, International Young Men's Christian Association College, Springfield, Mass., 1931), 134–37.

46. Lee, *History*, 182–86; Lupcho, "Professionalization," 271–86; and Paula D. Welch, *History of American Physical Education and Sport*, 3rd ed. (Springfield, Ill.: Charles C. Thomas, 2004), 139–40.

47. Elmer Berry, "Problems in the Recruiting of Teachers of Physical Education," *APER* 25 (1920): 233–39; W. P. Bowen, "The Preparation of Teachers of Physical Education," *APER* 19 (1914): 421–25; and Hanna, "Present Status," 296–97.

48. Armstead A. Pierro, "History of Professional Preparation for Physical Education in Some Selected Negro Colleges and Universities" (Ph.D. diss., University of Michigan, 1962), 37n3, 40n1, and 51.

49. Ibid., 130, 136–37.

50. Michael Fultz, "Teacher Training and African American Education in the South, 1900–1940," *JNE* 64 (1995): 201–2; and Pierro, "History" (diss.), 28–31, 50–51, 54–58.

51. Herman Newman Neilson, "An Evaluation of the Physical Education of Negro Professional Schools" (master's [Ed.] thesis, International Young Men's Christian Association College, Springfield, Mass., 1936), 28–30.

52. Brandford, "Training," 10–11; Burr, "Survey," 134–37; and Frances C. Haddock, "A Study of Physical Education for Women in Accredited Negro Colleges and Universities," 26, 33-b, 58–59 (Special Study Project, Hygiene 323: Graduate Seminar, Department of Hygiene and Physical Education, Wellesley College, May 1938; copy in WCA).

53. Earle F. Zeigler, "A History of Undergraduate Professional Preparation for Physical Education in the United States, 1861–1961," in *A History of Physical Education and Sport in the United States and Canada: Selected Topics*, ed. Earle F. Zeigler (Champaign, Ill.: Stipes, 1975), 233, 241–42.

54. Debbie M. Cottrell, "The Sargent School for Physical Education," *JOPERD* 65 (March 1994): 35.

55. Betty Spears, *Leading the Way: Amy Morris Homans and the Beginnings of Professional Education for Women* (New York: Greenwood Press, 1986), 53–54, 65, 85–86; and Verbrugge, *Able-Bodied Womanhood*, 171–72.

56. Barbara Miller Solomon, *In the Company of Educated Women: A History of Women and Higher Education in America* (New Haven, Conn.: Yale University Press, 1985), 62–77, 141–56.

57. Alice Towne Deweese, "Life and Times of a Physical Education Major, 1897–1909," 25, typed manuscript, Box 1, Records of Teachers College: Women's Physical Education—Memoirs and Theses (Collection 23/18/7), University Archives and Special Collections, University of Nebraska at Lincoln, Lincoln, Neb.

58. "M. Gladys Scott (1905–1990): Teacher, Researcher, Friend," 2, in Files of Active Fellows in Memoria, Papers of the American Academy of Physical Education, Archives, AAHPERD.

59. Weston, *Making of American Physical Education*, 76–77; and Zeigler, "Undergraduate," 231–37, 241–47.

60. Neilson, "Evaluation"; and Pierro, "History" (diss.), 58–65.

61. Zeigler, "Undergraduate," 234–36, 242–45.

62. From the title of a handbook prepared by and for physical education majors at the University of Wisconsin, October 1946; copy found in Box 12, Folder I-21, Trilling Files, SA-UW (82/50).

63. Letter from Charlotte (Mrs. U. L.) Blatchly McCall to Prof. Elmo A. Robinson, October 27, 1939, in Folder: Elmo Robinson Article and Correspondence, 1936–1953, Collection 3P: Amy Morris Homans, WCA. See also Spears, *Leading the Way*, 53–62, 72–74; and Verbrugge, *Able-Bodied Womanhood*, 175–76.

64. Quoted in Umstead, "Coleman," 63; see also 191–97.

65. "Recommendations of Committee Appointed by Major Committee to Prepare Statement Regarding Costumes," Box 2: Faculty Meeting Minutes, Folder: 1942–43, in Papers of School of Education: Department of Women's Physical Education (Acc. 16/82), SA-UW. Hereafter, collection cited as DWPE Papers, SA-UW (16/82).

66. Ruth Diamond Levinson, interview by author, tape recording, November 11, 1991, Lincoln, Neb. Levinson attended the University of Nebraska in 1927–31 and directed women's physical education at the Omaha branch from 1931 to 1942. After an interlude for war work and marriage, she returned to the Lincoln campus as a teacher (1951–72).

67. "Delphine Hanna & Physical Education in Oberlin, 1885–1920," in Box 7, Folder 21, Oberlin Files, College Archives, Oberlin College, Oberlin, Ohio. (Hereafter, depository cited as OCA.)

68. Comments by Class of 1942 alumna, on graduate questionnaire, in Series 4: Moulton, Folder 2, Records of Physical Education Department, Subgroup 6: Physical Education for Women, OCA. (Hereafter, collection cited as PEW Records.)

69. Comments by Class of 1926 alumna, on graduate questionnaire, in Series 4: Moulton, Folder 2; and Staff meeting minutes, vol. 1: October 13, 1926, in Box 1: 1925–1942, Series 1: Minutes, PEW Records, OCA.

70. Staff meeting minutes, vol. 1: May 6, 1930, in Box 1: 1925–1942, Series 1: Minutes, PEW Records, OCA.

71. "Vital Statistics for Alumnae Breakfast, November 18, 1939," 2, in Box 8, Folder I-38: Alumnae Reports, Trilling Files, SA-UW (82/50).

72. Minutes, February 25, 1932, Box 2: Faculty Meeting Minutes, Folder: 1931–1932, DWPE Papers, SA-UW (16/82).

73. Quotations from Minutes, May 13, 1947, and "Ratings of Major Students, January, 1950," Box 11, Folder I-16: Majors Rating, Trilling Files, SA-UW (82/50).

74. Minutes, January 16, 1929, Box 2: Faculty Meeting Minutes, Folder: 1928–1929, DWPE Papers, SA-UW (16/82).

75. Minutes, June 2, 1927, Box 2: Faculty Meeting Minutes, Folder: 1927–1928, DWPE Papers, SA-UW (16/82).

76. From "Personal and Professional Rating Chart," meeting of March 16, 1948, Box 7, Folder: Staff Meeting Minutes, 1946/47–1947/48, in Papers of Department of Physical Education for Women, Bentley Historical Library, University of Michigan, Ann Arbor, Mich. (Hereafter, collection cited as DPEW Papers, BHL-UM.)

77. Examples from minutes, March 5, 1940: 2–3, in Box 1, Folder: WPE Staff Meeting Minutes, 1937–38 through 1939–40, Papers of Department of Physical Education for Women (SC 144), Special Collections, Green Library, Stanford University, Stanford, Calif. (Hereafter, collection cited as DPEW Papers, SC-SU.)

78. "Personality Questionnaire," Box 7, Folder: Minutes of Staff Meetings, 1952–53, DPEW Papers, BHL-UM.

79. "An Outline Treatment of the Essential Elements of Success in One's Occupation," ca. 1940, Box 9, Folder I-34: Career in P.E. for Women, Trilling Files, SA-UW (82/50).

80. "Vital Statistics for Alumnae Breakfast, November 18, 1939," Box 8, Folder I-38: Alumnae Reports, Trilling Files, SA-UW (82/50).

81. Examples include Margaret C. Brown, "A Study of Personality of College Students of Physical Education," *RQ* 6 (December 1935): 69–77; Anne Schley Duggan, "A Comparative Study of Undergraduate Women Majors and Non-Majors in Physical Education with Respect to Certain Personality Traits," *RQ* 8 (October 1937): 38–45; and C. E. Ragsdale, "Personality Traits of College Majors in Physical Education," *RQ* 3 (May 1932): 243–48.

82. Spears, *Leading the Way*, 73; and Smith, "'Out of Adversity,'" 21–22.

83. Cottrell, "Women's Minds, Women's Bodies," 205.

84. On graduates' sentiments, see Smith, "'Out of Adversity,'" 160, 161, 202–3.

85. Letter signed by "Assistant Professor of Physical Education," April 8, 1936, Box 1, Folder 6, Papers of Laura J. Huelster (Coll. 16/4/22) in Papers of College of Applied Life Studies: Physical Education for Women Department, University Archives, University of Illinois at Urbana-Champaign, Urbana, Ill. (Hereafter, depository cited as UA-UI.)

86. Comments by Connie (Mrs. Carl) Davis, Class of 1940, on graduate questionnaire, in Series 4: Moulton, Folder 2, PEW Records, OCA.

87. Training programs kept close tabs on their alumnae and regularly described their activities in alumnae publications or annual department reports.

88. Howard University and the University of Michigan were typical. See Maryrose Reeves Allen, "Department of Physical Education for Women," in *College of Liberal Arts Annual Report, Howard University, 1946–47*, 187–89; and "List of Graduates and Positions Held," vol. 1930–31: 240–43, and vol. 1940–41: 96–106, Box 4: Annual Reports, DPEW Papers, BHL-UM. The higher figures derive from the University of Wisconsin; see "Alumnae Placement," Folder I-37, and "Vital Statistics for Alumnae Breakfast, November 18, 1939," Folder I-38, in Box 8, and "Graduates of Dept. of P. E. for Women, 1910–1940," Folder I-70, in Box 10, Trilling Files, SA-UW (82/50).

89. Calculated from "Placement Study," *JOHPER* 22 (May 1951): 48–49.

90. Weston, *Making of American Physical Education*, 50.

91. Ambrose Caliver, "Education of Negro Teachers," in *National Survey of the Education of Teachers*, U.S. Office of Education Bulletin, 1933, no. 10 (Washington, D.C.: GPO, 1933; repr., Westport, Conn.: Greenwood Press, 1970), 4:30; and Linda M. Perkins, "The History of Blacks in Teaching: Growth and Decline Within the Profession," in Warren, *American Teachers*, 350.

92. Wayne Urban and Jennings Wagoner Jr., *American Education: A History* (New York: McGraw-Hill, 1996), 158–240.

93. Boykin, "Physical Training," 1:580–94; Edward M. Hartwell, "On Physical Training," in *Report of the [U.S.] Commissioner of Education for the Year 1897–98* (Washington, D.C.: GPO, 1899), 1: 550, 560–62; and Lee, *History*, 80, 83–86, 165–66.

94. Guy Lewis, "Adoption of the Sports Program, 1906–39: The Role of Accommodation in the Transformation of Physical Education," *Quest* 12 (May 1969): 38; and Thomas A. Storey, Willard S. Small, and Elon G. Salisbury, *Recent State Legislation for Physical Education*, Bureau of Education Bulletin, 1922, no.1 (Washington, D.C.: GPO, 1922), 5, 15.

95. Lewis, "Adoption," 38.

96. Marie M. Ready, *Physical Education in City Public Schools*, Bureau of Education Physical Education Series, no. 10 (Washington, D.C.: GPO, 1929), 98, and 2–3, 5–18, 22, 30–35 in general.

97. Brandford, "Training," 7–9.

98. Ready, *City Public Schools*, 1–2.

99. Lee, *History*, 174.

100. Ready, *City Public Schools*, 5–18.

101. Ibid., 1.

102. Lewis, "Adoption," 39. On their backgrounds and duties, see E. B. Stansbury, "The Status of State Directors of Health and Physical Education," *RQ* 12 (1941): 98–114.

103. Perkins, "Blacks in Teaching," 350–60.

104. Boykin, "Physical Training," 1:580, 582–89.

105. J. H. McCurdy, "A Study of the Characteristics of Physical Training in the Public Schools of the United States," *APER* 10 (1905): 204–5.

106. Brandford, "Training," 9–12.

107. Marie M. Ready, *Physical Education in American Colleges and Universities*, Bureau of Education Bulletin, 1927, no. 14 (Washington, D.C.: GPO, 1927), 11–14.

108. Ainsworth, *History of Physical Education*, 47–56; Gray, ed., *Century of Growth*, 10–12, 29–32; and Lee, *History*, 180.

109. Brandford, "Training," 9–12; Burr, "Survey," 41–46, 70, 84; and A. W. Ellis, "The Status of Health and Physical Education for Women in Negro Colleges and Universities," *RQ* 10 (May 1939): 137.

110. Haddock, "Study," 25–26, 51–52, 58.

111. Correspondence between Amy Morris Homans (BNSG director) and Hollis Burke Frissell (Hampton Principal) describes the arrangement; see Homans to Frissell, March 25, 1895, and December 3, 1907; and Frissell to Homans, June 6, 1901, and June 12, 1901, Papers of H. B. Frissell, Record Group 2.3, University Archives, Hampton University, Hampton, Va. (Hereafter, depository cited as HUA.) Information about early appointees is found in Biographical Data, Boxes 5–13, Records of the Alumnae Association: Hygiene and Physical Education Section, WCA, and in faculty information cards and Faculty Files, HUA.

112. Homans to Frissell, January 1, 1897, April 20, 1898, and April 28, 1898; and Frissell to Homans, April 23, 1898, and April 22, 1899, Frissell Papers.

113. The relationship waned for financial reasons; see Homans to Frissell, December 3, 1907, and March 16, 1908, Frissell Papers; and Spears, *Leading the Way*, 60–61.

114. Dean M. Florence Lawson to Dean William E. Stark, August 1, 1929; and Helen E. Luffman to Dean William E. Stark, July 31, 1929, in Faculty File: Mary Catherine Baker, HUA.

115. President Arthur Howe to Mary C. Baker, September 23, 1937; unsigned letter of recommendation to Teachers College, Columbia University, ca. 1936; Charles H. Williams to Bureau of Appointments, School of Education, New York University, July 1, 1937; and Mary C. Baker, "Social Conditions at Hampton," ca. 1935–36, in Faculty File: Mary C. Baker, HUA.

116. For example, Charles H. Williams to Bernice Miller (m. Smothers), May 25, 1931, in Faculty File: Bernice Miller, HUA.

117. Faculty File: Charlotte Moton Hubbard, HUA; and Box 54–1, Folder 1, Papers of Charlotte Moton Hubbard, Manuscript Division, MSRC.

118. On faculty and administrators, see Beverly Guy-Sheftall, "Black Women and Higher Education: Spelman and Bennett Colleges Revisited," *JNE* 51 (1982): 281. Information about physical educators from Marguerite Simon, interviewed by the author, May 28, 1996, Spelman College, Atlanta, Ga. On hiring a white gym teacher, see letter from Spelman administrator to principal of Posse Normal School, June 5, 1924, in Personnel Records, Box 40: Shirlie T. Pettee File, College Archives, Spelman College, Atlanta, Ga. (Hereafter, depository cited as SCA.)

119. Dean Edna E. Lamson to Mildred Churchill, May 6, 1925, in Personnel Records, Box 5: Churchill File, SCA.

120. Staff files in Personnel Records, SCA, contain copies of the form.

121. Shirlie T. Pettee to Dean Lamson, June 19, 1924, in Personnel Records, Box 40: Pettee File, SCA.

122. Edna B. Callahan to President Florence M. Read, July 18, 1927, Box 5: Callahan File; and Pauline to Aunt Angie, ca. 1922, Box 41: Evelyn Sargent File, in Personnel Records, SCA.

123. Dean Edna E. Lamson to Shirlie T. Pettee, June 26, 1924, in Personnel Records, Box 40: Pettee File, SCA.

124. [Yomans?] to President Read and Florence Warwick, December 7, 1937; and Warwick to Read, August 24, 1940, in Personnel Records, Box 43: Warwick File, SCA.

125. Dean Edna E. Lamson to Shirlie T. Pettee, June 23, 1924, and June 26, 1924, Personnel Records, Box 40: Pettee File, SCA.

126. On Wisconsin, see Blanche Trilling to William Skarstrom, April 15, 1924, Box 15, Folder I-74, Trilling Files, SA-UW (82/50). On the South, see President Florence Read to Evelyn Sargent, February 22, 1922, Box 41: Sargent File; and Read to Edna Callahan, August 5, 1947, Personnel Records, Box 5: Callahan File, SCA.

127. "As You Were, or Forty Years of 'Happenings' in the Department of Health and Physical Education, The Woman's College, Duke University, 1924–1964," 1, Folder: Writings "As You Were," Julia R. Grout Papers, University Archives, Duke University (hereafter, depository cited as UA-Duke); and "first letter from Durham," ca. September 1924, Box: Grout Family, North Brookfield, Mass. and Durham, NC—Correspondence, 1848–1982, and Addresses and Writings, 1883–1982, Folder 1: Correspondence, 1848–1928, Grout Family Papers, SC-Duke.

128. On the 1920s and 1930s, see Haddock, "Study," 26–27, 60; Kathro Kidwell and Dorothy Simpson, "A Study and Investigation of the Health of Women Teachers of Physical Education," *APER* 34 (1929): 85–86; and Bertha M. Kirk, "The Health of Women in the Physical Education Profession," *APER* 32 (1927): 295. On the 1940s and 1950s, see Kathleen Lowrie, "Teaching Load of Women in Physical Education in Colleges and Universities," *RQ* 26 (1955): 244–45. For directors' estimates, see Julia R. Grout to William Hane Wannamaker, March 21, 1935, in Personnel File, Wannamaker Papers, UA-Duke; Gertrude Moulton, "Annual Report, 1933–34," ms. version, Secretary Papers, OCA; and Mary Channing Coleman to Chancellor Julius Isaac Foust, January 22, 1924, Foust Papers, General Correspondence: 1924, University Archives, University of North Carolina at Greensboro, Greensboro, N.C. (hereafter, depository cited as UA-UNCG). On male staff, see Hyman Krakower, "National Survey of Teacher Loads in Departments of Physical Education in Institutions of Higher Learning," *RQ* 16 (1945): 288–92.

129. "Women as Leaders: 'Our Mentors, Our Foremothers, Our Friends,'" 7, Box 6, Folder: Iowa Seminar, June 1981, Huelster Papers, UA-UI.

130. For example, Allen, "Department of Physical Education for Women," in *College of Liberal Arts Annual Report, 1946–47*, 184–96; and *CLA Annual Report, 1947–48*, 204–16, 301.

131. "Annual Report, 1936–37," ms. version, Secretary Papers, OCA.

132. See weekly schedules in Box 1, Folder: Personal Correspondence, 1932–33, Bell Papers, BHL-UM.

133. "The History of Physical Education at Milwaukee-Downer College," (1960 rev. ed.), 5–6; copy provided by Archives, Lawrence University, Appleton, Wisc. See also Elizabeth Ludwig, "Swimming Without a Tank at Milwaukee-Downer College," *Sportswoman* 6 (September 1929): 18, 29.

134. "The Time Has Come," *Spelman Messenger* 66 (February 1950): 3–6; and Simon, interview.

135. Minnie Lynn, "Fifty Years of Physical Education—1885–1935," *Oberlin Alumni Magazine* 31 (April 1935): 204 (quotation); and Delphine Hanna, "Oberlin Begins Physical Education for Women," *Oberlin Alumni Magazine* 26 (March 1930): 168–69.

136. Unedited manuscript versions of Moulton's annual reports to the president for 1928–29:2–3, 1929–30:1, and 1931–32:1, Secretary Papers, OCA. An alumna recounted the splinter story on a graduate questionnaire; see Series 4: Moulton, Box 1, Folder 2, PEW Records, OCA.

137. Blanche Trilling, "History of Physical Education for Women at the University of Wisconsin, 1898–1946," 27, copy in University Archives, Memorial Library, University of Wisconsin, Madison, Wisc. (Hereafter, depository cited as UA-UW.)

138. Mary M. Yost, interview by the author, tape recording, July 7, 1994, Ohio State University, Columbus, Ohio. Yost taught at OSU from 1937 to 1982.

139. *A Report Concerning Physical Education at the University of Michigan, 1945*, 12, insert in Box 5, Volume: 1946–47, DPEW Papers, BHL-UM.

140. Quoted in Trekell, "Moulton," 91.

141. Trilling to President Clarence A. Dykstra, September 23, 1938, in Box 7 (General Subject Files), Papers of Chancellors of the University (4/0/2), UA-UW.

142. Trilling, Biennial Report for 1922, 7, Box 9, Folder: Biennial Report Material; and Trilling to Guy Lowman, April 26, 1922, April 2, 1924, and April 2, 1925, Box 15, Folder I-10: Facilities, Trilling Files, SA-UW (82/50).

143. Trilling to Dykstra, September 23, 1938, Chancellor Papers, UA-UW.

144. Minutes of the Athletic Committee, September 28, 1917, March 23, 1918, and October 13, 1920, in Box 20, Folder: Athletic Committee, Papers of Robert Stewart Darnaby, University Archives, Tuskegee University, Tuskegee, Ala. (Hereafter, depository cited as UA-TU.)

145. Handwritten notes about coaching and administration, Box 3, Folder: Speeches, Papers of Nell Cecilia Jackson, UA-TU.

146. See letters from J. Anna Norris to President L. D. Coffman, Winter 1936–Spring 1937, in Box 43, Folder: University of Minnesota, Physical Education for Women, 1918–1944, Papers of the President's Office, 1911–1945, UA-UMN; and "A Report to President Coffey from the Committee on Administrative Reorganization," 7, April 7, 1942, copy in UA-UMN.

147. "As You Were," 6, Julia R. Grout Papers, UA-Duke.

148. Margaret Bell, "The Need for a New Physical Education Plant with Swimming Pool for the Women of the University of Michigan, December 18, 1945 [rev. April 13, 1948]," 4 [p. 181 in volume], Box 5, vol. 1949–50, DPEW Papers, BHL-UM.

149. "Annual Report, 1949–1950," 4, Papers of the Department of Health and Physical Education: Annual Reports, The Woman's College, UA-Duke.

150. "Appendix," in collection of unpublished writings and speeches, Box 1, Folder: Selected Writings of Mary Channing Coleman, Records of the School of Health, Physical Education, Recreation, and Dance, UA-UNCG.

151. Gertrude E. Moulton to President Ernest Hatch Wilkins, October 1, 1928, 3 (ms. version), Box 8, Folder: J-M 1927–28, in Secretary Papers, OCA.

152. Elizabeth A. Wright, "The Radcliffe Gymnasium," *Radcliffe Quarterly* 6 (September 1922): 52–56.

153. "Report of the Director of the Gymnasium," in *Annual Report of Radcliffe College, 1907–08* (Cambridge, Mass.: The College, 1908), 35.

154. For example, see Box 15, Folder I-54, Trilling Files, SA-UW (82/50); Box 5, Folder: Department of Physical Education for Women-Required Physical Education, 1919–1938, Bell Papers, BHL-UM; and Dean J. B. Johnston to Prof. H. O. Crisler and Dr. J. Anna Norris, January 21, 1931; Johnston to President L. D. Coffman, May 29, 1933; and Coffman to Mr. P. O. Clapp, Lawrence College, December 22, 1933, Box 43, Folder: Physical Education for Women, 1918–1944, in Papers of the President's Office, 1911–1945, UA-UMN.

155. President L. D. Coffman to Mr. P. O. Clapp, December 22, 1933, Box 43, Folder: Physical Education for Women, 1918–1944, Papers of the President's Office, 1911–1945, UA-UMN.

156. Moulton to President Ernest Hatch Wilkins, October 1, 1928, 3 (ms. version); and Moulton, "Annual Report, 1940–41," 3–4 (ms. version), in Secretary Papers, OCA.

157. Grout to Dean Alice M. Baldwin, May 19, 1931, and May 28, 1940, in Alphabetical File: D-Duke University, Physical Education for Women, Papers of Alice Mary Baldwin, UA-Duke.

158. Grout to William Hane Wannamaker, June 24, 1942, Personnel File, Wannamaker Papers, UA-Duke.

159. Geraldine Jonçich Clifford, "Introduction," in *Lone Voyagers*, 1–46.

160. Moulton to President Ernest Hatch Wilkins, October 1, 1928, 3 (ms. version), Secretary Papers, OCA.

161. Speech to Dean and Counsellor staff of the Woman's College, Duke University, 1942, 4, Folder: Addresses-Untitled, Julia R. Grout Papers, UA-Duke.

162. See Wilbur P. Bowen, "The Evolution of Athletic Evils," *APER* 14 (1909): 151–56; Clark W. Hetherington, "Analysis of Problems in College Athletics," *APER* 12 (1907): 154–81; and Howard J. Savage et al., *American College Athletics* (New York: Carnegie Foundation for the Advancement of Teaching, 1929).

163. Levinson, interview.

164. Georgia Borg Johnson, *Organization of the Required Physical Education for Women in State Universities*, Contributions to Education, no. 253 (New York: Bureau of Publications, Teachers College, Columbia University, 1927), 83–89, 93.

165. Gertrude M. Baker, "A Survey of Administrative Relationships of Departments of Physical Education in Colleges and Universities," *RQ* 13 (1942): 221, 225.

166. Ruth E. Eckert, Associate Professor of Education, to Dean W. E. Peik, August 18, 1941, Box 1, Folder 2, Records of College of Education, 1917–1950 (Coll. AQ1.1), UA-UMN. (Hereafter, cited as Education Records.)

167. See Baker, "Survey," 226–28; Johnson, *Organization of the Required Physical Education*, 88–93; and Allen Ericson Weatherford II, "Professional Health Education, Physical Education, and Recreation in Negro Colleges and Universities in the United States" (Ph.D. diss., Pennsylvania State College, 1948), 84–86.

168. Trilling, "History," 17–18, UA-UW.

169. Trilling to Mabel Lee, March 26, 1925, Box 14, Folder I-37, Trilling Files, SA-UW (82/50).

170. Trilling's most cogent case was her letter to President Charles R. Van Hise, November 29, 1915, Box 15, Folder I-57, Trilling Files, SA-UW (82/50).

171. Trilling to Mr. George Little, July 16, 1926, Box 14, Folder I-56, Trilling Files, SA-UW (82/50).

172. Trilling to J. Anna Norris, January 21, 1925, Box 15, Folder I-57, Trilling Files, SA-UW (82/50).

173. Trilling to Van Hise, November 29, 1915, 2, Trilling Files.

174. Trilling to Norris, January 21, 1925, Trilling Files.

175. M. F. McCaffrey, Secretary, Board of Regents, to Blanche Trilling, June 26, 1930, Box 15, Folder I-57, Trilling Files, SA-UW (82/50). For staff discussions, see Box 1, Faculty Meeting Minutes, DWPE Papers, SA-UW (16/82).

176. President Guy Stanton Ford to Dean M. M. Willey, September 18, 1939; and Ford to Committee on Administrative Reorganization, November 6, 1940, Box 43, Folder: Administrative Reorganization Plan, 1939–41, Papers of the Office of the President, 1911–1945, UA-UMN.

177. "A Report to President Coffey from the Committee on Administrative Reorganization," April 7, 1942, copy in UA-UMN. See also letter from Gertrude M. Baker, Acting Director, to Committee on Administrative Reorganization, January 7, 1941, Box 1, Folder 1; and correspondence from other institutions in Box 1, Folder 3: Physical Education Reorganization, Education Records, UA-UMN.

178. Baker to Committee, January 7, 1941, Box 1, Folder 1, Education Records, UA-UMN.

179. "A Petition to the Board of Trustees of Smith College from the Physical Education Faculty," May 31, 1941, Box 1, Folder: Academic Departments-Physical Education, 1941–1946, n.d.; and Florence Gilman, M.D., to President Davis, June 3, 1941, Box 1, Folder: Academic Departments-Hygiene and Bacteriology, 1940–1947, Presidential Papers of Herbert John Davis (1940–1949), SCA-SC.

180. Roberta J. Park and Joan S. Hult, "Women as Leaders in Physical Education and School-Based Sports, 1865 to the 1930s," *JOPERD* 64 (March 1993): 36.

181. Estimate based on membership lists in *Proc. AAAPE* 10 (1895): 212–24; and *APER* 10 (1905): 344–64.

182. Joan S. Hult, "The Governance of Athletics for Girls and Women: Leadership by Women Physical Educators, 1899–1949," *RQES*, Centennial Issue (April 1985): 64–77; and Eline von Borries, *The History and Functions of the National Section on Women's Athletics* (Washington, D.C.: AAHPER, 1941).

183. Hult, "Governance," 66, 67.

184. Dorothy S. Ainsworth, "The National Association of Physical Education for College Women," *JOHPE* 17 (November 1946): 525–26, 575–76; Phyllis Hill, *"The Way We Were": A History of the Purposes of the NAPECW, 1924–1974* (n.p.: NAPECW, 1975); and "Women's College Directors' Societies," *JOHPE* 3 (May 1932): 3–8, 51–52.

185. Alice Allene Sefton, *The Women's Division, National Amateur Athletic Federation: Sixteen Years of Progress in Athletics for Girls and Women, 1923–1939* (Stanford, Calif.: Stanford University Press, 1941). The NSWA and WD-NAAF merged in 1940.

186. Park and Hult, "Leaders," 36, 39–40.

187. See Edwin B. Henderson, "Tolerance: An Objective," *JOHPE* 17 (February 1946): 76; and "Minority Groups and the AAHPER: A Talk with Melvin I. Evans," *JOHPER* 42 (November–December 1971): 22–23.

188. Information about the NPEA and black chapters of the APEA is scant. The NPEA's constitution is reprinted in Burr, "Survey," 100–103.

189. Higginbotham, "Employment," 74.

190. See correspondence of Julia R. Grout (especially her letters home, 1924–36), in Grout Family Papers, SC-Duke. Later reminiscences include Grout, "As You Were," Folder: Writings "As You Were"; and speech for Dean Baldwin's retirement, 1947, and "Pastorale: Andante," 1970, in Folder: Addresses-Retirements, Julia R. Grout Papers, UA-Duke; and Elizabeth Circle Bookhout, "Notes on Miss Grout's Accomplishments," Folder: Papers, 1964–65, 1984, addition (Acc. 86–20) to Julia R. Grout Papers, UA-Duke.

191. Speech for Dean Baldwin's retirement, 1947, 6, Folder: Addresses-Retirements, Julia R. Grout Papers, UA-Duke.

192. Based on Trilling, "History," 91–93, UA-UW. My calculations excluded ten deceased alumnae.

193. Calculations based on "Directory," in *Bulletin of the Physical Education Alumnae Association, Department of Physical Education for Women, University of Minnesota,* 1943: i–xvii; copy found in UA-UMN. "Instructor" was a common occupational listing with occasional references to specialty, such as English or mathematics; I assumed that, when unspecified, "instructor" meant physical educator.

194. Based on "List of Graduates and Positions Held," 96–106, Box 4, vol. 1940–41, DPEW Papers, BHL-UM. My figures are approximate because many entries were incomplete or ambiguous. Moreover, the list includes younger graduates who may have changed fields and/or married later in life.

195. Comparisons based on Clifford, "Introduction," in *Lone Voyagers,* 30–31; Nancy F. Cott, *The Grounding of Modern Feminism* (New Haven, Conn.: Yale University Press, 1987), 147–48; Morantz-Sanchez, *Sympathy and Science,* 135–38; Rossiter, *Women Scientists,* 139–42; and Solomon, *In the Company,* 119–22.

196. Florence Nightingale Mitchell, "A Survey of Physical Education Personnel for Women in Negro Colleges and Universities" (master's [Ed.] thesis, Springfield College, 1958), 44–45.

197. Alice Kessler-Harris, *In Pursuit of Equity: Women, Men, and the Quest for Economic Citizenship in 20th-Century America* (New York: Oxford University Press, 2001), 43.

198. Clifford, "Introduction," in *Lone Voyagers*, 30.

Chapter 2

1. Emily Martin, *The Woman in the Body: A Cultural Analysis of Reproduction* (Boston: Beacon Press, 1987), 27–53.

2. Overview based on historical studies by Hamilton Cravens, Carl N. Degler, Crista DeLuzio, Anne Fausto-Sterling, Thomas Laqueur, Rosalind Rosenberg, Cynthia Eagle Russett, Londa Schiebinger, and Nancy Leys Stepan.

3. Nelly Oudshoorn, *Beyond the Natural Body: An Archeology of Sex Hormones* (London: Routledge, 1994), 144–48.

4. Nancy L. Struna, "The Recreational Experiences of Early American Women," in *Women and Sport: Interdisciplinary Perspectives*, ed. D. Margaret Costa and Sharon R. Guthrie (Champaign, Ill.: Human Kinetics, 1994), 45–62; and Patricia Vertinsky, "Women, Sport, and Exercise in the 19th Century," in *Women and Sport*, 63–82.

5. Mark Dyreson, *Making the American Team: Sport, Culture, and the Olympic Experience* (Urbana: University of Illinois Press, 1998); and S. W. Pope, *Patriotic Games: Sporting Traditions in the American Imagination, 1876–1926* (New York: Oxford University Press, 1997).

6. T. J. Jackson Lears, "American Advertising and the Reconstruction of the Body, 1880–1930," in *Fitness in American Culture: Images of Health, Sport, and the Body, 1830–1940*, ed. Kathryn Grover (Amherst: University of Massachusetts Press; Rochester, N.Y.: Margaret Woodbury Strong Museum, 1989), 47–66; and Donald J. Mrozek, "Sport in American Life: From National Health to Personal Fulfillment, 1890–1940," in *Fitness in American Culture*, 18–46.

7. Harvey Green, *Fit for America: Health, Fitness, Sport, and American Society* (New York: Pantheon, 1986), 219–58; and Jan Todd, "Bernarr Macfadden: Reformer of Feminine Form," in *Sport and Exercise Science: Essays in the History of Sports Medicine*, ed. Jack W. Berryman and Roberta J. Park (Urbana: University of Illinois Press, 1992), 213–32.

8. Lears, "American Advertising"; Nancy Tomes, *The Gospel of Germs: Men, Women, and the Microbe in American Life* (Cambridge, Mass.: Harvard University Press, 1998), 157–233; and James C. Whorton, *Inner Hygiene: Constipation and the Pursuit of Health in Modern Society* (New York: Oxford University Press, 2000), 81–194.

9. Lois W. Banner, *American Beauty: A Social History Through Two Centuries of the American Idea, Ideal, and Image of the Beautiful Woman* (New York: Alfred A. Knopf, 1983), 175–201; John D'Emilio and Estelle B. Freedman, *Intimate Matters: A History of Sexuality in America* (New York: Harper and Row, 1988), 194–201; and Kathy Peiss, *Cheap Amusements: Working Women and Leisure in Turn-of-the-Century New York* (Philadelphia: Temple University Press, 1986), 88–114.

10. Joan Jacobs Brumberg, *The Body Project: An Intimate History of American Girls* (New York: Vintage Books, 1997); and Kathy Peiss, *Hope in a Jar: The Making of America's Beauty Culture* (New York: Henry Holt and Company, 1998).

11. Susan K. Cahn, *Coming on Strong: Gender and Sexuality in Twentieth-Century Women's Sport* (New York: Free Press, 1994), 17.

12. Banner, *American Beauty*, 128–225.

13. Ibid., 151.

14. Gail Bederman, *Manliness and Civilization: A Cultural History of Gender and Race in the United States, 1880–1917* (Chicago: University of Chicago Press, 1995); John F. Kasson, *Houdini, Tarzan, and the Perfect Man: The White Male Body and the Challenge of Modernity in America* (New York: Hill and Wang, 2001); and Donald J. Mrozek, *Sport and American Mentality, 1880–1910* (Knoxville: University of Tennessee Press, 1983), 28–66, 189–225.

15. D'Emilio and Freedman, *Intimate Matters*, 121–30, 188–94, 226–29, 288–95; and Jennifer Terry, *An American Obsession: Science, Medicine, and Homosexuality in Modern Society* (Chicago: University of Chicago Press, 1999), 27–119.

16. Thomas F. Gossett, *Race: The History of an Idea in America* (New York: Schocken Books, 1965), 253–408; and Grace Elizabeth Hale, *Making Whiteness: The Culture of Segregation in the South, 1890–1940* (New York: Pantheon, 1998).

17. Evelynn M. Hammonds and Rebecca M. Herzig, eds., *The Nature of Difference: Sciences of Race in the United States from Jefferson to Genomics* (Cambridge, Mass.: MIT Press, 2009), 103–11, 147–49, 197–200.

18. Bederman, *Manliness and Civilization*, 1–44; Cahn, *Coming on Strong*, 19–23, 51–53, 164–77; and Siobhan B. Somerville, *Queering the Color Line: Race and the Invention of Homosexuality in American Culture* (Durham, N.C.: Duke University Press, 2000), 1–38.

19. Galen Cranz, "Women in Urban Parks," *Signs* 5, no. 3 suppl. (1980): S87–S88.

20. Ibid., S89–S90; Stephen Hardy, *How Boston Played: Sport, Recreation, and Community, 1865–1915*, rev. ed. (Knoxville: University of Tennessee Press, 2003), 65–106; and Roy Rosenzweig, "Middle-Class Parks and Working-Class Play: The Struggle over Recreational Space in Worcester, Massachusetts, 1870–1910," *Radical History Review* 21 (Fall 1979): 31–46.

21. John Bloom, *To Show What an Indian Can Do: Sports at Native American Boarding Schools* (Minneapolis: University of Minnesota Press, 2000); and Devon A. Mihesuah, *Cultivating the Rosebuds: The Education of Women at the Cherokee Female Seminary, 1851–1909* (Urbana: University of Illinois Press, 1993), 85–94.

22. Bloom, *To Show What an Indian Can Do*, 96.

23. Cahn, *Coming on Strong*, 36–47, 72–73, 92–96, 141–47.

24. Peiss, *Cheap Amusements*.

25. Susan G. Zieff, "From Badminton to the Bolero: Sport and Recreation in San Francisco's Chinatown, 1895–1950," *JSH* 27 (2000): 1–29.

26. Linda J. Borish, "'Athletic Activities of Various Kinds': Physical Health and Sport Programs for Jewish American Women," *JSH* 26 (1999): 240–70; and George Eisen, "Sport, Recreation and Gender: Jewish Immigrant Women in Turn-of-the-Century America (1880–1920)," *JSH* 18 (1991): 103–20.

27. Agnes R. Wayman, *Education through Physical Education: Its Organization and Administration for Girls and Women*, 2nd ed. (Philadelphia: Lea and Febiger, 1928), 60.

28. Examples from Margaret Bell, "Why, from the Health Point of View, We Urge Girls' Rules for Girls," in *A Handbook of Basketball for Women*, ed. Eline von Borries (Baltimore,

Md.: Sutherland, 1929), 14; Ethel Bowers, *Recreation for Girls and Women* (New York: A. S. Barnes, 1934), xiii; Elizabeth Burchenal, "A Constructive Program of Athletics for School Girls: Policy, Method and Activities," *APER* 24 (1919): 272; Helen Frost and Charles Digby Wardlaw, *Basket Ball and Indoor Baseball for Women* (New York: Scribner, 1936), 10–11, 13, 14; Alice W. Frymir, *Track and Field for Women* (New York: A. S. Barnes, 1930), 82; Gertrude Hawley, *An Anatomical Analysis of Sports* (New York: A. S. Barnes, 1940), 32, 41–48; Mabel Lee, "A Consideration of the Fundamental Differences between Boys and Girls as They Affect the Girls' Program of Physical Education," *Education* 53 (1933): 467–68; and Agnes R. Wayman, *A Modern Philosophy of Physical Education with Special Implications for Girls and Women and for the College Freshman Program* (Philadelphia: W. B. Saunders, 1938), 165–66.

29. Examples from Marjorie Bateman, "Health Aspects of Girls' Basketball," *Mind and Body* 42 (April 1935): 22; Frymir, *Track and Field*, 18–19; Mabel Lee, *The Conduct of Physical Education: Its Organization and Administration for Girls and Women* (New York: A. S. Barnes, 1937), 70, 437; and Emma Fuller Waterman, "The Physiologic and Anatomic Basis for the Selection and Limitation of Women's Motor Activities" (master's thesis, Department of Hygiene and Physical Education, Wellesley College, 1925), 44–62, 73.

30. Helen Frost, "Soccer—Introductory," in *Official Handbook of the National Committee on Women's Athletics of the American Physical Education Association, Containing the General Policies of the Committee and the Official Rules for Swimming, Track and Field [and] Soccer* (New York: American Sports Publishing, 1923), 107.

31. Lee, "Fundamental Differences," 468.

32. Conclusion based on my survey of fifty scientific articles about physical sex differences published in the United States and abroad between 1900 and 1940. Sources included the *American Journal of Physiology*, *American Journal of Physical Anthropology*, *Journal of the American Medical Association*, and *Journal of Physiology*.

33. For example, Lee, "Fundamental Differences," 467–68; and Wayman, *Education through Physical Education*, 201–2.

34. Helen McKinstry, "Introduction," in *Spalding's Official Basket Ball Guide for Women, 1917–18* (New York: American Sports Publishing, 1917), 4.

35. For example, Harriet I. Ballintine, "The Value of Athletics to College Girls," *APER* 6 (1901): 151–53. Sports advocates were especially liberal; see Anne Pugh, "Interscholastic Squad Competition," in *Spalding's Official Field Hockey Guide, 1930* (New York: American Sports Publishing, 1930), 23–25.

36. Wayman, *Modern Philosophy*, 166.

37. McKinstry, "Introduction," 4.

38. On divergent personalities, see Lee, "Fundamental Differences," 468–69; and Wayman, *Education through Physical Education*, 128–29. On unitary human psychology, see Gertrude Dudley and Frances A. Kellor, *Athletic Games in the Education of Women* (New York: Henry Holt, 1909), 24–25; Ina E. Gittings, "Why Cramp Competition?" *JOHPE* 2 (January 1931): 10–12, 54; and Helen Norman Smith and Helen Leslie Coops, *Physical and Health Education: Principles and Procedures* (New York: American Book, 1938), 72–78.

39. Blanche M. Trilling, "The Playtime of a Million Girls or an Olympic Victory— Which?" *Nation's Schools* 4 (August 1929): 54.

40. Frances A. Kellor, "Ethical Value of Sports for Women," *APER* 11 (1906): 164.

41. Florence D. Alden, "Basket Ball for Girls in Recreation Centers," in *Basket Ball for Women: A Guide for Player, Coach and Official*, ed. Dorothy Bocker (New York: Thos. E. Wilson, 1920), 96–97.

42. Lois Pedersen Broady, *Health and Physical Education for Small Schools* (Lincoln: Teachers College and the University Extension Division, University of Nebraska, 1937), 104.

43. Wayman, *Education through Physical Education*, 170.

44. Helen M. McKinstry, "Athletics for Girls," *Playground* 3 (July 1909): 6–7.

45. Ethel Perrin, "Outdoor Recreation as a Factor in Child Welfare," *Playground* 18 (July 1924): 242.

46. Ibid.

47. Ibid., 241.

48. Carol Lee Bacchi, *Same Difference: Feminism and Sexual Difference* (Sydney: Allen and Unwin, 1990), 6–28; Nancy F. Cott, "Feminist Theory and Feminist Movements: The Past Before Us," in *What Is Feminism? A Re-Examination*, ed. Juliet Mitchell and Ann Oakley (New York: Pantheon, 1986), 49–62; and Regina Markell Morantz-Sanchez, *Sympathy and Science: Women Physicians in American Medicine* (New York: Oxford University Press, 1985), 56–61, 184–202.

49. Helen W. Hazelton, "Outdoor Baseball for Girls," *APER* 34 (1929): 241.

50. Helen N. Smith, "Athletic Education," *APER* 32 (1927): 610.

51. Frymir, *Track and Field*, 34.

52. Hazel H. Pratt, "Women's versus Men's Basket Ball Rules," in *Spalding's Official Basket Ball Guide for Women Containing the Revised Rules 1919–20* (New York: American Sports Publishing, 1919), 66.

53. On evolution, see Lillia Belle Otto, "The Demands for the Twentieth Century Girl—Are We Prepared for Them?" *APER* 21 (1916): 363–68. On endocrinology, see Wayman, *Modern Philosophy*, 62, and "Concepts of Physical Education for Girls and Women," *Sportswoman* 11 (May 1935): 10.

54. Beulah Kennard, "What the Playground Can Do for Girls," in *Proceedings of the Second Annual Playground Congress* (New York: Playground Association of America, 1908), 95–101.

55. Quotations from Smith and Coops, *Physical and Health Education*, 66, and Bowers, *Recreation*, xiii.

56. Alden, "Basket Ball," 97.

57. Kathryn E. Darnell, "Abuse of Basket Ball," in *Spalding's Official Basket Ball Guide for Women, 1913–14* (New York: American Sports Publishing, 1913), 56.

58. Roberta J. Park, "High-Protein Diets, 'Damaged Hearts,' and Rowing Men: Antecedents of Modern Sports Medicine and Exercise Science, 1867–1928," *ESSR* 25 (1997): 137–69; and Roberta J. Park, "Physiologists, Physicians, and Physical Educators: Nineteenth-Century Biology and Exercise, *Hygienic* and *Educative*," in Berryman and Park, *Sport and Exercise Science*, 137–81.

59. Luther H. Gulick, "The Problem of Physical Training in the Modern City," *APER* 8 (1903): 30.

60. On paradigm shifts, see Patricia A. Vertinsky, "Science, Social Science, and the 'Hunger for Wonders' in Physical Education: Moving Toward a Future Healthy Society," in *New Possibilities, New Paradigms?*, American Academy of Physical Education Papers, no. 24 (Champaign, Ill.: Human Kinetics, 1991), 71–83.

61. Mrozek, *Sport and American Mentality*, 67–102.
62. Perrin, "Outdoor Recreation," 241.
63. Wayman, *Education through Physical Education*, 128.

Chapter 3

1. Katharine F. Wells, "Overcoming Periodic Pain," *Parents Magazine* 14 (February 1939): 48.
2. For example, Mabel Lee, *The Conduct of Physical Education: Its Organization and Administration for Girls and Women* (New York: A. S. Barnes, 1937), 259.
3. Helen McKinstry, "The Hygiene of Menstruation," *MHAAB* (1916–17): 18.
4. Ibid., 20.
5. Margaret Bell, "Why Girls Should Play Girls' Basketball Rules—Discussed from the Physiological Angle," in *Spalding's Official Basketball Guide for Women, 1925–26* (New York: American Sports Publishing, 1925), 66.
6. For example, Margaret Bell and Eloise Parsons, "Dysmenorrhea in College Women," *Medical Woman's Journal* 38 (February 1931): 31–35; Marjorie Carolyn Hamer, "Dysmenorrhea and Its Relation to Abdominal Strength as Tested by the Wisconsin Method," *RQ* 4 (1933): 229–37; and Ruth E. Boynton, "A Study of the Menstrual Histories of 2,282 University Women," *American Journal of Obstetrics and Gynecology* 23 (1932): 516–24.
7. Joan Jacobs Brumberg, "'Something Happens to Girls': Menarche and the Emergence of the Modern American Hygienic Imperative," *Journal of the History of Sexuality* 4 (1993): 111–17, 122–25.
8. Agnes R. Wayman, *Education through Physical Education: Its Organization and Administration for Girls and Women* (Philadelphia: Lea and Febiger, 1925), 154.
9. Margaret Bell, "Answers to Practical Questions on Menstruation," *Hygeia* 20 (1942): 208.
10. Alice W. Frymir, *Track and Field for Women* (New York: A. S. Barnes, 1930), 22. Women doctors made similar arguments; for example, Margaret Castex Sturgis, "Menstruation and Menstrual Hygiene in Relation to Physical Education," *Proceedings of the Eleventh Annual Meeting of the American Student Health Association*, Bulletin no. 14 (1930): 84 (and rejoinders on 85–87).
11. Joan Cadden, *Meanings of Sex Difference in the Middle Ages: Medicine, Science, and Culture* (Cambridge: Cambridge University Press, 1993), 21–26; and Nancy Tuana, "The Weaker Seed: The Sexist Bias of Reproductive Theory," in *Feminism and Science*, ed. Nancy Tuana (Bloomington: Indiana University Press, 1989), 147–53.
12. Cadden, *Meanings of Sex Difference in the Middle Ages*, 30–37; and Tuana, "Weaker Seed," 153–56.
13. Janice Delaney, Mary Jane Lupton, and Emily Toth, *The Curse: A Cultural History of Menstruation*, rev. ed. (Urbana: University of Illinois Press, 1988), 47–52; and John G. Gruhn and Ralph R. Kazer, *Hormonal Regulation of the Menstrual Cycle: The Evolution of Concepts* (New York: Plenum Medical, 1989), 3–94.
14. Alexandra Lord, "'The Great *Arcana* of the Deity': Menstruation and Menstrual Disorders in Eighteenth-Century British Medical Thought," *Bulletin of the History of Medicine* 73 (1999): 38–63.
15. Ronald O. Valdiserri, "Menstruation and Medical Theory: An Historical Overview," *Journal of the American Medical Woman's Association* 38 (May–June 1983): 69.

16. Emily Martin, *The Woman in the Body: A Cultural Analysis of Reproduction* (Boston: Beacon Press, 1987), 32–67.

17. Reviews by eminent gynecologists included George W. Corner, "The Nature of the Menstrual Cycle," *Medicine* 12 (1933): 61–82; Emil Novak, "Recent Advances in the Physiology of Menstruation," *JAMA* 94 (1930): 833–39; and Emil Novak, "The Biologic Significance of the Female Reproductive Cycle," *JAMA* 96 (1931): 2173–76.

18. Joan Jacobs Brumberg, *The Body Project: An Intimate History of American Girls* (New York: Random House, 1997), 27–55; and Lara Freidenfelds, *The Modern Period: Menstruation in Twentieth-Century America* (Baltimore, Md.: Johns Hopkins University Press, 2009).

19. Orthodox views included George J. Engelmann, "What is Normal Menstruation?" *New York Medical Journal* 72 (1900): 986–88; and Hugo Ehrenfest, "Menstruation and Its Disorders," *American Journal of Obstetrics and Gynecology* 34 (1937): 541–44, 699–713, 1053–63.

20. Freidenfelds, *Modern Period*, 38–73, 120–69.

21. Jane Farrell-Beck and Laura Klosterman Kidd, "The Roles of Health Professionals in the Development and Dissemination of Women's Sanitary Products, 1880–1940," *Journal of the History of Medicine and Allied Sciences* 51 (1996): 325–52; and Freidenfelds, *Modern Period*, 74–94.

22. See Ehrenfest, "Menstruation," 719–27; and Robert T. Frank, "Hormonal Disturbances as a Cause of Functional Menstrual Disorders," *Proceedings of the Thirteenth Annual Meeting of the American Student Health Association*, Bulletin no. 16 (1932): 69–77.

23. See Norman F. Miller, "Additional Light on the Dysmenorrhea Problem," *JAMA* 95 (1930): 1796–1803.

24. Alice W. Frymir, *Basket Ball for Women: How to Coach and Play the Game* (New York: A. S. Barnes, 1930), 26, 239–40; and Florence Somers, *Principles of Women's Athletics* (New York: A. S. Barnes, 1930), 131–32.

25. This lack of consensus was evident in my examination of numerous scientific articles. For one doctor's balanced review, see Ehrenfest, "Menstruation," 713–15.

26. Marjorie Bateman, "Health Aspects of Girls' Basketball," *Mind and Body* 42 (April 1935): 23.

27. Ibid.; and Helen N. Smith, "Athletic Education," *APER* 32 (1927): 608–11.

28. Margaret Bell, Memo to the House Heads, June 15, 1945, Box 2, Folder: Articles 1930–1944, Papers of Margaret Bell, Bentley Historical Library, University of Michigan, Ann Arbor, Mich.

29. Frymir, *Basket Ball*, 26–27; Elizabeth Richards, "Everyday Problems in Girls Basket Ball," *APER* 25 (1920): 408; and Somers, *Principles*, 28, 118–19.

30. Helen Leslie Coops, *High School Standards in Girls Athletics in the State of Ohio* (New York: Teachers College, Columbia University, 1933), 52–53.

31. For example, J. Anna Norris, "Dangers in Basket Ball: Popular Sport Should be Made Safe for Girls," *Child Health* 5 (1924): 513; and J. Anna Norris, "The Necessity for Supervision of Basket Ball," in *Spalding's Official Basket Ball Guide for Women, 1914–15* (New York: American Sports Publishing, 1914), 72.

32. Minutes of Staff Meeting, October 26, 1939, in Box 1, Folder: WPE Staff Meeting Minutes, 1937–38 through 1939–40, Records of Department of Women's Physical Education, Department of Special Collections, Green Library, Stanford University, Stanford, Calif.

33. This section emphasizes individual teachers; organizational statements are listed in the bibliography.

34. Quoted phrase from Clara G. Baer, "Therapeutic Gymnastics as an Aid in College Work. With Some Observations of Specific Cases," *APER* 21 (1916): 519. Bell and Parsons insisted that exercise and hygiene outperformed drugs; see "Dysmenorrhea," 31, 34–35. Clelia Duel Mosher devised popular exercises; see "A Physiologic Treatment of Congestive Dysmenorrhea and Kindred Disorders Associated with the Menstrual Function," *JAMA* 62 (1914): 1297–1301.

35. Quoted in Elizabeth Burchenal, "Athletics for Girls," in *Spalding's Official Basket Ball Guide for Women, 1916–17* (New York: American Sports Publishing, 1916), 86.

36. Ethel Perrin, "Athletics for Women and Girls," *Playground* 17 (March 1924): 658–59.

37. Frances A. Hellebrandt and Margaret H. Meyer, "Physiological Data Significant to Participation by Women in Physical Activities," *RQ* 10 (1939): 19.

38. Letter to Dr. Margaret Tyler, March 25, 1927, Box 19, Folder: Menstruation, Papers of the Department of Hygiene and Physical Education, Wellesley College Archives, Wellesley College, Wellesley, Mass.

39. Helen F. Cochran, "Basket Ball for High School Girls?" *Publication of the Physical Education Alumnae Association of Oberlin College* 4 (December 1917): 7.

40. Mary Channing Coleman, "Games and Athletics in the School Program," *North Carolina Parent-Teacher Bulletin* 8 (1930): 108. Here, Coleman's metaphor referred to children's recreation; other iterations specified puberty.

41. Elizabeth A. Wright, "The Physical Training of Post-Adolescent Girls," *APNEA* (1910): 942–46.

42. Emma Fuller Waterman, "The Physiologic and Anatomic Basis for the Selection and Limitation of Women's Motor Activities" (master's thesis, Department of Hygiene and Physical Education, Wellesley College, 1925), 139.

43. Kathro Kidwell and Dorothy Simpson, "A Study and Investigation of the Health of Women Teachers of Physical Education," *APER* 34 (1929): 88–89; and Elizabeth Stoner, "Report of the Effect of Teaching Gymnastics During the Menstrual Period," *MHAAB* (1917–18): 70–72.

44. Quoted phrases from Perrin, "Athletics," 660; and Elizabeth Halsey, "The College Curriculum in Physical Education for Women," *APER* 30 (1925): 495.

45. For example, Sturgis, "Menstruation," 84.

46. Tracking menstrual policies at ground level is no easy task. The historian must excavate diverse archival materials, including individual and departmental records along with student handbooks and other institutional publications. There is no guarantee, however, that such documents include the desired information. Many institutions probably did not codify their informal rules about exercise and menstruation; others wrote down their regulations, but extant documents have not preserved them. My research in more than fifty libraries uncovered relatively few accounts of explicit menstrual policies. My efforts were most successful at colleges and universities where national leaders worked. I also relied on my interviews with older physical educators as well as a dozen published and unpublished surveys of high school and collegiate policies.

47. The archival record of Smith's policies is especially complete and detailed. My analysis derives primarily from the Records of the Physical Education Department, Smith

College Archives, Smith College, Northampton, Mass. (Hereafter, cited as PE Records, SCA-SC.)

48. *Regulations of the Department of Hygiene and Physical Education* (three undated versions, ca. 1912–15), and *Regulations of the Department of Hygiene and Physical Education* (1915, 1916, 1918, 1920), in Box: Undergraduate Bulletins and Scrapbooks, 1920–1967; and Box 1206, Folder: Regulations, PE Records, SCA-SC.

49. *Regulations*, ca. 1913–14.

50. *Regulations*, ca. 1912–13 and 1915.

51. Quotation from *Regulations*, ca. 1912–13.

52. *Regulations*, ca. 1912–13, ca. 1913–14, and 1915.

53. *Regulations*, 1916 and 1918.

54. *Regulations*, 1916, 1918, and 1920.

55. See *Regulations*, 1921, 1922, 1923, 1924–25; and *Department of Hygiene and Physical Education. Regulations and Instructions*, 1926–27, 1927–28, 1928–29, 1929–30, and 1930–31. Copies found in Box 1206, Folder: Regulations, and Box: Undergraduate Bulletins and Scrapbooks, 1920–1967, PE Records, SCA-SC.

56. The following list indicates the year by which some institutions required class attendance during menstruation, according to my archival research: Stanford University (1910); University of North Carolina at Greensboro (1917–18); University of Wisconsin (1923); Wellesley College (1924); University of Michigan (ca. 1924); Radcliffe College (1924–25); State Normal Schools of Massachusetts (1925); University of Nebraska (1926–27); and Pembroke College of Brown University (1931–32).

57. Letter from J. Anna Norris to Blanche Trilling, December 13, 1924, Box 11, Folder I-18: Menstruation, Papers of School of Education: Department of Women's Physical Education—Blanche Trilling Files (Acc. 82/50), Steenbock Archives, Steenbock Memorial Library, University of Wisconsin, Madison, Wisc. Hereafter, collection cited as Trilling Files, SA-UW (82/50).

58. Gertrude Dudley to Blanche Trilling, December 15, 1924, Box 11, Folder I-18: Menstruation, Trilling Files, SA-UW (82/50).

59. See letter from Mabel Lee to Blanche Trilling, December 15, 1924; Mabel Cummings to Blanche Trilling, December 17, 1924; and Blanche Trilling to J. Anna Norris, December 20, 1924, Box 11, Folder I-18: Menstruation, Trilling Files, SA-UW (82/50).

60. *Physical Education Bulletin*, 1931–32 through September 1936, in Box 1206; and Box: Undergraduate Bulletins and Scrapbooks, 1920–1967, PE Records, SCA-SC.

61. *Physical Education Bulletin*, 1932–33 through 1965–66. Two retired Smith teachers confirmed this (Helen Russell and Rita Benson, interview by author, Northampton, Mass., March 1, 1996).

62. See Bell, "Answers," 187, 208; and Margaret Bell, *The Doctor Answers Some Practical Questions on Menstruation* (Washington, D.C.: NSWA of AAHPER, 1938), 5–6.

63. By mid-century, some teachers were more open-minded. See Grace Thwing, "Swimming During the Menstrual Period," *JOHPE* 14 (1943): 154; and successive editions of Bell, *Doctor Answers*, 1938:5, 1951:5, and 1955:8.

64. I examined several dozen studies on the effects of "periodicity." Some reported cyclic variations in motor functions; for example, Lillian M. Moore and J. Lucile Barker, "Monthly Variations in Muscular Efficiency in Women," *American Journal of Physiology* 64 (May 1923): 405–15. Others argued that such effects were minimal or unrelated to menstruation;

classic studies include Gertrude Bilhuber, "The Effect of Functional Periodicity on the Motor Ability of Women in Sports" (D.P.H. diss., University of Michigan, 1926); and Leta Stetter Hollingworth, *Functional Periodicity: An Experimental Study of the Mental and Motor Abilities of Women During Menstruation*, Contributions to Education, no. 69 (New York: Bureau of Publications, Teachers College, Columbia University, 1914).

65. McKinstry, "Hygiene," 22.

66. For Smith's procedures, see *Physical Education Bulletin*, 1931–32 and 1939–40.

67. Barbara Miller Solomon, *In the Company of Educated Women: A History of Women and Higher Education in America* (New Haven, Conn.: Yale University Press, 1985), 142–44, 146–48, 150–51, 157–71.

68. Florence Gilman, M.D., to President William H. Neilson, August 11, 1918, and May 12, 1919; and Neilson to Gilman, February 21, 1926, and March 11, 1938, in Box 373, Folder: Gilman; and Florence Meredith, M.D., to President Neilson, May 11, 1925, and January 10, 1926, Box 380, Folder: Meredith, in Presidential Papers: Neilson, SCA-SC.

69. Letter from Florence Gilman, M.D., to President Herbert John Davis, June 3, 1941, Box 1, Folder: Academic Departments—Hygiene and Bacteriology, 1940–1947; and "A Petition to the Board of Trustees of Smith College from the Physical Education Faculty," May 31, 1941, Box 1, Folder: Academic Departments—Physical Education, 1941–1946, n.d., in Presidential Papers: Davis, SCA-SC.

70. Heather Munro Prescott, *Student Bodies: The Influence of Student Health Services in American Society and Medicine* (Ann Arbor: University of Michigan Press, 2007), 11–92.

Chapter 4

1. R. McLaran Sawyer, *The Modern University, 1920–1969*, vol. 2 of *Centennial History of the University of Nebraska* (Lincoln: Centennial Press, 1973), 47.

2. Brief accounts are H. L. Ray and Ruth Schellberg, "Mabel Lee: The Alliance's First Lady," *JOPERD* 56 (April 1985): 67–68; and Celeste Ulrich, "In Memoriam: Mabel Lee, August 18, 1886–December 3, 1985," *JOPERD* 57 (March 1986): 24–26. The key manuscript collection is Mabel Lee Papers, Archives, American Alliance for Health, Physical Education, Recreation and Dance. I examined the collection (hereafter, cited as Lee Papers) at its former location, the AAHPERD headquarters in Reston, Va. My citations use original box designations, not those assigned since reprocessing.

3. Lee wrote a two-volume autobiography: *Memories of a Bloomer Girl (1894–1924)* (Washington, D.C.: AAHPER, 1977) and *Memories Beyond Bloomers (1924–1954)* (Washington, D.C.: AAHPER, 1978); hereafter, cited as *MBG* and *MBB*. Her diaries are contained in the Lee Papers; I assigned numbers to the documents (bound volumes, notebooks, desk calendars, and other formats) in chronological order. Although Lee's autobiography and diaries are essential to any analysis of her career, they also raise questions of accuracy for the scholar. Given Lee's obsession with her professional reputation and legacy, her memoirs represented her life in carefully constructed, often self-serving ways. Lee also altered various diary entries weeks, even years after the date she originally recorded them. A historian must keep these complications in mind when interpreting Lee's autobiography and private writings.

4. Transcript, "Groundbreakers Interview [November 12, 1979]," 18–19, Lincoln-Lancaster County Commission on the Status of Women, in Diaries, Box 3, Lee Papers; and Lee, *MBG*, 49–79.

5. *MBG*, 70–77; and "Groundbreakers," 7, Lee Papers.

6. Obituary, *Washington Post*, January 17, 1992; and Box 160–1, Folders 1–2, Papers of Maryrose Reeves Allen, Manuscripts Division, Moorland-Spingarn Research Center, Howard University, Washington, D.C. Hereafter, cited as Allen Papers.

7. Ted Chambers, *The History of Athletics and Physical Education at Howard University* (New York: Vantage Press, 1986), 25.

8. Lee, "A Consideration of the Fundamental Differences Between Boys and Girls as They Affect the Girls' Program of Physical Education," *Education* 53 (1933): 470–71.

9. Quotations from article prepared for *New York Times*, 1933; and speech, "The Underlying Principles in Athletics for Girls and Women," 10, WD-NAAF, Los Angeles, 1932, Box: Speeches and Writings, 1922–1977, Folder: 1932–1938, Lee Papers. This box contains all cited speeches and radio talks.

10. Mabel Lee to Leslie E. Edmonds, January 21, 1933, Correspondence Box "Pro-Notes," Folder: NSWA, Lee Papers.

11. See *The Conduct of Physical Education: Its Organization and Administration for Girls and Women* (New York: A. S. Barnes, 1937), 68–70, 101–2, 122–23, 436–39; "Fundamental Differences," 467–68; speech, "The Modern Trend of Girl's Athletics," 7–8, Indiana High School Athletic Association, Indianapolis, 1933, Lee Papers; and speech, "What Men Physical Educators and School Men Should Know About Physical Education for Girls," 6–7, Mid West Society of Physical Education, Milwaukee, 1935, Lee Papers.

12. *Conduct of Physical Education*, 437.

13. Ibid., 39.

14. *MBG*, 26.

15. Ibid., 113, 361–62.

16. Class Notes, Collin's Swedish Gymnastics (1908), 13; and Class Notes, Collin's Theory of Gymnastics (1909–10), 17, 18, and January 1910 (n.p.), Box "1908–1932," Lee Papers.

17. "Views of Parents on the Physical Education Program for Their Daughters," *JOHPE* 4 (April 1933): 13–14.

18. *MBB*, 227; and speech, "N.A.A.F.," 8, Beloit College, February 1924, Lee Papers.

19. Representative diary entries (see n3 above) include no. 3: July 30, 1902; no. 5: January 23, 1903; no. 16: January 28, 1905; no. 17: February 18, 1905 and April 1, 1905; no. 27: May 29, 1907; and no. 30: January 7, 1910, October 1912, and January 1, 1913, Lee Papers. For published examples, see *MBG*, 64–66, 137–39.

20. *MBB*, 82, and 80–83, 122–37 in general.

21. "Groundbreakers," 2–3, Lee Papers.

22. Phrases from diary, no. 22: May 17, 1906, Lee Papers.

23. "Groundbreakers," 2–3, Lee Papers; and *MBG*, 69–70.

24. *MBG*, 62–63; and diary, no. 26: February 28, 1907, Lee Papers.

25. Diary, no. 20: October 7–9, 1905; no. 26: March 27, 1907; no. 28: February 10, 1908; no. 28: March 14, 1908; and no. 30: May 9, 1910, Lee Papers.

26. *MBG*, 110–11, 227–28.

27. "Menstrual Period Regulations," ca. 1924–26; and *Handbook of the Department of Physical Education for Women, 1926–1927*, 12, in Correspondence Box CB4, Folder: Public N.S., Lee Papers.

28. Mabel Lee to Blanche Trilling, December 15, 1924, Box 11, Folder I-18: Menstruation, Records of School of Education: Department of Women's Physical Education—Blanche

Trilling Files (Acc. 82/50), Archives, Steenbock Memorial Library, University of Wisconsin, Madison, Wisc.

29. Lee to Dr. Ben Miller, August 19, 1944; and Lee to Dr. J. Milton Singleton, September 20, 1944, Correspondence Box CB1, Lee Papers.

30. Speech, "Comparison of the Physical-Activity Load for Men and Women," 4–5, East Tennessee Education Association Program for Section on HPER, Knoxville, 1953, Lee Papers.

31. "Groundbreakers," 12, Lee Papers.

32. *MBG*, 38, and 24–38 in general.

33. Lee's recollections of basketball are especially interesting. Invented in 1896, the sport reached Iowa by 1902; see *MBG*, 36, 41–43; and diary, nos. 2–4, 6, 11, Lee Papers.

34. Diary, no. 16: January 28, 1905, and no. 27: May 13, 1907, Lee Papers.

35. "Sports and Games—An Educational Dynamic Force," *Playground and Recreation* 23 (July 1929): 223; and speech, "Coeducational Physical Education," 15, Kansas Health and Physical Education Association, Wichita, 1936, Lee Papers.

36. "Beauty More Than Skin Deep, U. of N. Physical Expert Avers," *Omaha Bee*, November 1, 1935, Box: Scrapbooks and Clippings #1, Folder: Scrapbook, 1924–1930, Lee Papers; and speech, "The Physical Educator's Role as a Member of the Teaching Team," 6–13, Tennessee State Education Association, Nashville, 1951, Lee Papers.

37. See *Conduct of Physical Education*, 69, 74–77, 438–39; "Fundamental Differences," 468–69; "Views of Parents," 12–14; speech, "Modern Trend," 8, Lee Papers; and speech, "Coeducational," 19, Lee Papers.

38. Speech, "Modern Trend," 11, Lee Papers.

39. *MBG* 33, 55, 81–108 passim, 127–35, 155–97 passim.

40. Diary, no. 25: November 1, 1906, Lee Papers; and *MBG*, 52.

41. Diary, no. 22: April 23, 1906; no. 22: April 28, 1906; and no. 25: October 5, 1906, Lee Papers.

42. Diary, no. 30: January 12, 1910, Lee Papers.

43. Examples in diary no. 30 include December 17, 1908; year-end summary for 1908; January 7, January 13, March 30, May 24, and June 3, 1909; and January 3, January 7, and March 2, 1910, Lee Papers. For published accounts, see *MBG*, 86–108, 127–35, 155–58, 191.

44. *MBG*, 98.

45. Based on conversations with physical educators whom I met during interviews, conferences, and archival work.

46. *MBG*, 193, 231 (quoted phrases); *MBB*, 41; and in Lee Papers: Correspondence Box "Nebraska," Folder: "Confidential for ML's personal files" (quoted phrase); "12 Years of Trouble," Correspondence Box CB1, Folder 1; and diary, no. 33 (July 11, 1916–July 4, 1917).

47. *Conduct of Physical Education*, 20.

48. "The Modern Movement in Athletics for Women," *Club Woman* 15 (December 1926): 14–15; and *MBB*, 320–23.

49. "Modern Movement," 15.

50. Phrases from *MBB*, 223; and Lee to Edmonds, January 21, 1933, Lee Papers.

51. Diary, no. 1: December 3, 1900, and no. 26: April 16, 1907, Lee Papers.

52. Lee to Manager, Bowl Mor Lanes, February 16, 1950, Correspondence Box CB1, Folder: "UMT article," Lee Papers; also *MBB*, 158, 369–70, 386.

53. On racial discourse and silences, see Evelyn Brooks Higginbotham, "African-American Women's History and the Metalanguage of Race," *Signs* 17 (Winter 1992): 251–53.

54. Speech, "Modern Trend," 7–8; and speech, "What Men," 6–7, Lee Papers.

55. *Conduct of Physical Education*, 437.

56. "Sports and Games," 224.

57. *MBB*, 46.

58. Sawyer, *Modern University*, 34–45.

59. *MBB*, 46.

60. John R. Thelin, *A History of American Higher Education* (Baltimore, Md.: Johns Hopkins University Press, 2004), 205.

61. Ibid., 232.

62. Allen to Mr. Goodman, February 5, 1957, 5, Box 160–7, Folder 13, Allen Papers. Goodman probably authored the story on women's physical education that Howard University published in 1957; see n151 below.

63. "The Program and Budget for Intra-Mural and Intercollegiate Activities for Women," 1, ca. 1941, Box 160–8, Folder 9, Allen Papers.

64. Outline of "The Development of Beauty in College Women Through Health and Physical Education" (master's [Ed.] thesis, Boston University, 1938), 1, Box 160–4, Folder 4, Allen Papers.

65. "The Development of Beauty in College Women Through Health and Physical Education," *Report of the Twenty-Fourth Annual Meeting of the Eastern Society of Directors of Physical Education for College Women*, n.p., ca. 1938.

66. Thesis outline, 4 (quotation); "Program and Budget," 1; and letter from Department of Physical Education for Women to Dr. Charles H. Thompson, Dean, College of Liberal Arts, October 14, 1939, 2, 5 (quotation), Box 160–8, Folder 9, Allen Papers.

67. "Beauty," 5, n.d., Box 160–7, Folder 10, Allen Papers. Allen probably authored this.

68. "Program and Budget," 1, Allen Papers.

69. Thesis outline, 19; and "The Measurement and Relationship Between Beauty, Physical, Mental and Character Traits," 154, term paper for Dr. Donald D. Durrell, First Semester, 1938–39, Box 160–6, Folder 4, Allen Papers.

70. Quotations from Allen to Goodman, 3, February 5, 1957; and "A Study of the Health Problems of the Teacher and the Child," 21, Health Workshop, Hampton Institute Summer School, 1944, Box 160–9, Folder 13, Allen Papers.

71. "Study of Health Problems," 24, Allen Papers.

72. Leonie B. Harper, "Corrective and Remedial Physical Education Area," *CLA Annual Report, 1948–49*, 223.

73. "Study of Health Problems," 23, Allen Papers (quotation); and Nora Lee Banks, F. Irene Ford, and Frances C. Haddock, "Expressionistic Gymnastics Area Report," *CLA Annual Report, 1948–49*, 204. (The authors were physical education staff members.)

74. *CLA Annual Report, 1939–40*, lxiii (quotation); and *CLA Annual Report, 1944–45*, 114.

75. *CLA Annual Report, 1944–45*, 115.

76. Lola Young, "Racializing Femininity," in *Women's Bodies: Discipline and Transgression*, ed. Jane Arthurs and Jean Grimshaw (London: Cassell, 1999), 67–90.

77. Carla L. Peterson, "Foreword: Eccentric Bodies," in *Recovering the Black Female Body: Self-Representations by African American Women*, ed. Michael Bennett and Vanessa D. Dickerson (New Brunswick, N.J.: Rutgers University Press, 2000), xi–xv.

78. Banks, Ford, and Haddock, "Expressionistic Gymnastics," 207.

79. Handwritten notes, "Introduction—You," 8–10, n.d., Box 160–7, Folder 11, Allen Papers.

80. Maxine Leeds Craig, *Ain't I a Beauty Queen? Black Women, Beauty, and the Politics of Race* (New York: Oxford University Press, 2002), 23–64; Paula Giddings, *When and Where I Enter: The Impact of Black Women on Race and Sex in America*, 2nd ed. (New York: William Morrow, 1996), 46–55, 85–89, 183–93; and Margaret A. Lowe, *Looking Good: College Women and Body Image, 1875–1930* (Baltimore, Md.: Johns Hopkins University Press, 2003), 40–42, 57–61, 73–74, 99–102, 156–57.

81. "Body Aesthetics," 5, Box 160–7, Folder 10, Allen Papers.

82. See Leonie B. Harper, *CLA Annual Report, 1968–69*, 149, 156.

83. Allen, *CLA Annual Report, 1947–48*, 209; and *CLA Annual Report, 1950–51*, 123, 128–29.

84. Stephanie J. Shaw, *What a Woman Ought to Be and to Do: Black Professional Women Workers During the Jim Crow Era* (Chicago: University of Chicago Press, 1996).

85. Handwritten notes on "How Racism Affects Our Social Order in Health," 9, Box 160–7, Folder 11, Allen Papers.

86. Vinna Vinyard, "Dance Area Report," *CLA Annual Report, 1948–49*, 232–33.

87. See bell hooks, "Loving Blackness as Political Resistance," in *Black Looks: Race and Representation* (Boston: South End Press, 1992), 9–20.

88. Radio talk, "The Woman's Division of N.A.A.F.," 8, 1928, Lee Papers.

89. Speech, "Trend of Athletics for Women Today," 4–5, Coe College, 1925, Lee Papers.

90. Speech, "Modern Trend," 8, Lee Papers.

91. Speech, "What Men," 14, Lee Papers.

92. Ibid., 15.

93. On Coe, see *MBG*, 199–308; "Story of Troubles at OAC," handwritten MS, 14, in Scrapbook and Clippings Box 3, Folder: 1910s, Lee Papers; and diary, nos. 30–34 (Fall 1908–Spring 1919), Lee Papers.

94. Diary, no. 34: November 2, 1918, Lee Papers. Lee's published recollections about OAC (*MBG*, 310–25) are a tepid version of private accounts in her diary and correspondence.

95. Diary, no. 34: January 20, 1919, Lee Papers.

96. Mabel Lee to James M. Wood, May 15, 1924, Correspondence Box CG2, Folder 8, Lee Papers.

97. Ibid. Also *MBG*, 327–56, 374–77.

98. See *MBB*, 3–15, 30–73.

99. On structure, see Mabel Lee et al., *Seventy-Five Years of Professional Preparation in Physical Education for Women at the University of Nebraska–Lincoln, 1898–1973* (Lincoln: University of Nebraska, 1973), 3–47; and Mabel Lee, "History of Relation of Department of Physical Education for Women to the Department of Physical Education for Men," in Memoirs and Theses, Box 2, Records of Teachers College: Department of Physical Education for Women, University Archives, University of Nebraska–Lincoln, Neb. (Hereafter,

depository cited as UA-UNL.) On Lee's dealings with the chairman in 1924–25, see Correspondence Box "Nebraska," Folder: "Un. of Neb.," Lee Papers.

100. Mabel Lee to Mrs. R. N. Westover, June 17, 1925, Correspondence Box "Nebraska," Folder: "Un. of Neb.," Lee Papers.

101. Mabel Lee to Chancellor Samuel Avery, March 26, 1925, Correspondence Box "Nebraska," Folder: "Un. of Neb. Personal Correspondence, 1924–30," Lee Papers.

102. Ibid.

103. Handwritten MSS (year-by-year notes, 1924–30), Correspondence Box "Pro Notes," Folder 1, Lee Papers.

104. Lee to Avery, March 26, 1925, Lee Papers.

105. Ibid. On salaries, see *MBB*, 107–8.

106. *MBB*, 44–46, 50–57; and handwritten MSS (quoted phrase), Lee Papers.

107. A general account is *MBB*, 41–73. On departmental separation, see Minutes of Meetings, May 8, 1925, Papers of Board of Regents, UA-UNL; and Mabel Lee to Mabel Cummings, May 19, 1925, Correspondence Box "Nebraska," Folder: "Un. of Neb.," Lee Papers. On professional programs, see Mabel Lee to E. A. Burnett, November 28, 1928, and E. A. Burnett to Mabel Lee and R. G. Clapp, December 4, 1928, Papers of the Office of the Chancellor, UA-UNL. On facilities, see Mabel Lee to Vera Barger, October 12, 1926, Correspondence Box "Nebraska," Folder: "Un. of Neb.," Lee Papers.

108. Speech, "Modern Trend," 2, Lee Papers. Lee's reference was "that spectacle in Los Angeles" (the 1932 Olympiad).

109. On the 1930s–1950s, see *MBB*, 242–65, 386–91; professional correspondence, 1930s–1940s, Correspondence Box CB1, Lee Papers; and Correspondence Box CB5, Folder: "Trouble with Staff," Lee Papers.

110. Sawyer, *Modern University*, 34–48, 85–99, 139–54.

111. Patrick B. Miller, "To 'Bring the Race along Rapidly': Sport, Student Culture, and Educational Mission at Historically Black Colleges during the Interwar Years," *History of Education Quarterly* 35 (1995): 111–33.

112. Ibid., 122.

113. Ibid., 126–30; and Rayford W. Logan, *Howard University: The First Hundred Years, 1867–1967* (New York: New York University Press, 1969), 211–16, 231–44, 254, 277–78.

114. Louis L. Watson, Clarence W. Davis, and John H. Burr had studied at Springfield College.

115. Armstead A. Pierro, "A History of Professional Preparation for Physical Education in Some Selected Negro Colleges and Universities, 1924–1958" (Ph.D. diss., University of Michigan, 1962), 74–77, 114–15.

116. Howard University, *Catalogue, 1929–30*, 231; and *Catalogue, 1930–31*, 249, 254. Forty years later, the departments merged again, in the wake of Allen's retirement and Title IX.

117. Allen's summaries in *CLA Annual Reports* described these difficulties.

118. Pierro, "History," 237; and Leonie B. Harper, *CLA Annual Report, 1950–51*, 131.

119. Department to Thompson, October 14, 1939, 8, Allen Papers.

120. Quotations from Allen, untitled three-page description of department, 1, ca. 1930s, Box 160–7, Folder 13; and "Program and Budget," 6, Allen Papers.

121. Chambers, *History of Athletics and Physical Education*, 45–46.

122. "Program and Budget," 1, Allen Papers.

123. Ibid., 5; and Department to Thompson, October 14, 1939, 4, 10, Allen Papers.

124. Department to Thompson, October 14, 1939, 4 (quotation), 9; and "Program and Budget," 3–4, Allen Papers.

125. The men's department head also opposed the merger; see letter from John H. Burr to Dean Charles H. Thompson, October 14, 1939, Box 160–8, Folder 9, Allen Papers.

126. *Conduct of Physical Education*, 102, and 21–62 passim, 262–63.

127. Speech, "What Men," 3 (quotation); and speech, "'To Thine Own Self Be True,'" 22–23, Otterbein College, Westerville, Ohio, 1966, Lee Papers.

128. Speech, "Recreation for College Women," 9, NAAF, Chicago, April 1925, Lee Papers.

129. Radio talk, "Woman's Division," 5, Lee Papers.

130. Lee to J. Lyman Bingham, January 23, 1933, Correspondence Box CB5, Folder: "Correspondence 1930s, Women's Athletics," Lee Papers. Bingham was assistant to the president of the AAU.

131. Quotations from speech, "The Meaning of Performance in Physical Education," 2, Amsterdam, 1939, Lee Papers; and "Athletics and the American University," *Lincoln State Journal*, March 28, 1926.

132. For example, Wilbur P. Bowen, "The Evolution of Athletic Evils," *APER* 14 (1909): 151–56; and Clark W. Hetherington, "Analysis of Problems in College Athletics," *APER* 12 (1907): 154–81. A classic critique is Howard J. Savage et al., *American College Athletics* (New York: Carnegie Foundation for the Advancement of Teaching, 1929).

133. *MBG*, 34–35, 43; and in Lee Papers: "Groundbreakers," 13–15; speech, "'To Thine Own Self,'" 18–20; speech, "Modern Trend," 10; and article for *New York Times*, May 1933.

134. Diary, no. 22: April 28, 1906; no. 25: October 5, 1906; no. 26: February 28, 1907; no. 27: June 1, 1907; and no. 28: September 19, 1907, Lee Papers.

135. *MBG*, 112–14, 361–62.

136. Class Notes, 1909–10, n.p. (quotation); and diary, no. 30: January 25, 1912, no. 30: March 7–8, 1912, and no. 31: November 1914, Lee Papers.

137. Diary, no. 34: October 25, 1918, Lee Papers.

138. Lee to Wood, May 15, 1924, Lee Papers.

139. Speech, "Underlying Principles," 2, Lee Papers.

140. See *MBB*, 30–41; and Lee et al., *Seventy-Five Years*, 29–47.

141. Phrase from speech, "Coeducational," 15, Lee Papers; also *Conduct of Physical Education*, 512–15.

142. *MBG*, 240–42, 250–53; and *MBB*, 236–41.

143. *Handbook of the Department of Physical Education for Women, The University of Nebraska, 1926–1927*, 8, 10–12, (copy in Correspondence Box CB4, Folder: "Public. N.S.," Lee Papers).

144. Phyllis Kay Wilke, "The History of Physical Education for Women at the University of Nebraska from the Early Beginnings to 1952" (master's [Ed.] thesis, University of Nebraska, 1973), 178, 186–208. Nebraska sponsored women's intercollegiate sports at the turn of the century but banned them in 1908.

145. President's Report for 1931/32, 2, Box 3, Folder: President's Reports, Subseries 13 (Women's Athletic Association), in Records of Teachers College: Department of Physical Education for Women, UA-UNL. (Hereafter, collection cited as WAA Records.)

146. Reports of Points and Awards Chairman, 1936/37–1938/39, in Box 3; President's Report, 1931/32, 1937/38, and 1941/42, in Box 3, Folder: President's Reports; Minutes of Executive Council Meetings: October 17, 1929, November 21, 1929, January 16, 1930, January 23, 1930, and March 6, 1930, in Box 4, Folder 2; Minutes of Council Meetings: April 20, 1937, September 30, 1937, October 28, 1937, and November 18, 1937, in Box 4, Folder 3; Minutes of Council Meetings: April 30, 1940, May 14, 1940, and February 14, 1941, in Box 4, Folder 4; Minutes of Council Meetings: November 17, 1950, October 26, 1951, and November 9, 1951, in Box 4, Folder 6, WAA Records, UA-UNL.

147. *Conduct of Physical Education*, 434.

148. See President's Report for 1931/32, Box 3, Folder: President's Reports; Minutes of Council Meetings: December 16, 1937, Box 4, Folder 3; and Minutes of Council Meetings: May 14, 1940, Box 4, Folder 4, WAA Records, UA-UNL.

149. Quotations from department description, 1, n.d., Box 160–7, Folder 13; and thesis outline, 24, Allen Papers.

150. Examples from thesis outline, 23; "Beauty," 5–6; and department description, 3, n.d., Allen Papers.

151. Besides departmental *Catalogue* entries, good descriptions include Allen, *CLA Annual Report, 1944–45*, 115–16; Allen et al., *CLA Annual Report, 1948–49*, 193–228; and "Women's Physical Education Stresses Body Sculpture Through Movement," *Howard University Bulletin* (March 15, 1957): 5–7.

152. On beauty workshops, see Nora Lee Banks, "Expressionistic Gymnastics Area Report," *CLA Annual Report, 1948–49*, 205–7. During the 1940s the physical education staff included a licensed cosmetologist.

153. "Program and Budget," 1, Allen Papers.

154. On sports, see Wilhelmina O. Clark, "Intramural Area Report," *CLA Annual Report, 1948–49*, 234–37; and Cereta Perry, "Major Sports Area," *CLA Annual Report, 1948–49*, 239–43. On the May Festival, see Allen, *CLA Annual Report, 1939–40*, lxiv–lxvi. On dance, see Allen, *CLA Annual Report, 1945–46*, 95–96; and Vinna Vinyard, "Dance Area Report," *CLA Annual Report, 1948–49*, 229–33.

155. Perry, "Major Sports," 241, 243.

156. Women's Sports Day Association, *Constitution*, Article II, 31; copy in Box 160–10, Folder 27, Allen Papers.

157. On Howard and the WSDA, see Allen, *CLA Annual Report*: 1942–43, 176; 1950–51, 130; 1951–52, 150; and 1953–54, I:86.

158. See editions of *Catalogue*; and Pierro, "History," 144–46, 158–60.

159. Leonie B. Harper, *CLA Annual Report, 1950–51*, 130.

Chapter 5

1. Norris to President L. D. Coffman, May 9, 1927, Box 43, Folder: University of Minnesota, Physical Education for Women, 1918–1944, Papers of the President's Office, 1911–1945, University Archives, University of Minnesota, Minneapolis, Minn. (Hereafter, depository cited as UA-UMN.)

2. The moniker comes from Joan S. Hult, quoted in Sheryl Marie Szady, "The History of Intercollegiate Athletics for Women at the University of Michigan" (Ed.D. diss., University of Michigan, 1987), 32.

3. David O. Levine, *The American College and the Culture of Aspiration, 1915–1940* (Ithaca, N.Y.: Cornell University Press, 1986); and John R. Thelin, *A History of American Higher Education* (Baltimore, Md.: Johns Hopkins University Press, 2004), 205–59.

4. Levine, *American College*, 191–93; and Thelin, *History*, 205–8.

5. Levine, *American College*, 38.

6. Thelin, *History*, 245–49.

7. Levine, *American College*, 158–59, 201–2; Barbara Miller Solomon, *In the Company of Educated Women: A History of Women and Higher Education in America* (New Haven, Conn.: Yale University Press, 1985), 62–77, 141–49; and Thelin, *History*, 226–34.

8. Thelin, *History*, 226.

9. Ibid., 232.

10. Helen Lefkowitz Horowitz, *Campus Life: Undergraduate Cultures from the End of the Eighteenth Century to the Present* (New York: Knopf, 1987), 100–108; Levine, *American College*, 45–67, 89–112; and Thelin, *History*, 234–43.

11. Thelin, *History*, 234.

12. Ibid., 103–7, 243–49.

13. Horowitz, *Campus Life*, 134; and Levine, *American College*, 119.

14. Paula S. Fass, *The Damned and the Beautiful: American Youth in the 1920s* (New York: Oxford University Press, 1977); Horowitz, *Campus Life*, 98–150; Levine, *American College*, 113–23; and Thelin, *History*, 208–26 (quotation, 211).

15. Fass, *Damned and the Beautiful*, 260–326; Helen Lefkowitz Horowitz, *Alma Mater: Design and Experience in the Women's Colleges from Their Nineteenth-Century Beginnings to the 1930s*, 2nd ed. (Amherst: University of Massachusetts Press, 1993), 65–68, 166–67, 281–86; Horowitz, *Campus Life*, 208–13; and Solomon, *In the Company of Educated Women*, 98–102, 161–63.

16. Lynn D. Gordon, *Gender and Higher Education in the Progressive Era* (New Haven, Conn.: Yale University Press, 1990), 4–5, 33–40; Horowitz, *Alma Mater*, 147–78, 279–94; Horowitz, *Campus Life*, 193–219; Margaret A. Lowe, *Looking Good: College Women and Body Image, 1875–1930* (Baltimore, Md.: Johns Hopkins University Press, 2003), 103–54; and Solomon, *In the Company of Educated Women*, 157–71.

17. Horowitz, *Alma Mater*, 287.

18. Horowitz, *Campus Life*, 108–12, 119.

19. Solomon, *In the Company of Educated Women*, 141.

20. Blanche Trilling, "Talk at Pittsburgh Play Day," 4, n.d., Box 14, Folder I-7, Papers of School of Education: Department of Women's Physical Education—Blanche Trilling Files (Acc. 82/50), Archives, Steenbock Memorial Library, University of Wisconsin, Madison, Wisc. Hereafter, collection and depository cited as Trilling Files, SA-UW (82/50).

21. Senda Berenson, "Basket Ball for Women," n.d., in typed speeches (Item 29, p. 99), Box 706.1, Folder 34a, Papers of Senda Berenson, General Faculty Files, Smith College Archives, Smith College, Northampton, Mass. (Hereafter, depository cited as SCA-SC.)

22. This early-twentieth-century warning about "misdirected" attachments indicates that gym teachers' homophobia surfaced considerably earlier than other scholars have suggested.

23. Berenson, "Basket Ball," 99.

24. Mary Channing Coleman, "Today's Trends in Sports," radio address, n.d., Box 1, Folder: Speeches/Articles I, Records of the School of Health, Physical Education, Recreation, and Dance, Special Collections, Walter Clinton Jackson Library, University of North Carolina at Greensboro, Greensboro, N.C. (Hereafter, cited as HPERD Records, SC-UNCG.)

25. Mabel Cummings to Evelyn Abrams, March 17, 1927, and Cummings to M. Connell, November 7, 1923, Box 14, Folder: Competition 1945–1959 and Policies, 1920–1961; and Josephine Rathbone to Director of Hygiene and Social Schedule Committee, May 30, 1930 (quotation), Box 37, Folder: General to Modern Dance, Records of the Department of Hygiene and Physical Education, Wellesley College Archives, Margaret Clapp Library, Wellesley College, Wellesley, Mass. (Hereafter, cited as HPE Papers, WCA.)

26. Program for March 27, 1915, Competitive Gymnastic Exhibition, 2, in Papers of Althea Heimbach, Milwaukee-Downer Archives, in University Archives, Seeley G. Mudd Library, Lawrence University, Appleton, Wisc. (Hereafter, cited as Heimbach Papers, MDA-LU.)

27. Jessie Godfrey, "The Organization and Administration of Women's Athletic and Recreation Associations" (master's thesis, Wellesley College, 1951), 91–92; and M. Gladys Scott, "Competition for Women in American Colleges and Universities," *RQ* 16 (1945): 58–59, 62–63.

28. Letter to Chancellor Julius Isaac Foust, March 22, 1928, Foust Papers, General Correspondence: 1928, SC-UNCG.

29. Julia R. Grout, "Annual Report of the Department of Physical Education for Women," 4, 1937–38, Papers of President W. P. Few, Subject File: Duke University, Physical Education for Women, University Archives, William R. Perkins Library, Duke University, Durham, N.C. (Hereafter, depository cited as UA-Duke.)

30. Cummings to Connell, November 7, 1923, HPE Papers, WCA.

31. "Trends in Physical Education," 5, speech for Ohio State Education Association, 1931, Box 14, Folder I-12, Trilling Files, SA-UW (82/50).

32. "Dr. Bell Declares Intercollegiate Athletics Need Secure Foundation," *Michigan Daily*, December 10, 1926; copy in vol. 1, Box 1: Scrapbooks, 1923–1936, Papers of the Department of Physical Education for Women, 1923–1972, Bentley Historical Library, University of Michigan, Ann Arbor, Mich. (Hereafter, depository cited as BHL-UM.)

33. Godfrey, "Organization," surveyed 227 predominantly white four-year institutions.

34. Marguerite Schwarz, "The Athletic Federation of College Women," *JOHPE* 7 (May 1936): 297, 345–46.

35. Godfrey, "Organization," 69–98, 106–11.

36. Minutes of WAA, March 4, 1926 (quotation), March 5, 1926, January 4, 1927, January 18, 1927, February 8, 1927, October 10, 1928, November 6, 1928, and November 13, 1928, Box 4, Folder 4–3: Women's Athletic Association, Minutes, April 1925–November 1927 (*sic*), Records of Women's Recreation and Intramural Sports (1922–75), in Papers of Student Services: Director of Athletics, University Archives, Ohio State University, Columbus, Ohio. (Hereafter, depository cited as UA-OSU.) See also "Amendment to the W.A.A. Constitution," *W.A.A. Quarterly* (February 24, 1927): 3 (quotation); and *Women's Athletic Association of the Ohio State University Revised Constitution and By-Laws with Appendix*, 1922–23 and 1927, in Records of Women's Athletics (Coll. 9/e-5a, unprocessed acc. 124/89), UA-OSU.

37. *Women's Athletic Bulletin* (April 1931): 2; copy in UA-UMN.

38. Pauline Hodgson, "The Development of Intramural Athletics for College Women," *APER* 32 (1927): 496.

39. Gordon, *Gender and Higher Education*, 44–51; Horowitz, *Alma Mater*, 147–78; Lowe, *Looking Good*, 31–38, 96–99; and Thelin, *History*, 180–82, 228.

40. Horowitz, *Alma Mater*, 282–94; and Lowe, *Looking Good*, 103–33.

41. Information gleaned from file on "Physical Education Department," Archives, McCain Library, Agnes Scott College, Decatur, Ga.; annual issues of *Silhouette*, 1920–40; and Kate McKemie and Kay Manuel, interview by author, tape recording, Decatur, Ga., August 3, 1994.

42. *Silhouette* 28 (1932): 199; and *Silhouette* 30 (1934): 166.

43. Gordon, *Gender and Higher Education*, 165–66, 169–72, 181–88.

44. *Silhouette* 18 (1921), 24 (1927), 26 (1929), and 36 (1940): 126–27, 138, 141, 144.

45. Solomon, *In the Company of Educated Women*, 47–48, 65, 70, 76.

46. *Annual Report of the President of Smith College*, 1899–1900: 16, and 1900–01: 16. Accounts of later decades are Dorothy S. Ainsworth, "Recreational Trends in Physical Education at Smith College," *Smith Alumnae Quarterly* 27 (May 1936): 255–57; and Rita Benson and Helen Russell, interview with author, Northampton, Mass., March 1, 1996.

47. Ainsworth, "The Sportswoman Prior to 1920," 1, NAPECW speech, December 1963, Box 6, Folder: Speeches, 1928–1963, Papers of Dorothy S. Ainsworth, SCA-SC.

48. Ainsworth, "Speech given at the Springfield College Women's Physical Education Club, November 1956," 4–5, Box 6, Folder: Speeches, 1964–1969, Ainsworth Papers.

49. Dorothy S. Ainsworth, "Report of the Director of Physical Education," in *Annual Report of the President of Smith College, 1939–40*, 24–25.

50. Minutes, February 23, 1937, Box 1292, Folder: Athletic Association, Minutes, 1935–1942, Records of the Athletic Association, in Collection 80: Students–Athletics and Activities, SCA-SC. (Hereafter, collection cited as AA Records.)

51. Quotations from "Thoughts and Reflections of a Marvelously Rewarding Year as President of the Athletic Association," 1965–66, Box 1292.1, Folder: Athletic Association, Records, President's, 1960s; and "The Constitution and By-Laws of the Smith College Athletic Association, 1924–1925," 13, Box 1291, Folder: Constitutions, By-Laws, and Handbooks, 1911–Present, AA Records.

52. Minutes, October 9, 1941, Box 1292, Folder: Athletic Association, Minutes, 1935–1942, AA Records.

53. See Box 1295.1, Folder: Basketball, 1923, and Box 1295.2, Folder: Basketball Record Book, 1913–14 through 1930–31, in Coll. 80: Students–Athletics and Activities; quotation from 1925–26.

54. Marilyn Gardner, "After 41 Years, She Won't Plan Ahead," *Milwaukee Journal*, May 20, 1960, 8; and Althea Heimbach, "History of Physical Education at Milwaukee-Downer College" (rev. ed., 1960).

55. Elizabeth Dickerson, 14, typed records for 1908–1913, and Beatrice J. Pearson, 13, handwritten records for 1913–1919, in volume: "Department of Physical Education," Heimbach Papers.

56. Programs for annual regattas, June 9, 1928, and June 12, 1937, Heimbach Papers.

57. *Constitution and By-Laws of the Athletic Association of Milwaukee-Downer College, 1919*, 6–7; *Constitution and By-Laws of the Athletic Association of Milwaukee-Downer College, 1936*, 8, 10; and Class Books: Sports and Activities, in Heimbach Papers.

58. Elizabeth Ludwig, "Swimming without a Tank at Milwaukee-Downer College," *Sportswoman* 6 (September 1929): 18, 29.

59. Examples from WAA Minutes, 2 (December 4, 1914): 20; 3 (October 19, 1931): 64 (quotation); 3 (February 12, 1934): 134; 3 (May 21, 1934): 141; and 3 (November 16, 1934): 158, Heimbach Papers.

60. WAA Minutes, letter from Louise Marty and Dorothy Richmond to Milwaukee-Downer Seminary, 2: March 20, 1919, Heimbach Papers.

61. WAA Minutes, 3 (October 26, 1931): 65, Heimbach Papers.

62. WAA Minutes, 3 (September 24, 1934): 155–56; and 3 (November 14, 1934): 157, Heimbach Papers.

63. WAA Minutes, 3 (September 24, 1934): 154–55; 3 (September 30, 1934): 156; 3 (February 12, 1935): 166; 3 (November 16, 1937): 235–36; 3 (January 10, 1941): 297; 3 (February 27, 1941): 298; 4 (November 4, 1941): 13–15; and 4 (November 11, 1948): 77, Heimbach Papers.

64. "W.A.A. Awards," typed and handwritten report, Box 1, vol. 1926–1928, WAA Records, BHL-UM.

65. Godfrey, "Organization," 20–29; and Boxes 8 and 14, Trilling Files, SA-UW (82/50).

66. Godfrey, "Organization," 93–94, 108–10; Norma M. Leavitt and Margaret M. Duncan, "The Status of Intramural Programs for Women," *RQ* 8 (March 1937): 77; and Scott, "Competition," 62.

67. Mabel Lee, "The Case For and Against Intercollegiate Athletics for Women and the Situation as It Stands To-Day," *APER* 29 (1924): 120–21; and Janet Owen, *Sports in Women's Colleges* (New York: New York Tribune, 1932).

68. Stephen Isaac St. Clair, "The Play Day/Sport Day Movement in Selected Colleges of the South" (Ed.D. diss., University of North Carolina at Greensboro, 1984), 93–117.

69. Owen, *Sports*, 19; and Solomon, *In the Company of Educated Women*, 142.

70. James B. Munn, "The Washington Square College," in *New York University: 1832–1932*, ed. Theodore Francis Jones (New York: New York University Press, 1933), 379–90; and Owen, *Sports*, 23–24.

71. Basketball folders (2.5–7); and "Athletics for Girls," ca. 1934, Folder: Bessie Rudd and Other Staff, Radio Scripts and Speeches (6.12), in Records of the Department of Physical Education of Pembroke College, University Archives, John Hay Library, Brown University, Providence, R.I.

72. Owen, *Sports*, 40–41; and Terri Dean Riffe, "A History of Women's Sports at the University of Arizona" (Ph.D. diss., University of Arizona, 1986).

73. Horowitz, *Alma Mater*, 105–33; and Helen Lefkowitz Horowitz, *The Power and Passion of M. Carey Thomas* (New York: Knopf, 1994).

74. Horowitz, *Power and Passion*, 226–27, 230–32, 341–43, 364–65, 381–83, 397–99, 422–23, 428–29, 448; and Linda M. Perkins, "The African American Female Elite: The Early History of African American Women in the Seven Sister Colleges, 1880–1960," *Harvard Educational Review* 67 (Winter 1997): 733–37.

75. Examples from Thomas's letters to Applebee; see Reel 107 (LB 31): 10 (November 16, 1904), and 419 (March 21, 1905); Reel 108 (LB 32): 22 (April 7, 1905), 42 (April 14, 1905), and 307 (June 5, 1905); Reel 109 (LB 33): 53 (October 12, 1905) and 483 (February 19, 1906); Reel 117 (LB 42): 174 (December 1, 1908); and Reel 121 (LB 46): 494 (November 21, 1910), microfilm correspondence, Papers of M. Carey Thomas, College Archives, Mariam Coffin Canaday Library, Bryn Mawr College, Bryn Mawr, Penn. (Hereafter, depository cited as BMC.)

76. Horowitz, *Power and Passion*, 11–17, 297–98, 309–11.

77. Cynthia Wesson, "Miss C. M. K. Applebee: A Sketch of Forty Years of Service," *RQ* 12, suppl. (October 1941): 696–99; and "Constance Applebee," in *Encyclopedia of World Biography Supplement* 24 (Thomson Gale, 2005), http://galenet.galegroup.com/servlet/BioRC, document no. K1631008233.

78. Athletic Association annual reports, 1913–14 and 1917–18, Box 1, vols. 1 (1891–1916) and 2 (1916–30); and Board minutes, January 21, 1921, Box 2, Volume: AA Board Meeting Minutes, 1917–26, in Records of Physical Education Department (PED), BMC.

79. Godfrey, "Organization," 93–94; and Scott, "Competition," 63.

80. Susan K. Cahn, *Coming on Strong: Gender and Sexuality in Twentieth-Century Women's Sport* (New York: Free Press, 1994), 96–98, 129–30.

81. "Regulations Concerning Basket Ball," Reel 107 (LB 31): 419 (March 21, 1905); Thomas to Applebee, Reel 108 (LB 32): 307 (June 5, 1905); and Thomas to Applebee, Reel 114 (LB 38): 406 (March 14, 1908), Thomas Papers.

82. See obituary, *New York Times*, May 7, 1960; and Cornelia Meigs, *What Makes a College? A History of Bryn Mawr* (New York: Macmillan, 1956), 121–78.

83. Fass, *Damned and the Beautiful*, 294–95; and Perkins, "Female Elite," 735–36.

84. Minutes, May 22, 1924, and May 26, 1924, Box 2, Volume: AA Board Meeting Minutes, 1917–26, PED Records, BMC.

85. Thelin, *History*, 183; and Gordon, *Gender and Higher Education*, 25. Though describing earlier decades, these phrases apply equally well to the interwar years.

86. Horowitz, *Campus Life*, 205–15; Solomon, *In the Company of Educated Women*, 164–69; and Thelin, *History*, 228–31.

87. Thelin, *History*, 243–45.

88. Orrin Leslie Elliott, *Stanford University: The First Twenty-Five Years* (1937; repr., New York: Arno, 1977), 187–98, 224–48; Elizabeth K. Zimmerli, "A History of Physical Education for Women at Stanford University and a Survey of the Department of Physical Education for Women in 1943–1944" (Ed.D. diss., Stanford University, 1945), 24–25, 51, 59–71, 101–6; and WAA Minutes, Box 4, vol. 1 (1902–1910), Records of WAA-WRA, Department of Special Collections, Stanford University Libraries, Stanford University, Stanford, Calif. (Hereafter, depository cited as SC-SU.)

89. Lynne Emery, "The First Intercollegiate Contest for Women: Basketball, April 4, 1896," in *Her Story in Sport: A Historical Anthology of Women in Sport*, ed. Reet Howell (West Point, N.Y.: Leisure Press, 1982), 417–23.

90. Elliott, *Stanford University*, 219–48.

91. WAA Minutes, February 17, 1903, Box 4, vol. 1 (1902–1910): 20, WAA-WRA Records, SC-SU.

92. Thelin, *History*, 183.

93. Larry Cuban, *How Scholars Trumped Teachers: Change Without Reform in University Curriculum, Teaching, and Research, 1890–1990* (New York: Teachers College Press, Columbia University, 1999), 16–21; and Thelin, *History*, 138–40.

94. Elliott, *Stanford University*, 132–36; Gordon, *Gender and Higher Education*, 43–44; Levine, *American College*, 123–25; and Solomon, *In the Company of Educated Women*, 58–59, 70.

95. Cuban, *How Scholars Trumped Teachers*, 21–27, 36; and Rebecca S. Lowen, *Creating the Cold War University: The Transformation of Stanford* (Berkeley: University of California Press, 1997), 18–26.

96. Thelin, *History*, 244.

97. Lowen, *Creating the Cold War University*, 20.

98. Thelin, *History*, 244.

99. J. Pearce Mitchell, *Stanford University, 1916–1941* (Stanford, Calif.: Stanford University Press, 1958), 123–35.

100. Florence C. Burrell, "Intercollegiate Athletics for Women in Coeducational Institutions," *APER* 22 (1917): 17–19.

101. *President's Report, 1915*, 101. The WAA disobeyed the ban by conducting extramural events (Zimmerli, "History," 109).

102. Helen Masters Bunting, Chairman, "Women's Athletics," in *President's Report, 1920*, 237.

103. Elizabeth Griego, "The Making of a 'Misfit': Clelia Duel Mosher, 1863–1940," in *Lone Voyagers: Academic Women in Coeducational Institutions, 1870–1937*, ed. Geraldine Jonçich Clifford (New York: Feminist Press, 1989), 147–82.

104. Zimmerli, "History," 4–8, 45, 81, 91–92.

105. Griego, "'Misfit,'" 161.

106. On her impatience with Bunting, see Mosher diary, May 26, 1926, Box 1, Folder 10, Papers of Clelia Duel Mosher, SC-SU.

107. See Box 1, Folder: Bunting, 1929–30; Box 2, Folder: B, 1930–31; Box 3, Folder: B, 1932–33; and Bertha S. Dyment to Robert E. Swaim, October 21, 1931, Box 3, Folder: President, 1931–32, Papers of the Department of Physical Education for Women, SC-SU. (Hereafter, collection cited as DPEW Papers.)

108. For example, "Stanford-U.C. Women's Hockey," *Stanford Illustrated Review* 25 (December 1923): 142.

109. "Minutes of the Triangle Conference," February 7, 1925, Box 9, Folder 13: Triangular Sports Days, 1919–1952, WAA-WRA Records, SC-SU.

110. See "Minutes of Triangle Conference," January 23, 1926, Box 9, Folder 13, WAA-WRA Records, SC-SU; and scrapbooks in Papers of the Women's Athletic Association, Bancroft Library, University of California at Berkeley, Berkeley, Calif. (Hereafter, depository cited as BL-UCB.)

111. See Helen Crane, "Inter-collegiate Athletics" (prepared for ACACW newsletter, 1926), Folder: ARFCW-Miscellaneous, Papers of the Women's Division of the National Amateur Athletic Federation, BL-UCB.

112. FCWA annual reports in *President's Report*, 1925:245; 1926:225; 1927:242; 1928:254–55; and 1929:386; and Staff minutes, February 4, 1926, January 27, 1928, and February 24, 1928 (quotation), Box 1, Folder: Staff Minutes and Newsletters, 1924–25 through 1927–28, DPEW Papers, SC-SU. (Citations indicate date of meeting, not minutes preparation.)

113. Letter from Maxine Cushing, Stanford Sports Day Chairman, to Roberta Davenport, Berkeley, February 24, 1928, Box 9, Folder 13, WAA-WRA Records, SC-SU.

114. Staff minutes, February 24, 1928, Box 1, Folder: Staff Minutes and Newsletters, 1924–25 through 1927–28, DPEW Records, SC-SU.

115. Helen Masters Bunting, "Women's Athletics," in *President's Report*, 1929:386.

116. Cuban, *How Scholars Trumped Teachers*, 27–29; Lowen, *Creating the Cold War University*; and Thelin, *History*, 243–45.

117. Thelin, *History*, 244.

118. Zimmerli, "History," 9, 47.

119. "Report of Triangle Sports Day, November 2, 1929, submitted by Elisabeth Larsh, Stanford Manager," Box 9, Folder 13; and WAA Minutes, November 5, 1929, February 25, 1930, and April 8, 1930, Box 4, vol. 4 (1926–1935): 123, 135, 139–40 (quotation), WAA-WRA Records, SC-SU.

120. Minutes from WAA Council, November 19, 1929; "Review of W.A.A. Fall 1929," 2; and "Review of W.A.A. Spring 1930" (quotation), Folder: WAA Advisor's Reports, Fall 1925–Spring 1930, WAA Records, BL-UCB.

121. On the plan's adoption, see "Minutes of Triangular Sports Day Committee," February 14, 1931, Box 9, Folder 13, WAA-WRA Records, SC-SU. On Stanford's position, see WAA Minutes, February 24, 1931, Box 4, vol. 4 (1926–1935): 158, WAA-WRA Records; and "The Triangular Athletic Meet for Women" (probably October 31, 1931), Box 3, Folder: T, 1931–32, DPEW Papers, SC-SU.

122. See letter from Barbara Ross (Berkeley WAA) to Gertrude (Stanford WAA), April 8, 1931, Box 9, Folder 13, WAA-WRA Records, SC-SU; and "Review of W.A.A. Spring 1931," "Review of W.A.A. Fall 1931," and WAA Council notes, October 20, 1931, November 10, 1931, and November 1, 1932 (quotation), Folder: WAA Advisor's Reports, Fall 1930–Spring 1935, WAA Records, BL-UCB.

123. See letters from Mary C. Walker (TSD Manager, Mills) to Ruth Fisher (WAA President, Stanford), October 11, 1932, and October 25, 1932, Box 9, Folder 13, WAA-WRA Records, SC-SU.

124. For Stanford's proposal, see letter from Babe Dear (WAA President, Stanford) to Nat (Berkeley or Mills), ca. 1932–34, Box 9, Folder 13, WAA-WRA Records, SC-SU. For Berkeley's objections, see WAA Council notes, October 11, 1932, and November 9, 1932 (quotation), Folder: WAA Advisor's Reports, Fall 1930–Spring 1935, WAA Records, BL-UCB.

125. WAA Minutes, April 5, 1932, April 19, 1932, and April 26, 1932, Box 4, vol. 4 (1926–1935): 184, 187, 188; and letter from Ruth Fisher to Miss Gertrude Hawley, February 5, 1933, Box 9, Folder 13, WAA-WRA Records; and letter from Ruth Fisher to Dr. Dyment, April 5, 1933, Box 4, Folder: W, 1932–33, DPEW Papers, SC-SU.

126. Typical discussions are Staff minutes, January 6, 1932, January 23, 1932, April 22, 1932, and May 6, 1932, Box 3, Folder: Staff, 1931–32; and Staff minutes, March 18, 1933, April 7, 1933, and April 14, 1933, Box 4, Folder: Minutes of Staff Meetings, 1932–33, DPEW Papers, SC-SU. Professional consultations include letter from Gertrude Hawley to Agnes R. Wayman, May 4, 1932; Wayman to Hawley, May 11, 1932; Hawley to Blanche Trilling, May 12, 1932; Hawley to Rosalind Cassidy (Mills College), May 13, 1932; and Trilling to Hawley, May 27, 1932, Box 3, Folder: Director, Roble Gym, 1931–32, DPEW Papers, SC-SU.

127. "Annual Report to the President, 1933," 10–11, Box 4, Folder: President, 1932–33, DPEW Papers, SC-SU.

128. On Stanford's proposal, see Dear to Nat, ca. 1932–34; "Minutes for the Triangular Sports-Day Conference, October 20, 1934"; and letter from Jane Dearing to Marjorie McLaren, November 3, 1934, Box 9, Folder 13, WAA-WRA Records, SC-SU. On Berkeley, see WAA Council notes, January 30, 1934, October 23, 1934, and October 30, 1934, Folder: WAA Advisor's Reports, Fall 1930–Spring 1935, WAA Records, BL-UCB; and letter from Helen Avilla to Jane Dearing, November 2, 1934, Box 9, Folder 13, WAA-WRA Records, SC-SU. On Mills, see WAA Minutes, January 17, 1934, October 31, 1934, and November 14, 1934, Box 4, vol. 4 (1926–1935): 242, 265, 268; and letter from Marjorie McLaren to Jane Dearing, October 29, 1934, and McLaren to Dearing, November 7, 1934, Box 9, Folder 13, WAA-WRA Records, SC-SU.

129. On non-TSD overtures, see WAA Minutes, December 5, 1934, January 16, 1935, and February 6, 1935, Box 4, vol. 4 (1926–1935): 272, 276, 279–80, WAA-WRA Records, SC-SU. On TSD efforts, see WAA Minutes, March 3, 1937, November (n.d.) 1939, and January 8, 1941, Box 4, vol. 5 (May 1935–1941): 97–98, 213, 259; "Minutes of Tri-Sports Day Committee Meeting," November 27, 1941, Box 6, Folder 2: Correspondence, 1940–43; and Minutes of TSD meeting, February 27, 1937, October 12, 1940, and November 27, 1943, Box 9, Folder 13, WAA-WRA Records, SC-SU.

130. Staff minutes, March 27, 1947, November 25, 1947, and December 9, 1947, Box 1, Folder: WPE Staff meeting minutes, 1946–47 through 1948–49, DPEW Papers, SC-SU.

131. Roberta J. Park, "History and Structure of the Department of Physical Education at the University of California, with Special Reference to Women's Sports," in Howell, *Her Story in Sport*, 413–15.

132. Levine, *American College*, 158–60; and Solomon, *In the Company of Educated Women*, 147.

133. Thelin, *History*, 232.

134. Perkins, "Female Elite," 719.

135. Henry N. Drewry and Humphrey Doermann, *Stand and Prosper: Private Black Colleges and Their Students* (Princeton, N.J.: Princeton University Press, 2001), 45–53, 70–98; Solomon, *In the Company of Educated Women*, 144–45; and Thelin, *History*, 232–33.

136. James D. Anderson, "The Hampton Model of Normal School Industrial Education, 1868–1900," in *New Perspectives on Black Educational History*, ed. Vincent P. Franklin and James D. Anderson (Boston: G. K. Hall, 1978), 61, 62. As nurses, teachers, and community volunteers, however, many alumnae improved the lives of ordinary blacks in ways that Hampton's leaders never intended.

137. Ibid., 85–90.

138. *Hampton Institute Annual Report, 1912*, 10; Thomas Jesse Jones, *Negro Education: A Study of the Private and Higher Schools for Colored People in the United States*, Bureau of Education Bulletin, 1916, no. 39 (Washington, D.C.: GPO, 1917), 2:625; and Arthur J. Klein, *Survey of Negro Colleges and Universities*, Bureau of Education Bulletin, 1928, no. 7 (Washington, D.C.: GPO, 1926; repr., New York: Negro Universities Press, 1969), 884, 894.

139. I based this conclusion on Biographical Data, Boxes 5–13, Records of the Alumnae Association (7H): Hygiene and Physical Education Section, WCA; and faculty cards and personnel files of Hampton staff members, Archives, Hampton University, Hampton, Va. (Hereafter, depository cited as HUA.)

140. Summary based on Hampton's *Annual Report*, annual *Catalogue*, student yearbook, and faculty publications from the 1880s–1920s. Unpublished sources include the annual reports of the girls' physical education department, available in Box: "Physical Education, 1893, Box 4," Folder C, Records of School of Education: Division of Physical Education (Series 19, Subgroup 11), HUA. (Hereafter, collection cited as PE Records.)

141. *Catalogue of the Hampton Normal and Agricultural Institute, 1913*, 79.

142. Lucy Agnes Pratt, "Rational Physical Training," *Southern Workman* 31 (March 1902): 160. A BNSG graduate (1895), Pratt taught at Hampton in 1897–1904 and then at private schools in Boston.

143. Jessie Coope to Principal Frissell, January 13, 1911, Box: "Physical Education, 1893, Box 4," Folder C, PE Records; and Jessie Coope, "Gymnastic Games," *Southern Workman* 33 (February 1904): 82. A BNSG graduate (1897), Coope taught at Hampton in 1897–1900 and 1901–12, and then worked for thirty-one years in the public schools of Washington, D.C.

144. Grace H. Howes to Principal Frissell, May 1, 1895, 3, Box: "Physical Education, 1893, Box 4," Folder C, PE Records. A BNSG graduate (1896), Howes taught at Hampton in 1893–95.

145. Jessie Coope to Principal Frissell, January 12, 1903, Box: "Physical Education, 1893, Box 4," Folder C, PE Records.

146. Olive B. Rowell, "Report of the Director of Physical Training for Girls, February 1, 1920," 5, Box: "Physical Education, 1893, Box 4," Folder C, PE Records. A Vassar alumna, Rowell earned an HPE certificate at Wellesley (1919) and taught at Hampton in 1919–23.

147. Quoted phrases from *Forty-Ninth Annual Report of the Principal, 1917*, 14; and Pratt, "Rational," 160.

148. Rowell, "Report, 1920," 4, PE Records.

149. Howes to Frissell, May 1, 1895, 4 (quotation); Rowell, "Report, 1920"; and Jessie Coope to Dr. Frissell, February 1, 1912, Box: "Physical Education, 1893, Box 4," Folder C, PE Records.

150. Poem by Naomi Reed, quoted in Elizabeth D. Dunham, "Hampton Institute, Virginia," *APER* 30 (1925): 40–41.

151. Coope to Frissell, January 13, 1911, PE Records (quotation); and Elizabeth D. Dunham, "Physical Education of Women at Hampton Institute," *Southern Workman* 53 (April 1924): 166–67.

152. Klein, *Survey*, 885, 888–94; and William Hannibal Robinson, "The History of Hampton Institute, 1868–1948" (Ph.D. diss., New York University, 1954), 134–64.

153. Eric Anderson and Alfred A. Moss Jr., *Dangerous Donations: Northern Philanthropy and Southern Black Education, 1902–1930* (Columbia: University of Missouri Press, 1999), 191–218; and Drewry and Doermann, *Stand and Prosper*, 70–98.

154. Drewry and Doermann, *Stand and Prosper*, 59–60, 81–84, 88; and Raymond Wolters, *The New Negro on Campus: Black College Rebellions of the 1920s* (Princeton, N.J.: Princeton University Press, 1975), 16–18.

155. Drewry and Doermann, *Stand and Prosper*, 86–88; and Monroe H. Little, "The Extra-Curricular Activities of Black College Students, 1868–1940," *Journal of Negro History* 65 (1980): 135–48.

156. Quoted in Thelin, *History*, 187.

157. Solomon, *In the Company of Educated Women*, 159.

158. James D. Anderson, *The Education of Blacks in the South, 1860–1935* (Chapel Hill: University of North Carolina Press, 1988), 274 (quotation); and Wolters, *New Negro*, 253–69.

159. Robinson, "History," 148–64; and Wolters, *New Negro*, 230–75.

160. Wolters, *New Negro*, 273–75.

161. Robinson, "History," 174–221.

162. Williams later earned a physical education diploma and M.Ed. at Harvard.

163. Charles H. Williams, "Report of the Department of Physical Education, February 10, 1931," 15, Box: "PE Syllabus; FR and SO Classes; PE Dept; PE Medical Excuses; Annual Reports," PE Records. (Hereafter, box cited as Syllabi and Reports.)

164. Based on *Annual Catalogue*, faculty cards, faculty files, and student/graduate cards and alumnae files for teachers who were Hampton alumnae, HUA.

165. Baker's faculty card and faculty file, HUA, strongly suggest that Baker was white.

166. *Annual Catalogue* (1920s–1940s) and Wood's faculty card and faculty file, HUA, strongly suggest that Wood was white.

167. I based this conclusion on Hampton's *Annual Catalogue*, and faculty cards and personnel files, HUA, especially each teacher's baccalaureate institution.

168. From faculty card and faculty file, HUA; *Tuskegee Messenger* 10 (July 1934): 2; obituary, *New York Times*, December 21, 1994; and Papers of Charlotte Moton Hubbard, Manuscript Division, Moorland-Spingarn Research Center, Howard University, Washington, D.C. After teaching at Hampton in 1934–41, Moton became a sought-after expert in human relations and public affairs.

169. From Hampton Institute *Annual Catalogue;* and Nina Jo Woolley Smith, "'Out of Adversity, We Survived': Oral Histories of Seven Black Women Physical Educators" (master's thesis, San Francisco State University, 1992), 123.

170. Robinson, "History," 168–69, 178–85, 197–98, 200–201, 203–5.

171. Extant copies of annual reports are found in Box: Syllabi and Reports, PE Records, HUA.

172. Earl Henry Duvall Jr., "An Historical Analysis of the Central Intercollegiate Athletic Association and Its Influence on the Development of Black Intercollegiate Athletics: 1912–1984" (Ph.D. diss., Kent State University, 1985), 104.

173. Annual Report, 1938:6, PE Records.

174. Annual Report, 1931:1–2, PE Records.

175. Annual Report, 1936:7–8; and 1937:5–6, PE Records.

176. Annual Report, 1931:5–6 (quotation); 1938:1–2; 1939:1–2; 1940:1–3; and 1941:15–17, PE Records.

177. Quoted phrases from Annual Report, 1938:1; and 1939:2, PE Records.

178. Patrick B. Miller, "To 'Bring the Race along Rapidly': Sport, Student Culture, and Educational Mission at Historically Black Colleges during the Interwar Years," *History of Education Quarterly* 35 (1995): 111–33.

179. Information gleaned from the Institute's *Annual Catalogue*, student yearbook (*Log* and *Hamptonian*), and Williams's annual reports.

180. Baker, "Department of Physical Education, Women, 1934–35," 2, included in Williams, Annual Report, 1935; and Williams, Annual Report, 1939:7, PE Records.

181. Annual Report, 1936:11–12; and 1937:8, PE Records.

182. Baker, "Department of Physical Education-Women, 1931–1932," in Williams, Annual Report, 1932:9, PE Records.

183. Arthur Howe to Mary C. Baker, June 3, 1937; Howe to Baker, September 23, 1937; Charles H. Williams to Bureau of Appointments, School of Education, New York University, July 13, 1937; and unsigned, undated letter to Teachers College, Columbia University, in Baker faculty file, HUA.

184. Williams, Annual Report, 1939:6, PE Records.

185. *Hamptonian*, 1941, 99.

186. Williams, Annual Report, 1941:8, PE Records.

187. John O. Perpener III, *African-American Concert Dance: The Harlem Renaissance and Beyond* (Urbana: University of Illinois Press, 2001), 78–100.

188. Ibid., 80–81, 83.

189. Ibid., 84, 89–90; and Wolters, *New Negro*, 240.

190. Perpener, *African-American Concert Dance*, 84–86, 92.

191. Ibid., 91–93, 98–99; and Charles H. Williams, "The Hampton Institute Creative Dance Group," *Dance Observer* 4 (October 1937): 97–98. The ensemble's first off-campus concert at the Mosque Theatre in Richmond, Virginia, in 1935 was legendary.

192. "Statement of Plan of Work" (application to Rosenwald Fund, 1941), 2, 3, in Moton faculty file, HUA.

193. Ibid., 3.

194. This negotiation explains the restraint that many dance critics, especially white reviewers, observed in Institute performances; see Perpener, *African-American Concert Dance*, 93–97.

195. Ibid., 87, 91.

196. Ramsay Burt, "The Trouble with the Male Dancer . . . ," in *The Male Dancer: Bodies, Spectacle, Sexualities* (London: Routledge, 1995), 13.

197. Jennifer Terry, *An American Obsession: Science, Medicine, and Homosexuality in Modern Society* (Chicago: University of Chicago Press, 1999), 87–97, 114–19.

198. Perpener, *African-American Concert Dance*, 87, 88. Other black male dancers and choreographers were less conventional.

199. Jones, *Negro Education*, 2:62, 66–67.

200. Jones, *Negro Education*, 2:62–67; and Cynthia Neverdon-Morton, *Afro-American Women of the South and the Advancement of the Race, 1895–1925* (Knoxville: University of Tennessee Press, 1989), 32–38.

201. Stephanie J. Shaw, *What a Woman Ought to Be and to Do: Black Professional Women Workers During the Jim Crow Era* (Chicago: University of Chicago Press, 1996), 84–85, 128–29; and Donald Spivey, *Schooling for the New Slavery: Black Industrial Education, 1868–1915* (Westport, Conn.: Greenwood Press, 1978), 52–63.

202. Anderson, *Education of Blacks*, 102–5.

203. Jones, *Negro Education*, 2:65; Klein, *Survey*, 99–100; and Neverdon-Morton, *Afro-American Women*, 122–38.

204. Anderson, *Education of Blacks*, 102–9, 245–49, 270–72.

205. *Annual Catalogue*, 1887–88:n.p. (boys); 1895–96:40 (girls); and 1905–06:47 (girls).

206. Typical announcements in the *Tuskegee Student* include 18 (January 20, 1906); 20 (January 18, 1908); and 20 (May 23, 1908).

207. *Annual Catalogue*, 1898–99:20, and 1905–06:45.

208. *Annual Catalogue*, 1887–88 (boys), and 1905–06:46 (girls).

209. *Annual Catalogue*, 1905–06:46–47.

210. From Thomas's forms in student records of HPE Papers, WCA; and Biographical Data: Classes 1891–1900, in Records of the Alumnae Association: HPE, WCA.

211. *Annual Catalogue*, 1933–34:14; and Armstead A. Pierro, "A History of Professional Preparation for Physical Education in Some Selected Negro Colleges and Universities, 1924–1958" (Ph.D. diss., University of Michigan, 1962), 45, 67. In about 1909, Cromwell married Ezra Roberts, who directed the Institute's Academic Studies division.

212. For example, *Annual Catalogue*, 1915–16:45, and 1921–22:51–52.

213. Numerous reports appeared in the school newspaper and student yearbook; for instance, *Tuskegee Student* 34 (March 1924): 6; *Tuskegee Messenger* 2 (February 27, 1926): 3; and *The Crimson and Gold, 1927*: Owen J. Duncan, "Athletics at Tuskegee," and Hattie Lindsay, "Girls' Basketball."

214. Cahn, *Coming on Strong*, 36–41, 117–39; and Grundy, *Learning to Win*, 136–40, 234–45.

215. "All Work and No Play," *Tuskegee Messenger* 9 (October 1933): 1. The male icon probably alluded to handsome bodies rather than the ancient god of music and poetry. The female image invoked the Roman goddess of animals, forests, and hunting, as well as women teachers' Diana Athletic Club.

216. Pierro, "History," 45.

217. "Interview with Jessie Abbott," in *Black Women Oral History Project*, ed. Ruth Edmonds Hill (Westport, Conn.: Meckler, 1991), 1:1–37. (Hereafter, cited as *BWOHP*.) The Abbotts's daughter was a talented athlete as well; a Tuskegee graduate, she was instrumental in developing women's track and field at Tennessee State during the mid-1940s.

218. See *Annual Catalogue*, 1933–34:4; and Nolan A. Thaxton, "A Documentary Analysis of Competitive Track and Field for Women at Tennessee State A&I University and Tuskegee Institute" (Ph.D. diss., Springfield College, 1970), 71–72, 86–87.

219. "Coach Abbott Addresses Y.M.C.A.," *Tuskegee Student* 34 (March 1924): 7; Cleve Abbott, "A Close Up of Physical Education and Athletics at Tuskegee," n.d., in Box 31: Abbott, Papers of Ross C. Owen, Archives, Tuskegee University, Tuskegee, Ala. (hereafter, cited as UA-TU); and untitled handwritten notes, n.d., Box 3, Papers of Nell Cecilia Jackson, UA-TU.

220. Cahn, *Coming on Strong*, 134–35.

221. "Department of Physical Education for Boys," in *Annual Catalogue*, 1925–26:84–85.

222. Amelia C. Roberts, letter to editor, *Chicago Defender*, March 12, 1927, Part 1:9.

223. *Annual Catalogue*, 1930–31:77–78.

224. Cahn, *Coming on Strong*, 121–23; and Cindy Himes Gissendanner, "African-American Women and Competitive Sport, 1920–1960," in *Women, Sport, and Culture*, ed. Susan Birrell and Cheryl L. Cole (Champaign, Ill.: Human Kinetics, 1994), 88.

225. See "All Work," 1, 8; and "Hats Off to the Tennis Champions and Runners-Up," *Tuskegee Messenger* 10 (September 1934): 2, 8.

226. "Hats Off," 2, 8; and Gissendanner, "Competitive Sport," 88.

227. G. Lake Imes, "To Tuskegee," in *Robert Russa Moton of Hampton and Tuskegee*, ed. William Hardin Hughes and Frederick D. Patterson (Chapel Hill: University of North Carolina Press, 1956), 91–92; and "Hats Off," 2.

228. Typescript, ca. 1934–35, in Local Correspondence folder: A-Cleve Abbott, Box LC 62, Papers of Robert Russa Moton, UA-TU.

229. Wolters, *New Negro*, 142.

230. Anderson, *Education of Blacks*, 34, 257–61.

231. Miller, "To 'Bring the Race,'" 122n21.

232. Anderson, *Education of Blacks*, 270–73; Imes, "To Tuskegee," 81, 96–97; and Wolters, *New Negro*, 145.

233. Anderson, *Education of Blacks*, 253–63, 272–78.

234. Wolters, *New Negro*, 146.

235. Ibid., 151–91; and *Chronicles of Faith: The Autobiography of Frederick D. Patterson*, ed. Martia Graham Goodson (Tuscaloosa: The University of Alabama Press, 1991), 50–51, 111–12.

236. Obituary, *New York Times*, April 27, 1988; and *Chronicles of Faith*.

237. *Chronicles of Faith*, 30, 45, 66–82, 84–100.

238. Ibid., 28–29, 110–11.

239. Pierro, "History," 259. According to Whitney Van Cleve, a student-athlete of the late 1940s who later joined Tuskegee's staff, Patterson neither obstructed nor encouraged varsity sports (interview by author, tape recording, Tuskegee, Ala., July 28, 1994).

240. See *Annual Catalogue*, 1936–37:150–55; *Loganite, 1936–37*, 86; and Frances Davis, "Tuskegee's Crack Girls Team Writes New Saga of Cinder Path Conquest for the Race," *Tuskegee Service* 4 (November 1939): 28–30. Ballard graduated with a B.S. in Physical Education in 1936.

241. Thaxton, "Documentary Analysis," 86–87, 110, 154, 156, 187–89.

242. Abbott, "Close Up," in Owen Papers; Pierro, "History," 259–61, 339; Van Cleve, interview; and Henry Hooten, interview by author, tape recording, Tuskegee, Ala., July 28, 1994.

243. Hooten, interview.

244. Cahn, *Coming on Strong*, 110–11 (quotation), 119–20; Gissendanner, "Competitive Sport," 85–86; and Thaxton, "Documentary Analysis," 77–78, 93, 98–99, 102, 105, 108, 165, 168, 208–9.

245. Davis, "Crack Girls Team," 30.

246. Cahn, *Coming on Strong*, 117, 118. This neglect lasted until the Cold War, when white Americans hailed black athletes as symbols of national pride and social equality.

247. Quotations from Davis, "Crack Girls Team," 29, 30.

248. Handwritten notes for speeches and articles in Box 3, Jackson Papers, UA-TU.

249. Cahn, *Coming on Strong*, 121–25; "Abbott," *BWOHP*, 1:15–16 (quotations), 34; and Nolan A. Thaxton, "Tuskegee Institute: Pioneer in Women's Track & Field," *PE* 29 (May 1972): 78.

250. Thaxton, "Documentary Analysis," 163, 176, 190, 204.

251. Ibid., 73–74, 87–90, 157–63. As Thaxton emphasizes, available data usually represent budget requests, not actual allocations or expenses. Moreover, Abbott had a knack for securing additional funds.

252. *Chronicles of Faith*, 62–64, 82–83; and Wolters, *New Negro*, 141–42.

253. *Chronicles of Faith*, 49, and 49–50, 138–40 in general.

254. Evelyn Brooks Higginbotham, *Righteous Discontent: The Women's Movement in the Black Baptist Church, 1880–1920* (Cambridge, Mass.: Harvard University Press, 1993), 24–31, 114 (quotation); and James M. McPherson, "White Liberals and Black Power in Negro Education, 1865–1915," *American Historical Review* 75 (1970): 1370–74, 1382–83.

255. Higginbotham, *Righteous Discontent*, 24–31, 111–19.

256. Lowe, *Looking Good*, 74 (quotation); and Shaw, *What a Woman*, 69–76, 101–3.

257. Higginbotham, *Righteous Discontent*, 31–33; Lowe, *Looking Good*, 6, 58–59; McPherson, "White Liberals and Black Power," 1383; and Neverdon-Morton, *Afro-American Women*, 42–43, 48.

258. Primary accounts are *Annual Catalogue, 1921–22*, 14 (quotation); and Mabel H. Parsons, "A Day at Spelman," *Spelman Messenger* 25 (November 1908): 2–3.

259. Higginbotham, *Righteous Discontent*, 33–39; and Neverdon-Morton, *Afro-American Women*, 48–53.

260. Klein, *Survey*, 296.

261. Higginbotham, *Righteous Discontent*, 22–23, 32, 241n45; Klein, *Survey*, 296–97; and James M. McPherson, *The Abolitionist Legacy: From Reconstruction to the NAACP*, 2nd ed. (Princeton, N.J.: Princeton University Press, 1995), 157. In 1884 the school was renamed Spelman Seminary to honor Rockefeller's wife and her family.

262. Florence Matilda Read, *The Story of Spelman College* (Princeton, N.J.: Princeton University Press, 1961), 77–81, 229–42; and Patricia Bell Scott, "Schoolin' 'Respectable' Ladies of Color: Issues in the History of Black Women's Higher Education," *Journal of the National Association of Women's Deans, Administrators, and Counselors* 43 (Winter 1979): 24.

263. Higginbotham, *Righteous Discontent*, 47–63; McPherson, "White Liberals and Black Power," 1370–74; and McPherson, *Abolitionist Legacy*, 149, 284–91.

264. McPherson, "White Liberals and Black Power," 1372; and Klein, *Survey*, 295.

265. Jones, *Negro Education*, 2:223; McPherson, "White Liberals and Black Power," 1383; Neverdon-Morton, *Afro-American Women*, 43; and Read, *Story of Spelman College*, 86–87, 310.

266. Information gleaned from the *Athenaeum* (joint Spelman and Atlanta Baptist College student newspaper until 1924), Spelman's *Annual Catalogue*, the *Spelman Messenger*, and Fred Douglas Pullum, "Professional Preparation in Physical Education at Historically Black Institutions in Georgia" (Ed.D. diss., University of Georgia, 1974), 110–16.

267. Dr. J. H. Hanford, "Health Department," *Spelman Messenger* 1 (March 1885): 7.

268. Jane A. Ganderson (English), "College Athletics," *Spelman Messenger* 15 (June 1899): 6.

269. See Hanford, "Health Department"; Fannie L. Showers (Class of 1893), "Physical Culture," *Spelman Messenger* 10 (March 1894): 1–2; and Lucy Hale Tapley (President), "Annual Report," *Spelman Messenger* 41 (April 1925): 5–6.

270. *Athenaeum* 25, no. 7 (April 1923): 153.

271. "Annual Report," *Spelman Messenger* 34, no. 7 (April 1918): 3.

272. Letter from [Dean Lamson?] to principal of Posse Normal School, June 5, 1924, in Personnel Records, Box #40: Shirlie T. Pettee, Archives, Spelman College, Atlanta, Ga. (hereafter, cited as SCA); and letter from President Tapley to Evelyn Sargent, March 11, 1922 (quotation), in Personnel Records, Box #41: Evelyn Sargent, SCA.

273. H.A.M., "Our Leisure Hours," *Spelman Messenger Supplement* 30, no. 5 (February 1914): 3–4.

274. Documents in Personnel Records, SCA, often revealed a teacher's race, directly or indirectly; I found other clues in the *Spelman Messenger* and *Annual Catalogue*.

275. Samples of the application form are found in Personnel Records, SCA.

276. Letter from Ruth Stevens to Lucy Tapley, August 22, 1921, in Personnel Records, Box #42: Stevens, SCA.

277. Neverdon-Morton, *Afro-American Women*, 48.

278. Lowe, *Looking Good*, 125–31.

279. Klein, *Survey*, 296; and Read, *Story of Spelman College*, 190–93, 210–16.

280. Klein, *Survey*, 302; and Read, *Story of Spelman College*, 202, 217, 307–10.

281. Summary based on the *Spelman Messenger*, *Annual Catalogue* entries, and files in Personnel Records, SCA.

282. Lowe, *Looking Good*, 9–10, 103–4, 112–13, 125–31, 149–54.

283. Ibid., 129.

284. Read, *Story of Spelman College*, 248–54.

285. *Annual Catalogue, 1927–28*, 34; see also Jean E. Taylor (1932), "From Gymnastics to Athletics," *Campus Mirror* 7 (May 15, 1931): 1.

286. Marguerite Simon, interview by author, tape recording, Atlanta, Ga., May 28, 1996.

287. *Campus Mirror* 23 (May 1947): 14, and 24 (May 1948): 18.

288. "Walking," *Campus Mirror* 5 (April 1929): 7.

289. *Annual Catalogue, 1927–28*, 47; *Annual Catalogue, 1928–29*, 54; and "Founders Day," *Campus Mirror* 5 (April 1929): 4.

290. *Campus Mirror* 18 (November 15, 1941): 8; 20 (May–June 1944): 31; 21 (January 1945): 4; and "Athletic Council Awards," *Spelman Messenger* 65 (August 1949): 21.

291. Annie Hudson, "The 'Tigers and Lions' Big Thanksgiving Game," *Campus Mirror* 4 (December 15, 1927): 5.

292. Klein, *Survey*, 305.

293. *Campus Mirror* 7 (May 15, 1931): 2; *Campus Mirror* 8 (May–June 1932): 2; and "Spelman at the Tuskegee Relays," *Spelman Messenger* 48 (July 1932): 24.

294. *Campus Mirror* 9 (May–June 1933): 17.

295. "May Day Celebration," *Spelman Messenger* 51 (May 1935): 26.

296. Read to Mr. Favrot, April 27, 1935, in Personnel Records, Box #43: Florence Mae Warwick, SCA.

297. *Annual Catalogue, 1935–36,* 60; *Campus Mirror* 13 (April 15, 1937): 1; and Read, *Story of Spelman College,* 267–68.

298. On the dismissal, see Dean Yomans to President Read and Florence Warwick, December 7, 1937; and Warwick to Read, August 24, 1940, in Personnel Records, Box #43: Warwick. For Read's assessment of Denham, see letter to Credential Secretary, National Foundation for Infantile Paralysis, July 3, 1945, in Personnel Records, Box #6: Denham. In all likelihood, Denham was white; see "An Interview with Miss Julia Denham," *Campus Mirror* 17 (March 1, 1941): 4, 7; and documents in Personnel Records, Box #6: Denham.

299. "Naming of the Health and Recreation Building," *Spelman Messenger* 71 (May 1955): 14.

300. *Annual Catalogue, 1951–52,* 52.

Chapter 6

1. Board Minutes, 2 (November 4, 1903): 4–5, in records of the District of Columbia Public Schools, Charles Sumner School Museum and Archives, Washington, D.C. (hereafter, cited as CSSMA).

2. "Report of Director of Physical Training," *Board Report, 1896–97,* 161–64.

3. Hattie B. George, "Physical Training," *Board Report, 1897–98,* 242.

4. Anita J. Turner, "Report of the Assistant Director of Physical Training," *Board Report, 1916–17,* 270–71.

5. David Tyack and Elisabeth Hansot, *Learning Together: A History of Coeducation in American Public Schools* (New Haven, Conn.: Yale University Press; New York: Russell Sage Foundation, 1990), 99–110, 138, 227–34, 242; and Wayne Urban and Jennings Wagoner Jr., *American Education: A History* (New York: McGraw-Hill, 1996), 168–69.

6. William Dove Thompson, "The Development of Physical Education in the District of Columbia Public Schools" (Ed.D. diss., New York University, 1941), 99–102, 108.

7. Phrase from Philip D. R. Corrigan, "The Making of the Boy: Meditations on What Grammar School Did With, To, and For My Body," *Journal of Education* 170 (1988): 153.

8. Manuscript minutes of Board of Education meetings are available from 1902 on; citations are standardized as Board Minutes, volume (date): pages, CSSMA. Published annual reports of the Board of Trustees to the D.C. Commissioners (1886–99), succeeded by Board of Education reports, are cited as *Board Report, Year,* pages.

9. See Martha Strayer, "Physical Education Pioneer Retires," newspaper clipping, January 14, 1935 (copy obtained from the Washingtoniana Division, Martin Luther King Jr. Memorial Library, Washington, D.C.); and Thompson, "Development," 95–145 passim. On race, see Stoneroad's awkward, often condescending remarks in her reports to the Board of Education: 1900–1901: 131; 1901–02: 138; 1902–03: 160; and 1903–04: 162.

10. Quotations from Stoneroad, "Physical Education of Girls During Childhood and Pubescent Period, or Upper-Grammar and Lower-High-School Age," *APNEA*, 1910: 936–41.

11. Thompson, "Development," 269–79, 309–50, 420–52, 678–96.

12. Chronology gleaned from P. M. Hughes, *Board Report, 1901–02*, 178; Thompson, "Development," 679–80, 690–91; and Board Minutes, 25 (November 9, 1934): 40; 53 (March 6, 1946): 76; 64 (April 20, 1949): 41–42; 64 (May 4, 1949): A9–A15; and 65 (July 1, 1949): 114–16, CSSMA.

13. Turner, "Report," *Board Report, 1916–17*, 271.

14. Thompson, "Development," 170–76, 187–92, 199–207, 661–72.

15. Ibid., 362–73.

16. Examples from ibid., 203–5, 314–16, 430–33, 439, 455, 459, 462–63, 477, 485–86.

17. Board Minutes, 53 (May 1, 1946): 27, CSSMA.

18. Board Minutes, 55 (September 18, 1946): 60–61.

19. Board Minutes, 25 (December 12, 1934): 30. Preliminary discussions, including the football incident, are Board Minutes, 25 (November 7, 1934): 33–34; and 25 (November 9, 1934): 35–48.

20. Board Minutes, 25 (January 9, 1935): 28–29 (quotation); 25 (January 16, 1935): 33; and 25 (May 1–8, 1935): 22–23.

21. Board Minutes, 25 (May 1–8, 1935): 22–23; and 26 (July 1, 1935): 36.

22. Obituary, *New York Times*, August 27, 1971; and Indiana State Athletics Hall of Fame entry, http://www.indstate.edu/athletics/bbayh.html (accessed January 29, 2004). Bayh headed the District's program for nearly three decades. His son, Birch Bayh Jr., was instrumental in passing Title IX while serving as a U.S. Senator (D-Ind.) during the 1970s.

23. Board Minutes, 25 (January 16, 1935): 33; and 26 (July 1, 1935): 36–37.

24. Board Minutes, 36 (September 11, 1940): 109–11; and 36 (September 18, 1940): 41–42.

25. A distinguished member of the District's black elite, Henderson was a lifelong civil rights activist and NAACP leader, a scholar and organizer of sports for African Americans, and prolific writer of opinion pieces.

26. On player and spectator conduct, see Board Minutes, 25 (November 7, 1934): 33–34; 25 (November 9, 1934): 35–48; and 72 (December 6, 1950): 88–91.

27. Bettie G. Francis, "Report of Committee on Industrial Education and Special Instruction," *Board Report, 1902–03*, 37.

28. The instigator probably was Elizabeth Walton, a physical educator in the white secondary schools; see Thompson, "Development," 281, 351–52, 359, 379. One commentary is Emory M. Wilson, "Report of the Principal of Central High School," *Board Report, 1906–07*, 164.

29. On competition, see *Central Review* 18 (February 1907): 12; *Central Review* 18 (March 1907): 11–12; and Emory M. Wilson, "Report of the Principal of Central High School," *Board Report, 1910–11*, 179. On white programs, see Marguerite Florence Steis, "How Washington Equips School Girls for Health," *Nation's Schools* 5 (February 1930): 45–52. On older black girls, see Mary P. Evans, "Physical Culture," *Board Report, 1893–94*, 189; Hattie B. George, "Health Exercises," *Board Report, 1894–95*, 181; and R. H. Terrell, *Board Report, 1898–99*, 289–90.

30. Edith C. Westcott, "Report of the Principal of Western High School," *Board Report, 1913–14*, 196.

31. Representative comments by white administrators include Emory M. Wilson, "Report of Principal of Central High School," *Board Report, 1907–08*, 170–71; and Willard S. Small, "Report of Principal of Eastern High School," *Board Report, 1908–09*, 185. Their superiors also expressed concern; see Ernest L. Thurston, "Annual Report of the Superintendent," *Board Report, 1917–18*, 52–53; and Frank W. Ballou, "Annual Report of the Superintendent," *Board Report, 1920–21*, 108–09.

32. Quoted in Thompson, "Development," 311.

33. On 1885–1919, see ibid., 104–7, 124–28, 269–79, 309–42; on 1920–37, see 136–38, 140–43, 406–11, 413–15, 420–46.

34. Ibid., 444–45.

35. Westcott, "Report of Principal of Western High School," *Board Report, 1909–10*, 181–82.

36. Board Minutes, 51 (October 17, 1945): 2; 52 (December 5, 1945): 47–49; and 53 (March 20, 1946): 51.

37. Tyack and Hansot, *Learning Together*, 83–88, 163–64.

38. Ibid., 155–64; and Victoria Bissell Brown, "The Fear of Feminization: Los Angeles High Schools in the Progressive Era," *Feminist Studies* 16 (1990): 493–518.

39. David L. Angus, "The Origins of Urban Schools in Comparative Perspective," in *Southern Cities, Southern Schools*, ed. David N. Plank and Rick Ginsberg (Westport, Conn.: Greenwood Press, 1990), 59–78; David B. Tyack, *The One Best System: A History of American Urban Education* (Cambridge, Mass.: Harvard University Press, 1974), 72–77, 177–216; Tyack and Hansot, *Learning Together*, 114–24; and Urban and Wagoner, *American Education*, 185–214.

40. Tyack and Hansot, *Learning Together*, 201–42.

41. Ibid., 165–200; and Brown, "Fear of Feminization."

42. Timothy P. O'Hanlon, "Interscholastic Athletics, 1900–1940: Shaping Citizens for Unequal Roles in the Modern Industrial State" (Ph.D. diss., University of Illinois, Urbana-Champaign, 1979), 98–101; and Jeffrey L. Mirel, "Progressive School Reform in Comparative Perspective," in Plank and Ginsberg, *Southern Cities*, 161–62.

43. David L. Angus and Jeffrey E. Mirel, *The Failed Promise of the American High School, 1890–1995* (New York: Teachers College Press, 1999), 57–58, 67–83.

44. Paula S. Fass, *Outside In: Minorities and the Transformation of American Education* (New York: Oxford University Press, 1989), 73–111; and Tyack and Hansot, *Learning Together*, 229–30, 232.

45. O'Hanlon, "Interscholastic Athletics," 2, 5, and 2–11, 174–77 in general.

46. Paul R. Mills, "The Place of Interscholastic Sport in American Society, 1920–1939," in *Sport in American Education: History and Perspective*, ed. Wayne M. Ladd and Angela Lumpkin (Washington, D.C.: AAHPERD, 1979), 37–38; and O'Hanlon, "Interscholastic Athletics," 217–28.

47. Jeffrey Mirel, "From Student Control to Institutional Control of High School Athletics: Three Michigan Cities, 1883–1905," *Journal of Social History* 16 (1982): 83–100; and O'Hanlon, "Interscholastic Athletics," 137–70.

48. Tyack and Hansot, *Learning Together*, 200.

49. Emory M. Wilson, "Report," *Board Report, 1907–08*, 170.

50. Edward C. Wilson, "Report," *Board Report, 1909–10*, 241.

51. Stoneroad, "Report," *Board Report, 1909–10*, 154; Stoneroad, "Report," *Board Report, 1914–15*, 155–56; and Thompson, "Development," 293–97, 344–45, 348, 495. For summaries from a white secondary school, see reports by Elmer S. Newton, principal of Western High School, in *Board Report, 1916–17*, 221–24; and *Board Report, 1918–19*, 215–16.

52. Quoted in Thompson, "Development," 647.

53. See Stoneroad's updates in *Board Report: 1916–17*, 187–89; *1917–18*, 232–33; *1918–19*, 172–73; and *1919–20*, 239–40.

54. Newton, "Report," *Board Report, 1916–17*, 221.

55. Quotations from Stoneroad, "Report of the Director of Physical Training," *Board Report, 1913–14*, 134; "Report," *Board Report, 1917–18*, 232; "Report," *Board Report, 1919–20*, 240; and "Report," *Board Report, 1909–10*, 154.

56. Stoneroad, "Report," *Board Report, 1914–15*, 155.

57. See Stoneroad's entries in *Board Report: 1914–15*, 155–56; *1915–16*, 193; *1916–17*, 187–88; *1917–18*, 232; and *1919–20*, 239; also Thompson, "Development," 648–56.

58. See Stoneroad's reports in *Board Report: 1913–14*, 131–32; *1914–15*, 153–54; *1915–16*, 192; and *1918–19*, 170–72; Turner's reports in *Board Report, 1915–16*, 266, and *Board Report, 1918–19*, 266; and Frank W. Ballou, "Annual Report of the Superintendent, V: Physical Welfare of Pupils," *Board Report, 1920–21*, 108–20.

59. Cora Grant, "Report of the Modern Health Crusade," *Board Report, 1918–19*, 174–77.

60. Stoneroad, "Report," *Board Report, 1919–20*, 239.

61. Grant, "Modern Health Crusade," 176.

62. Ibid., 175.

63. Guy Lewis, "Adoption of the Sports Program, 1906–39: The Role of Accommodation in the Transformation of Physical Education," *Quest* 12 (May 1969): 34–46; and O'Hanlon, "Interscholastic Athletics," 170–95, 330–32.

64. Roberta J. Park, *Measurement of Physical Fitness: A Historical Perspective*, Office of Disease Prevention and Health Promotion Monograph Series (Washington, D.C.: U.S. Department of Health and Human Services, Public Health Service, 1989), 3–9.

65. Susan G. Zieff, "The American 'Alliance' of Health and Physical Education: Scholastic Programs and Professional Organizations, 1920–1950," *RQES* 77 (2006): 437–50.

66. On the paradox of marginality and limits of dissent, see Leslie Gotfrit, "Women Dancing Back: Disruption and the Politics of Pleasure," in *Postmodernism, Feminism, and Cultural Politics: Redrawing Educational Boundaries*, ed. Henry A. Giroux (Albany: State University of New York Press, 1991), 191–95; and David Kirk, "Physical Education, Discourse, and Ideology: Bringing the Hidden Curriculum Into View," *Quest* 44 (1992): 46–48.

67. "Report of the Physical Training Department," *Board Report, 1910–11*, 256.

68. Jervis Anderson, "A Very Special Monument: The Dunbar High School on First Street," *New Yorker* 54 (March 20, 1978): 94–96, 100–102, 104–08, 110–21; and Mary Church Terrell, "History of the High School for Negroes in Washington," *Journal of Negro History* 2 (July 1917): 258–66.

69. W. T. S. Jackson, "Report of Principal of M Street High School," *Board Report, 1908–09*, 212.

70. P. M. Hughes, "Report of Director of High Schools," *Board Report, 1903–04*, 191–92.

71. Edward C. Wilson, "Report of Principal of M Street High School," *Board Report, 1909–10*, 241.

72. Terrell, "History," 252–53; G. C. Wilkinson, "Report of the Principal of Dunbar High School," *Board Report, 1916–17*, 279; and Wilkinson, "Report of the Principal of Dunbar High School," *Board Report, 1917–18*, 320.

73. "Equal Facilities," *Star* (ca. September 1955), Box 44–15, Scrapbook #8, in Papers of Edwin B. Henderson, Manuscript Division, Moorland-Spingarn Research Center, Howard University, Washington, D.C. (Hereafter, collection cited as Henderson Papers.)

74. Thompson, "Development," 659–60.

75. Ibid., 153–54; and Paul Cooke, "The Cost of Segregated Public Schools in the District of Columbia," *JNE* 18 (1949): 96–97.

76. See Edwin B. Henderson, "Separate and Unequal" (letter to editor, ca. 1946–47), Box 44–15, Scrapbook #8, Henderson Papers; T. J. Anderson and E. B. Henderson, "Recreation and Race Adjustment in Washington, D.C. (Prepared for the Committee on Democracy Through Recreation)," 6, ca. 1942, Box 44–1, Folder 26, Henderson Papers; and Mary A. Morton, "The Education of Negroes in the District of Columbia," *JNE* 16 (1947): 333.

77. Edwin B. Henderson, *The Negro in Sports*, 2nd ed. (Washington, D.C.: Associated Publishers, 1949), 320.

78. Howard H. Long, "The Support and Control of Public Education in the District of Columbia," *JNE* 7 (1938): 397–98; and Morton, "Education of Negroes," 330–31.

79. Board Minutes, 47 (May 3, 1944): 42–43; and 48 (September 13, 1944): 203.

80. Board Minutes, 59 (November 19, 1947): 6–7; 59 (December 3, 1947): 10–11; 67 (November 16, 1949): 82–84; 68 (February 1, 1950): 100–101; 72 (November 1, 1950): 108–9; and 72 (December 20, 1950): 87.

81. Board Minutes, 59 (November 19, 1947): 6–7; and 67 (November 16, 1949): 82–84, 86.

82. Board Minutes, 63 (November 3, 1948): 56–58; 66 (November 2, 1949): 109–11; 67 (November 16, 1949): 82–84; 72 (November 1, 1950): 108–9; and 73 (March 7, 1951): 115–17.

83. Henderson, "Segregated School Systems Take Toll," *Journal and Guide (Norfolk, Va.)*, June 5, 1948; and "School Coaches Rebel Over 'Extra Duties,'" *Baltimore Afro-American*, May 8, 1948, Box 44–12, Scrapbook #5, Henderson Papers.

84. Board Minutes, 92 (November 17, 1954): 66–67.

85. Board Minutes, 92 (February 16, 1955): 91; and 95 (February 15, 1956): 56–58.

86. Edwin B. Henderson, "Progress and Problems in Health and Physical Education Among Colored Americans," *JOHPE* 6 (June 1935): 9.

87. Board Minutes, 16 (February 17, 1926): 7.

88. Board Minutes, 17 (May 4, 1927): 22–23; 17 (May 18, 1927): 21–22; 18 (December 7, 1927): 8; and 18 (December 21, 1927): 5–7.

89. Jacqueline M. Moore, *Leading the Race: The Transformation of the Black Elite in the Nation's Capital, 1880–1920* (Charlottesville: University Press of Virginia, 1999), 86–111.

90. For example, Board Minutes, 53 (May 1, 1946): 26–27, 31; and 54 (June 19, 1946): 132.

91. Tyack, *One Best System*, 217–25.

92. On intra- and interracial conflict, see Willard B. Gatewood, *Aristocrats of Color: The Black Elite, 1880–1920* (Bloomington: Indiana University Press, 1990), 59–60, 162–63,

166–67, 258–63, 325–26; Constance McLaughlin Green, *The Secret City: A History of Race Relations in the Nation's Capital* (Princeton, N.J.: Princeton University Press, 1967), 84–89, 99–102, 119–54, 210–12, 244–47; and Moore, *Leading the Race*, 86–111.

93. Linda M. Perkins, "The History of Blacks in Teaching: Growth and Decline Within the Profession," in *American Teachers: Histories of a Profession at Work*, ed. Donald Warren (New York: Macmillan, 1989), 344–69; and Michael W. Homel, "Two Worlds of Race? Urban Blacks and the Public Schools, North and South, 1865–1940," in Plank and Ginsberg, *Southern Cities*, 239–44.

94. Henderson, "Separate and Unequal," ca. 1946–47; and "Segregated School Systems," June 5, 1948, Henderson Papers.

95. David K. Wiggins, "Edwin Bancroft Henderson: Physical Educator, Civil Rights Activist, and Chronicler of African American Athletes," *RQES* 70 (1999): 94–95, 102–3; and "Edwin Bancroft Henderson, African American Athletes, and the Writing of Sport History," in *Glory Bound: Black Athletes in a White America* (Syracuse, N.Y.: Syracuse University Press, 1997), 228–30.

96. William A. Joiner and Edwin B. Henderson, eds., *Official Handbook of Inter-Scholastic Athletic Association of Middle Atlantic States* (New York: American Sports Publishing, 1910); and Edwin B. Henderson and Garnet C. Wilkinson, eds., *Official Handbook of Inter-Scholastic Athletic Association of Middle Atlantic States* (New York: American Sports Publishing, 1912; 1913); copies in Library of Congress, Washington, D.C.

97. Firsthand accounts include Edwin B. Henderson, "An Experiment in Elementary School Athletics," *JOHPER* 22 (June 1951): 22; Turner, "Report," *Board Report, 1910–11*, 255; J. E. Walker, "Supervising Principal's Report of 10th to 13th Division," *Board Report, 1913–14*, 225–26; "Report of the Secretary of the Public Schools Athletic League of Washington, D.C.," in *Official Handbook of ISAA* (1912), 17–39; and "Report of the Secretary of the PSAL of Washington, D.C.," in *Official Handbook of ISAA* (1913), 23–55.

98. Thompson, "Development," 294–96, 344–45, 348.

99. Henderson, "Experiment," 21–22; and items in Box 44–12, Scrapbook #5, Henderson Papers.

100. Leon N. Coursey, "The Life of Edwin Bancroft Henderson and His Professional Contributions to Physical Education" (Ph.D. diss., Ohio State University, 1971), 122–54.

101. Henderson, "Segregated School Systems," June 5, 1948, Henderson Papers.

102. Patrick Miller, "To 'Bring the Race along Rapidly': Sport, Student Culture, and Educational Mission at Historically Black Colleges during the Interwar Years," *History of Education Quarterly* 35 (1995): 111–33; and David K. Wiggins, "The Notion of Double-Consciousness and the Involvement of Black Athletes in American Sport," in *Glory Bound*, 200–220.

103. Turner, "Report," *Board Report, 1910–11*, 254; and Sharon Harley, "Beyond the Classroom: The Organizational Lives of Black Female Educators in the District of Columbia, 1890–1930," *JNE* 51 (1982): 254–65.

104. Turner, "Report," *Board Report, 1910–11*, 255.

105. Henderson, *Negro in Sports*, rev. ed., 230–33; and "Sports Comment," *Atlanta Daily World*, February 28, 1950, Box 44–12, Scrapbook #5, Henderson Papers.

106. Henderson, "Negro Women in Sports," *Negro History Bulletin* 15 (December 1951): 55.

107. Henderson, *Negro in Sports*, rev. ed., 242.

108. Ibid.

109. Henderson, "Sports Comment" (February 28, 1950), Henderson Papers.

110. Henderson, "Colored Boxers May Win Olympic Boxing Crown; Seven Negroes to Vie for USA," *Kansas City Call*, August 6, 1948, Box 44–12, Scrapbook #5, Henderson Papers.

111. Ibid.

112. "Henderson's Comments: Need of the Day—More Women Athletes," n.p., n.d., Box 44–12, Scrapbook #5, Henderson Papers.

113. Ibid.

114. Henderson, *Negro in Sports*, rev. ed., 242.

115. Henderson, "Need of the Day," n.p., n.d.

116. Henderson, "Negro Women in Sports," 55.

117. Green, *Secret City*, 298–310; and George D. Strayer et al., *Report of a Survey of the Public Schools of the District of Columbia* (Washington, D.C.: GPO, 1949).

Chapter 7

1. Quotations from Thomas J. Templin, "Some Considerations for Teaching Physical Education in the Future," in *Trends Toward the Future in Physical Education*, ed. John D. Massengale (Champaign, Ill.: Human Kinetics, 1987), 56; Nadine J. Maggard, "Upgrading Our Image," *JOPERD* 55 (January 1984): 17; and Judith H. Placek, "Conceptions of Success in Teaching: Busy, Happy and Good?" in *Teaching in Physical Education*, ed. Thomas J. Templin and Janice K. Olson, Big Ten Body of Knowledge Symposium Series, vol. 14 (Champaign, Ill.: Human Kinetics, 1983), 46.

2. Shirl J. Hoffman, "In My View: Therapy for an Ailing Profession," *JOPERD* 56 (November–December 1985): 17.

3. No comprehensive survey of female physical educators, coaches, and administrators in late twentieth-century America exists. I consulted archival materials, unpublished memoirs, biographical sketches, dissertations and theses, award announcements, obituaries, professional directories, and oral histories.

4. Robertha Abney, "The Effects of Role Models and Mentors on Career Patterns of Black Women Coaches and Athletic Administrators in Historically Black and Historically White Institutions of Higher Education" (Ph.D. diss., University of Iowa, 1988), 57–67. This dissertation profiles nearly one hundred women of color.

5. Charlene R. Burgeson et al., "Physical Education and Activity: Results from the School Health Policies and Programs Study 2000," *JOPERD* 74 (January 2003): 288.

6. Calculated from U.S. Census Bureau, *Statistical Abstract of the United States, 1951*, 124 (Table 149), http://www2.census.gov/prod2/statcomp/documents/1951-01.pdf (accessed March 19, 2006).

7. U. S. Census Bureau, *Statistical Abstract of the United States, 1976*, 147 (Table 247), http://www2.census.gov/prod2/statcomp/documents/1976-02.pdf (accessed March 19, 2006).

8. National Center for Education Statistics, "Bachelor's, master's, and doctor's degrees conferred by degree-granting institutions, by sex of student and field of study: 1997–98," Table 257, in *Digest of Education Statistics: Tables and Figures, 2000*, http://nces.ed.gov/programs/digest/d00 (accessed March 19, 2006).

9. Allen Ericson Weatherford II, "The Status of Graduate Offerings in Health Education, Physical Education, and Recreation Education in Negro Colleges and Universities, 1950–1951," *JNE* 21 (1952): 220–23.

10. Darrell Crase et al., "Perspectives on Physical Education in Traditionally Black Institutions," *JOPERD* 62 (September 1991): 28.

11. Darrell Crase and Michael H. Hamrick, "Gender and Race/Ethnicity Differentials Among Physical Education Doctorates," *PE* 51 (Fall 1994): 165; and Fred Douglas Pullum, "Professional Preparation in Physical Education at Historically Black Institutions in Georgia" (Ed.D. diss., University of Georgia, 1974), 133, 135.

12. Crase and Hamrick, "Differentials," 164–65; and Darrell Crase and Hollie Walker Jr., "The Black Physical Educator—An Endangered Species," *JOPERD* 59 (October 1988): 65–69.

13. Crase and Walker, "Black Physical Educator," 65; and Yevonne R. Smith, "Recruitment and Retention of African American and Other Multicultural Physical Educators," *JOPERD* 64 (March 1993): 66–69.

14. Dudley Ashton, "Recruiting Future Teachers," *JOHPER* 28 (October 1957): 25–26, 49; Rachel Bryant, "Opportunities in Physical Education and Sports for Girls," *JOHPER* 30 (April 1959): 73; and June Hackett, "It's Up to Us to Solve Our Teacher Shortage," *JOAAHPER* 24 (November 1953): 23–24.

15. "Summary, Follow-Up Study of Graduates, University of Illinois, April 1958," Box 4, Folder: "Graduates Follow-Up Study, 1957–1959," Papers of Laura J. Huelster, Records of Applied Life Studies: Physical Education for Women Department, University Archives, University of Illinois at Urbana-Champaign, Urbana, Ill. (Hereafter, cited as Huelster Papers.)

16. Gertrude M. Baker, "Survey of the Administration of Physical Education in Public Schools in the United States," *RQ* 33 (1962): 632–36; and Andrew Grieve, "State Legal Requirements for Physical Education," *JOHPER* 42 (April 1971): 19–23.

17. Helen T. Mackey, "Job Analysis of Women Supervisors of Physical Education in United States Public Schools," *RQ* 27 (1956): 32–40; Marjorie Phillips, "Compensation Practices and Extracurricular Responsibilities of Women High School Physical Education Teachers," *RQ* 28 (1957): 379–94; and "Summary," Huelster Papers.

18. Phillips, "Compensation Practices," 386; and AAHPER Vocational Guidance Committee, "Placement Study: Undergraduate Majors in Health, Physical Education, and Recreation in Selected Teacher-Education Institutions for 1949," *JOHPER* 22 (May 1951): 48–49.

19. Allen Ericson Weatherford II, "Professional Health, Physical Education, and Recreation Education in Negro Colleges, 1948–1949," *JNE* 22 (1953): 530.

20. Pullum, "Professional Preparation," 184.

21. Virden Evans and Charles D. Henry, "The Black High School Coach—Will He Become Extinct?" *PE* 30 (1973): 153.

22. Melvin I. Evans, "The Vanishing Americans," *JOHPER* 44 (October 1973): 57.

23. See articles by Ray C. Maul (Research Division, NEA): "Wanted: Physical Education Teachers," *JOAAHPER* 24 (May 1953): 12, 14; "Are There Future Teachers?" *JOAAHPER* 25 (May 1954): 29–30; and "Our Critical Need for Teachers," *JOHPER* 27 (October 1956): 29–30.

24. Angela Lumpkin and Jane Jenkins, "Basic Instruction Programs: A Brief History," *JOPERD* 64 (August 1993): 33–36; and Joseph B. Oxendine, "100 Years of Basic Instruction," *JOPERD* 56 (September 1985): 32–36.

25. Quotation from "Summary of Factors Leading to the Recommendation on Physical Education by the College of Arts and Sciences," appended to letter from Walter E. Militzer, Dean, to A. C. Breckenridge, Dean of Faculties, April 22, 1960, Box 4: Arts and Sciences, Folder: Arts and Sciences, College of—Women's Physical Education, 1960, Papers of Chancellor Clifford Hardin, University Archives, University of Nebraska, Lincoln, Neb. (Hereafter, depository cited as UA-UNL.)

26. Celeste Ulrich, interview by author, tape recording, Eugene, Ore., May 28, 1995.

27. Kate McKemie, interview by author, tape recording, Decatur, Ga., August 3, 1994.

28. Anna S. Espenschade, interview by author, tape recording, Laguna Hills, Calif., August 9, 1993; and Madge M. Phillips, interview by author, tape recording, Knoxville, Tenn., August 6, 1994.

29. Letter from Women's Staff, Physical Education Department to Dr. H. N. Neilson (Chair), November 9, 1970; and Neilson to Women of Physical Education Faculty, November 23, 1970, Box: "Job of Athletic Director and Chairman of PE-Neilson, 1957; Department of PE, 1966–69," Folder: 1972, Records of College of Education: Division of Physical Education, Hampton University Archives, Hampton University, Hampton, Va.

30. Letter from Ruth Schellberg to Chancellor R. G. Gustavson, April 4, 1952, Box 2, Folder: Physical Education for Women (Chairmanship), 1952, Papers of Chancellor Gustavson, UA-UNL; also Minnie Lynn to Dean Henzlik, Teachers College, January 19, 1952, and Minnie Lynn to Chancellor Gustavson, March 15, 1952, in same folder.

31. "Annual Report, 1954–55," 6, 8; and "Annual Report, 1960–61," 1, Box 1, Folders 16–17, Papers of the Woman's College: Department of Health and Physical Education, University Archives, Duke University, Durham, N.C.

32. Mrs. Charles I. Taylor to B. N. Greenberg, M.D., May 5, 1960, Box 4: Arts and Sciences, Folder: Arts and Sciences, College of—Women's Physical Education, 1960, Chancellor Hardin Papers, UA-UNL.

33. R. McLaran Sawyer, *The Modern University, 1920–1969*, vol. 2 of *Centennial History of the University of Nebraska* (Lincoln, Neb.: Centennial Press, 1973), 207–12.

34. Mary G. Jacobs, "An Evaluation of the Physical Education Service Program for Women in Certain Selected Colleges" (Ed.D. diss., New York University, 1957), 142–49, 198–99.

35. Rita J. Ashcraft, "Comparison of Employment Status of Men and Women in Four-Year Public Institutions," *JOHPER* 44 (April 1973): 60–62; and Charles H. Belanger and Peter W. Everett, "Salaries of Physical Education Faculty in Selected Four-Year Institutions," *JOHPER* 44 (April 1973): 58–60.

36. Jane S. McIlroy, "A Study of Degrees and Ranks Held and the Graduate Credit Offerings Taught by Men and by Women in Physical Education," *RQ* 21 (1950): 239–44.

37. Ashcraft, "Comparison," 60–61.

38. Robert H. Kirk, "The Posture of Predominantly Negro College and University Health and Physical Education Faculties," *JOHPER* 40 (February 1969): 83–84, 86; and Weatherford, "Professional Health," 532.

39. Jacobs, "Evaluation," 127–29; and Florence Nightingale Mitchell, "A Survey of Physical Education Personnel for Women in Negro Colleges and Universities" (master's [Ed.] thesis, Springfield College, 1958), 29–33.

40. Mitchell, "Survey," 23–26, 33–39; and Weatherford, "Professional Health," 531–32.

41. Lacey Bell, quoted in Nina Jo Woolley Smith, "'Out of Adversity, We Survived': Oral Histories of Seven Black Women Physical Educators" (master's thesis, San Francisco State University, 1992), 138.

42. John D'Emilio, *Sexual Politics, Sexual Communities: The Making of a Homosexual Minority in the United States, 1940–1970*, 2nd ed. (Chicago: University of Chicago Press, 1998), 38.

43. Quotation from Hackett, "It's Up to Us," 23.

44. Mary Jo Festle, *Playing Nice: Politics and Apologies in Women's Sports* (New York: Columbia University Press, 1996), 109–41, 165–91; Joan S. Hult, "The Philosophical Conflicts in Men's and Women's Collegiate Athletics," *Quest* 32 (1980): 77–94; and Ying Wushanley, *Playing Nice and Losing: The Struggle for Control of Women's Intercollegiate Athletics, 1960–2000* (Syracuse, N.Y.: Syracuse University Press, 2004), 33–152.

45. Linda Jean Carpenter and R. Vivian Acosta, *Title IX* (Champaign, Ill.: Human Kinetics, 2005), 3.

46. Ibid., 41, 47.

47. Ibid., 35–63; quotations from 47, 59.

48. See timeline in *Title IX*, 194–97.

49. Ibid., 193.

50. Information gaps exist because only postsecondary institutions are required to make data publicly available.

51. Becky L. Sisley and Susan A. Capel, "High School Coaching Filled With Gender Differences," *JOPERD* 57 (March 1986): 40.

52. Ibid., 39–43.

53. Mary C. Lydon, "Secondary School Programs: Diversity in Practice," in *Women in Sport: Issues and Controversies*, ed. Greta L. Cohen (Thousand Oaks, Calif.: Sage, 1993), 99.

54. James G. Ross et al., "What Are Kids Doing in School Physical Education?" *JOPERD* 56 (January 1985): 74; and James G. Ross et al., "What Is Going on in the Elementary Physical Education Program?" *JOPERD* 58 (November–December 1987): 79.

55. Quotation from Russell R. Pate et al., "School Physical Education," *Journal of School Health* 65 (October 1995): 317.

56. NASPE and American Heart Association, *2006 Shape of the Nation Report: Status of Physical Education in the USA* (Reston, Va.: NASPE, 2006), 1.

57. Catherine D. Ennis, "Curriculum: Forming and Reshaping the Vision of Physical Education in a High Need, Low Demand World of Schools," *Quest* 58 (2006): 51–55.

58. Calculation based on Lynda E. Randall, "Employment Statistics: A National Survey in Public School Physical Education," *JOPERD* 57 (January 1986): 23; and Russell R. Pate and Richard C. Hohn, "Introduction: A Contemporary Mission for Physical Education," in *Health and Fitness Through Physical Education*, ed. Russell R. Pate and Richard C. Hohn (Champaign, Ill.: Human Kinetics, 1994), 1.

59. Templin, "Considerations," 55.

60. Calculations based on National Center for Education Statistics, *Digest of Education Statistics: Tables and Figures, 2004*, Table 70, http://nces.ed.gov/programs/digest/d04/tables/dt04_070.asp (accessed March 19, 2006).

61. Bonnie J. Hultstrand, "Women in High School PE Teaching Positions—Diminishing Numbers," *JOPERD* 61 (November–December 1990): 20.

62. Smith, "Recruitment and Retention," 66–67.

63. Burgeson et al., "Physical Education," 284–85, 288, 291; Pate et al., "School Physical Education," 314, 316, 317; and Elba Stafford, "Middle Schools: Status of Physical Education Programs," *JOHPER* 45 (February 1974): 27–28.

64. Mary O'Sullivan, "Failing Gym is Like Failing Lunch or Recess: Two Beginning Teachers' Struggle for Legitimacy," *JTPE* 8 (1989): 227–42; and Sandra A. Stroot et al., "Contextual Hoops and Hurdles: Workplace Conditions in Secondary Physical Education," *JTPE* 13 (1994): 342–60.

65. Rory Suomi, Fred Hebert, and Scott E. Frazier, "Employment Trends for K–12 Physical Education Teachers in Wisconsin: 1987–96," *PE* 56 (Fall 1999): 121–25.

66. O'Sullivan, "Failing Gym"; and Deborah Tannehill et al., "Attitudes Toward Physical Education: Their Impact on How Physical Education Teachers Make Sense of Their Work," *JTPE* 13 (1994): 406–20.

67. Nell Faucette et al., "'I'd Rather Chew on Aluminum Foil': Overcoming Classroom Teachers' Resistance to Teaching Physical Education," *JTPE* 21 (2002): 287.

68. O'Sullivan, "Failing Gym," 242.

69. Andrew C. Sparkes, Thomas J. Templin, and Paul G. Schempp, "Exploring Dimensions of Marginality: Reflecting on the Life Histories of Physical Education Teachers," *JTPE* 12 (1993): 386–87.

70. Lumpkin and Jenkins, "Basic Instruction," 34, 36.

71. Oxendine, "100 Years," 33.

72. Larry D. Hensley, "Current Status of Basic Instruction Programs in Physical Education at American Colleges and Universities," *JOPERD* 71 (November–December 2000): 30–36; and William F. Stier, Jerome Quarterman, and Mark Martin Stier, "The Status of Physical Education Performance Classes Within Historically Black Colleges and Universities," *JOPERD* 64 (May–June 1993): 87–92.

73. Hensley, "Current Status," 33–35; Don Hilsendager and Tom Evaul, "Basic Instruction Programs: Issues and Answers," *JOPERD* 64 (August 1993): 37–38; and R. Thomas Trimble and Larry D. Hensley, "Basic Instruction Programs at Four-Year Colleges and Universities: II. Course Offerings and Administration," *JOPERD* 61 (August 1990): 69–73.

74. Aaron L. Banks and Ottley Wright, "The Top Five Employment Opportunities in Physical Education in Higher Education: 1993–1999," *PE* 58 (Fall 2001): 150–57; and Joanne Rowe, "Consumer Needs in Physical Education and Athletics in Higher Education," *PE* 53 (Late Winter 1996): 28–33.

75. Mary J. Hoferek, "At the Crossroad: Merger or—?" *Quest* 32 (1980): 95–102 (quotation, 99).

76. Margaret J. Safrit, "Women in Research in Physical Education," *Quest* 31 (1979): 158–71; Margaret J. Safrit, "Women in Research in Physical Education: A 1984 Update," *Quest* 36 (1984): 103–14; and Jayne Schuiteman and Annelies Knoppers, "An Examination of Gender Differences in Scholarly Productivity Among Physical Educators," *RQES* 58 (1987): 265–72.

77. R. Vivian Acosta and Linda Jean Carpenter, "As the Years Go By—Coaching Opportunities in the 1990s," *JOPERD* 63 (March 1992): 36; William F. Stier Jr., "Physical Education Faculty and Programs in Small Colleges and Universities," *PE* 39 (December 1982): 195–98; and Trimble and Hensley, "Basic Instruction, II," 72.

78. Abney, "Role Models," 57–62, 67–75, 142–43, 148–49; Crase and Walker, "Black Physical Educator," 66–67; Crase et al., "Perspectives," 28–32, 75; and Priscilla Rice and David K. Leslie, "Comparisons of Selected Characteristics of Faculty in Large and Small Black Colleges," *PE* 44 (Spring 1987): 321–24.

79. William F. Stier Jr., and Jerome Quarterman, "Characteristics of Physical Education Faculty in Historically Black Colleges and Universities (HBCUs)," *PE* 49 (Spring 1992): 73–80; and Marianne L. Woods, D. Allen Phillips, and Cynthia Carlisle, "Characteristics of Physical Education Teacher Educators," *PE* 54 (Fall 1997): 150–59.

80. Carpenter and Acosta, *Title IX*, 175.

81. Ibid., 173–76, 181–82nn8–9.

82. Abney, "Role Models," 15–21; Acosta and Carpenter, "As the Years Go By," 37; Alpha Alexander, "Status of Minority Women in the Association of Intercollegiate Athletics for Women" (master's [Ed.] thesis, Temple University, 1978), 54; and Margaret Dianne Murphy, "The Involvement of Blacks in Women's Athletics in Member Institutions of the Association of Intercollegiate Athletics for Women" (Ph.D. diss., Florida State University, 1980), 46–48.

83. Carpenter and Acosta, *Title IX*, 174.

84. Ibid., 175.

85. Sue Inglis, Karen E. Danylchuk, and Donna L. Pastore, "Multiple Realities of Women's Work Experiences in Coaching and Athletic Management," *WSPAJ* 9 (Fall 2000): 1–26; four of eleven interviewees were American.

86. Robertha Abney, "African American Women in Sport," *JOPERD* 70 (April 1999): 37; R. Vivian Acosta and Linda Jean Carpenter, "Women in Intercollegiate Sport: A Longitudinal, National Study—Twenty-Seven Year Update, 1977–2004," *WSPAJ* 13 (2004): 63, 75, 78–82; Richard Lapchick, "The 2005 Racial and Gender Report Card: College Sports," 4–5, 35–37, http://www.bus.ucf.edu/sport/public/downloads/2005_Racial_Gender_Report_Card_Colleges.pdf (accessed January 11, 2007); and National Coalition for Women and Girls in Education, "Title IX at 30: Report Card on Gender Equity (June 2002)," 17, www.aahperd.org/nagws/pdf_files/title930.pdf (accessed October 9, 2006).

87. NCWGE, "Title IX at 30," 18.

88. Calculated from National Collegiate Athletic Association, *NCAA Gender-Equity Report 2003–04*, 17, 22, http://ncaa.org/library/research/gender_equity_study/2003 04_gender_equity_report.pdf (accessed January 17, 2007).

89. Carpenter and Acosta, *Title IX*, 177.

90. Acosta and Carpenter, "As the Years Go By," 37.

91. Abney, "Role Models," 16–18; Alexander, "Status of Minority Women," 44–46; and Murphy, "Involvement of Blacks," 48–49.

92. Acosta and Carpenter, "As the Years Go By," 37.

93. Ray Anne Shrader and Jane Maver, interview by author, West Lafayette, Ind., June 29, 1994.

94. R. Vivian Acosta and Linda Jean Carpenter, "Women in Athletics—A Status Report," *JOPERD* 56 (August 1985): 32.

95. Robertha Abney and Dorothy Richey, "Barriers Encountered by Black Female Athletic Administrators and Coaches," *JOPERD* 62 (August 1991): 19.

96. Quotations from Abney, "Role Models," 83–84, 89, 91, 92.

97. Acosta and Carpenter, "Women in Intercollegiate Sport," 86.

98. Ibid., 85, 86.

99. Abney, "African American Women," 37; and Lapchick, "2005 Racial and Gender Report Card: College Sports," 6.

100. Acosta and Carpenter, "Women in Intercollegiate Sport," 75; and NCWGE, "Title IX at 30," 18 (quotation).

101. Acosta and Carpenter, "Women in Intercollegiate Sport," 76.

102. Elizabeth Murphey and Marilyn Vincent, "Status of Funding of Women's Intercollegiate Athletics in AIAW Charter Member Colleges and Universities," *JOHPER* 44 (October 1973): 11–12, 14–15.

103. Festle, *Playing Nice*, 180.

104. Handwritten loose notes (n.d.), Box: Speeches, Photos, and Articles, Folder: Speeches, Papers of Nell Cecilia Jackson, Archives, Tuskegee University, Tuskegee, Ala.

105. Kate McKemie (Chair) to President Perry and Dean Gary, October 4, 1979, Box: Correspondence and Academic Planning, Folder: Department Reports, Papers of Kate McKemie, Archives, Agnes Scott College, Decatur, Ga.

106. Carpenter and Acosta, *Title IX*, 66–72, 78–84.

107. Women's Sports Foundation, comp., *Women's Sports & Fitness Facts and Statistics* (Updated 3/26/09), 10, http://www.womenssportsfoundation.org/~/media/Files/PDFs%20 and%20other%20files%20by%20Topic/Issues/General/W/WSF%20FACTS%20March%20 2009.pdf (accessed October 16, 2009).

108. Carpenter and Acosta, *Title IX*, 136–37.

109. The federal Equity in Athletics Disclosure Act (EADA, 1994) requires institutions receiving Title IV funds for student aid to file annual reports on participants, staff, budgets, and other Title IX compliance areas (available via the Office of Postsecondary Education, http://ope.ed.gov/athletics).

110. Examples abound in the archival records. On the work of one leader near retirement, see Huelster Papers, UA-UI.

111. R. Vivian Acosta and Linda Jean Carpenter, "Status of Women in Athletics: Changes and Causes," *JOPERD* 56 (August 1985): 35–37; and *1989 NCAA Study of Perceived Barriers to Women's Intercollegiate Athletic Careers*, http://www.ncaa.org/library/research/ womens_barriers/1989WomensAthleticCareerBarriers.pdf (accessed February 1, 2007).

112. From oral histories; Acosta and Carpenter, "As the Years Go By," 38–40; and Safrit, "Research: Update," (1984), 105–6.

113. Reviews include Susan L. Greendorfer and Laurna Rubinson, "Homophobia and Heterosexism in Women's Sport and Physical Education," *WSPAJ* 6 (Fall 1997): 189–210; Helen J. Lenskyj, *Out on the Field: Gender, Sport and Sexualities* (Toronto: Women's Press, 2003), 103–15; and Heather Sykes, "Constr(i)(u)cting Lesbian Identities in Physical Education: Feminist and Poststructural Approaches to Researching Sexuality," *Quest* 48 (1996): 459–69.

114. Since the early 1990s, scholars have collected physical educators' life histories more systematically in England, Australia, and the United States; studies by Doune Macdonald and Andrew C. Sparkes are especially informative.

115. Pat Griffin, *Strong Women, Deep Closets: Lesbians and Homophobia in Sport* (Champaign, Ill.: Human Kinetics, 1998), 157–80; and Sarah L. Squires and Andrew C. Sparkes, "Circles of Silence: Sexual Identity in Physical Education and Sport," *Sport, Education and Society* 1 (1996): 77–101.

116. Mary B. Harris and Joy Griffin, "Stereotypes and Personal Beliefs about Women Physical Education Teachers," *WSPAJ* 6 (1997): 71–72; and Sherry E. Woods, "Describing the Experience of Lesbian Physical Educators: A Phenomenological Study," in *Research in Physical Education and Sport: Exploring Alternative Visions*, ed. Andrew C. Sparkes (London: Falmer, 1992), 98.

117. Pat Griffin, "Changing the Game: Homophobia, Sexism, and Lesbians in Sport," *Quest* 44 (1992): 256.

118. Ibid., 255.

119. Griffin, *Strong Women, Deep Closets*, 65–89; and Susan Wellman and Elaine Blinde, "Homophobia in Women's Intercollegiate Basketball," *WSPAJ* 6 (Fall 1997): 63–82. On students, see Elaine M. Blinde and Diane E. Taub, "Women Athletes as Falsely Accused Deviants: Managing the Lesbian Stigma," *Sociological Quarterly* 33 (1992): 521–33.

120. Vikki Krane and Heather Barber, "Identity Tensions in Lesbian Intercollegiate Coaches," *RQES* 76 (2005): 75, 79.

121. Jennifer Terry, *An American Obsession: Science, Medicine, and Homosexuality in Modern Society* (Chicago: University of Chicago Press, 1999), 367.

122. John D'Emilio and Estelle B. Freedman, *Intimate Matters: A History of Sexuality in America* (New York: Harper and Row, 1988), 358.

123. Terry, *American Obsession*, 378–95.

Chapter 8

1. Phrase from "Issues: How can you have an elective physical education program and maintain gender balance within the classes?" *JOPERD* 71 (February 2000): 11.

2. Ron French et al., "Revisiting Section 504, Physical Education, and Sport," *JOPERD* 69 (September 1998): 58.

3. Hans Kraus and Ruth P. Hirschland, "Muscular Fitness and Health," *JOAAHPER* 24 (December 1953): 17.

4. John Tunis, *Sport for the Fun of It: A Handbook of Information on Nineteen Sports Including the Official Rules for a Selected List of 18*, rev. ed. (New York: Ronald Press, 1958), v, 31–34, 40–41, 69–71, 222–23.

5. "Exercise and Fitness," *JOHPER* 29 (April 1958): 42.

6. Barbara E. Ainsworth and Catrine Tudor-Locke, "Health and Physical Activity Research as Represented in *RQES*," *RQES* 76, suppl. (June 2005): S-41, S-48.

7. A research review is Marion R. Broer, "For Physical Fitness Vary Your Program," *JOHPER* 27 (September 1956): 16–18, 80. On tests, see Paul Hunsicker, "Physical Fitness Tests," *JOHPER* 28 (September 1957): 21–22, 68–69.

8. Doris Soladay, "Functions and Purposes of NSGWS," *JOHPER* 27 (October 1956): 51.

9. Examples from Maryhelen Vannier and Hollis F. Fait, *Teaching Physical Education in Secondary Schools* (Philadelphia: W. B. Saunders, 1957), 248; Betty Hartman and H. June Hackett, "Softball," in *Team Sports for Girls*, ed. Ann Paterson (New York: Ronald Press, 1958), 300; and Jean M. Homewood, "Guarding Positions—Legal or Illegal?" in *Official Basketball and Officials Rating Guide for Girls and Women Containing Revised Rules, September 1957–September 1958* (Washington, D.C.: DGWS, 1957), 61–62.

10. *Basketball Bulletin, December 1953*, 2, prepared by the National Basketball Committee, NSGWS, in new Box 25: Rules and Editorial Committee—Basketball, 1949–1962, Folder: Basketball 1953, Subseries 6: Structures, Papers of NSWA/NSGWS/DGWS (AC 3:6:1), Archives, AAHPERD. Hereafter, collection and subseries cited as DGWS Papers (AC 3:6:1:6).

11. Letter from Anna S. Espenschade to G. Ed Adams, May 15, 1953, Folder: Competition-Women, Papers of Anna S. Espenschade, Bancroft Library, University of California at Berkeley, Berkeley, Calif.

12. Amy Louise Brown, "The Need for More Track and Field Clinics," in *Official Softball—Track and Field Guide with Official Rules and Standards, January 1958–January 1960* (Washington, D.C.: AAHPER, DGWS, 1958), 129–30.

13. Martha J. Haverstick, "Track and Field: Preface," in *Official Softball—Track and Field Guide with Official Rules, January 1952–January 1953* (Washington, D.C.: AAHPER, 1952), 117.

14. Brown, "Need," 129.

15. Pauline A. Hess, "Why Track and Field for Girls?" in *Official Softball—Track and Field Guide with Official Rules, January 1956–January 1958* (Washington, D.C.: AAHPER, 1956), 129 (first quotation); Nancy A. Lamp, "Volleyball Skills of Junior High School Students as a Function of Physical Size and Maturity," *RQ* 25 (1954): 189–200; and Donna Mae Miller and Katherine L. Ley, *Individual and Team Sports for Women* (New York: Prentice Hall, 1955), 58 (second quotation).

16. Margaret A. Bourne, "Basketball—Starvation Diet?" *JOAAHPER* 23 (December 1952): 23, 31; and Norma R. Diemert, "A Coach and Her Team," in *Official Basketball and Officials Rating Guide for Girls and Women, Containing Revised Rules, September 1956–September 1957* (Washington, D.C.: AAHPER, 1956), 23–24.

17. Staff of Department of Physical Education, University of California, Los Angeles, "Coeducational Classes: A Statement of Philosophy and Policy," *JOHPER* 26 (February 1955): 18.

18. Elizabeth Halsey and Lorena Porter, *Physical Education for Children: A Developmental Approach* (New York: Henry Holt, 1958), 392–93.

19. Examples from Staff, "Coeducational Classes"; and Madelyne Walker and Ray Hobbs, "Coeducational Physical Education: A Successful High School Program," *JOHPER* 27 (April 1956): 17–18.

20. Kathro Kidwell, "The 'New' Bowling Instructor—Welcome!" in *Bowling Fencing—Golf Guide* (Washington, D.C.: DGWS, 1958), 21.

21. Walker and Hobbs, "Coeducational," 18.

22. Carl N. Degler, *In Search of Human Nature: The Decline and Revival of Darwinism in American Social Thought* (New York: Oxford University Press, 1991), 215–24; Anne Fausto-Sterling, *Sexing the Body: Gender Politics and the Construction of Sexuality* (New York: Basic Books, 2000), 45–48, 66, 195–216; and Marianne van den Wijngaard, *Reinventing the Sexes: The Biomedical Construction of Femininity and Masculinity* (Bloomington: University of Indiana Press, 1997), 4–9.

23. Allan M. Brandt, "Behavior, Disease, and Health in the Twentieth-Century United States: The Moral Valence of Individual Risk," in *Morality and Health*, ed. Allan M. Brandt and Paul Rozin (New York: Routledge, 1997), 58–67.

24. Research reviews include "Exercise and Fitness: A Statement on the Role of Exercise in Fitness by a Joint Committee of the American Medical Association and the American Association for Health, Physical Education, and Recreation," *JOHPER* 35 (May 1964): 42–44, 82; and Leonard A. Larson, "Research Turns the Spotlight on Health and Fitness," *JOHPER* 36 (April 1965): 86–90.

25. Roberta J. Park, *Measurement of Physical Fitness: A Historical Perspective*, Office of Disease Prevention and Health Promotion Monograph Series (Washington, D.C.: U.S. Department of Health and Human Services, 1989), 17–18.

26. Joseph B. Oxendine, "100 Years of Basic Instruction," *JOPERD* 56 (September 1985): 35.

27. Degler, *In Search of Human Nature*, 215–44; Fausto-Sterling, *Sexing the Body*, 66–69, 217; and van den Wijngaard, *Reinventing the Sexes*, 4–6, 27–46, 99–101.

28. Peter G. Filene, *Him/Her/Self: Gender Identities in Modern America*, 3rd ed. (Baltimore, Md.: Johns Hopkins University Press, 1998), 191–246; Rosalind Rosenberg, *Divided Lives: American Women in the Twentieth Century* (New York: Noonday Press, Hill and Wang, 1992), 180–219; Mary P. Ryan, *Mysteries of Sex: Tracing Women and Men Through American History* (Chapel Hill: University of North Carolina Press, 2006), 248–65; and Chris Weedon, *Feminism, Theory, and the Politics of Difference* (Oxford, Eng.: Blackwell, 1999), 13–16, 19–23.

29. Anne F. Millan, "Sex Differences: Do They Make Any Difference?" *PE* 26 (1969): 114.

30. Laura J. Huelster, "Philosophy of Physical Education in the U.S.A.," in *Expanding Horizons in Physical Education: Proceedings of 4th International Congress on Physical Education and Sports for Girls and Women* (Washington, D.C.: International Association of Physical Education and Sports for Girls and Women, 1962), 101.

31. Letter from Alyce Cheska, Chairman, DGWS, to Ruth Lindsey, Chairman, Sports Guides and Official Rules Committee, April 30, 1968, new Box 32: Structures-SGOR, Folder: Football-Type Games, 1965–70, DGWS Papers (AC 3:6:1:6).

32. Phebe M. Scott to Tom Hamilton, June 30, 1965, Box 14: Executive Records, Folder: Football-Type Games, 1940–1969, Subseries 1: Executive Records, DGWS Papers (AC 3:6:1). Hereafter, subseries cited as AC 3:6:1:1.

33. Quotation from Phebe Scott, in "Excerpt from the Minutes of the Executive Council, Division for Girls and Women's Sports, November 12–14, 1965, Washington, D.C.," new Box 35: Structures, Folder: Touch Football Committee 1948, DGWS Papers (AC 3:6:1:6). On cancer studies, see new Box 32: Structures-SGOR, Folder: Football-Type Games, 1965–70, DGWS Papers (AC 3:6:1:6).

34. "Tabulation to Questionnaires on Touch Football for Girls, 12/5/66," 3, new Box 32: Structures-SGOR, Folder: Football-Type Games, 1965–70, DGWS Papers (AC 3:6:1:6).

35. "History of Council Action on Football-Type Games," 2, ca. 1969, new Box 32: Structures-SGOR, Folder: Football-Type Games, 1965–70, DGWS Papers (AC 3:6:1:6).

36. Cheska to Lindsey, 1, DGWS Papers (AC 3:6:1:6).

37. Camille Dorman and Betty Gena Blanton, "Flag Football for Girls: Does It Have a Place in Our Programs?" Box 14: Executive Records, Folder: Football-Type Games, 1940–1969, DGWS Papers (AC 3:6:1:1). *JOHPER* withdrew this heretical piece shortly before publication, explaining that an official DGWS statement on football was forthcoming.

38. Ibid., 4.

39. *Proceedings of the Second National Institute on Girls Sports* (Washington, D.C.: AAHPER, 1966), 119–23.

40. See Marcia Barratt et al., *Foundations for Movement* (Dubuque, Iowa: Wm. C. Brown, 1964); Marion R. Broer, *Efficiency of Human Movement* (Philadelphia: W. B. Saunders, 1966); Phebe M. Scott and Virginia R. Crafts, *Track and Field for Girls and Women* (New York: Appleton-Century-Crofts, 1964); and Celeste Ulrich, "The Tomorrow Mind," *JOHPER* 35 (October 1964): 17–18, 83–84.

41. Eleanor C. Rynda, "Physiological Aspects of Competition for Women," in *Track and Field Guide, January 1968–January 1970, with Official Rules and Standards* (Washington, D.C.: DGWS, 1968), 35.

4322 Notes to Pages 210–214

442. Virginia R. Crafts, "Building on Basics," in *Proceedings of Second National Institute,* 79; and Phebe M. Scott, "Reflections on Women in Sports," in *Proceedings of the Third National Institute on Girls Sports* (Washington, D.C.: AAHPER, 1966), 10.

43. Typical research included Vera Skubic and Jean Hodgkins, "Relative Strenuousness of Selected Sports as Performed by Women," *RQ* 38 (1967): 305–13.

44. Frances Todd, "Is the Sports Program Designed to Meet the Needs of Girls?" in *Current Administrative Problems: Athletics, Health Education, Physical Education, and Recreation,* ed. Elmon L. Vernier (Washington, D.C.: AAHPER, 1960), 138.

45. Anna S. Espenschade and Helen M. Eckert, *Motor Development* (Columbus, Ohio: Charles E. Merrill, 1967), 162.

46. Margaret H. Meyer and Marguerite M. Schwarz, *Team Sports for Girls and Women,* 4th ed. (Philadelphia: W. B. Saunders, 1965), 37, 58.

47. Hilda Clute Kozman, Rosalind Cassidy, and Chester O. Jackson, *Methods in Physical Education,* 4th ed. (Dubuque, Iowa: Wm. C. Brown, 1967), 12.

48. Patsy Neal, *Basketball Techniques for Women* (New York: Ronald Press, 1966), 16; and Patsy Neal, *Coaching Methods for Women* (Reading, Mass.: Addison-Wesley, 1969), 25.

49. Barratt et al., *Foundations,* 42, 44, 45.

50. Scott and Crafts, *Track and Field,* 109.

51. Dorothy Humiston and Dorothy Michel, *Fundamentals of Sports for Girls and Women: Team and Individual* (New York: Ronald Press, 1965), 72.

52. Kathryn Fossum, in "Basic Issues," *JOHPER* 33 (May–June 1962): 8.

53. Clara L. Hester, "Games in the Elementary School Program," *PE* 23 (1966): 59.

54. Gladys Andrews, Jeannette Saurborn, and Elsa Schneider, *Physical Education for Today's Boys and Girls* (Boston: Allyn and Bacon, 1960), 62–63.

55. Espenschade and Eckert, *Motor Development,* 225.

56. See Humiston and Michel, *Fundamentals,* 151–52; Shirley Jameson, "Smaller Balls for Smaller Hands?" in *Basketball Guide for Girls and Women with Official Rules and Standards, September 1960–September 1961* (Washington, D.C.: DGWS, 1960), 36–37; Maryhelen Vannier and Hally Beth Poindexter, *Physical Activities for College Women,* 2nd ed. (Philadelphia: W. B. Saunders, 1969), 93; and chapters in Betty Foster McCue, ed., *Physical Education Activities for Women* (New York: Macmillan, 1969): Jane M. Lloyd, "Golf," 122; Rita Narcisian, "Gymnastics," 154; and Evelyn F. Terhune, "Fencing," 111.

57. For example, Emily R. Andrews et al., *Physical Education for Girls and Women,* 2nd ed. (Englewood Cliffs, N.J.: Prentice-Hall, 1963), 96.

58. Evelyn L. Schurr, *Movement Experiences for Children: Curriculum and Methods for Elementary School Physical Education* (New York: Appleton-Century-Crofts, 1967), 25.

59. Andrews, Saurborn, and Schneider, *Physical Education,* 61; and Schurr, *Movement,* 548.

60. Neal, *Coaching,* vi, 18–20, 24–26.

61. Nell C. Jackson, "Track and Field," in McCue, *Physical Education Activities,* 202.

62. Espenschade and Eckert, *Motor Development,* 206–10.

63. Nell C. Jackson, "Contribution of Track and Field to the Development of Girls and Women," in *Proceedings of First National Institute,* 93–94.

64. Neal, *Coaching,* 105.

65. Ibid.

66. Patricia Vertinsky, "Science, Social Science, and the 'Hunger for Wonders' in Physical Education: Moving Toward a Future Healthy Society," in *New Possibilities, New Paradigms?,*

American Academy of Physical Education Papers, no. 24 (Champaign, Ill.: Human Kinetics, 1991), 77–80.

67. Degler, *In Search of Human Nature*, 224–27, 242–43, 293–309; Fausto-Sterling, *Sexing the Body*, 3, 68–70, 126–45, 216–27; and van den Wijngaard, *Reinventing the Sexes*, 5–6, 15–20, 62–78, 101–11.

68. Adjective from Linda Nicholson, "Interpreting Gender," *Signs* 20 (1994): 81.

69. Nancy Fraser, "Equality, Difference, and Democracy: Recent Feminist Debates in the United States," in *Feminism and the New Democracy: Resiting the Political*, ed. Jodi Dean (Thousand Oaks, Calif.: Sage, 1997), 99–101; Judith Squires, *Gender in Political Theory* (Malden, Mass.: Polity Press and Blackwell Publishers, 2000), 78–79, 116–122; and Weedon, *Feminism*, 13–16, 26–50.

70. Dorothy V. Harris, "What Are Little Girls Made Of?" (ca. 1981), 11, 16, Box 17, Folder: "What Are Little Girls," Papers of Dorothy V. Harris, Special Collections and University Archives, Penn State University, University Park, Pa. (Hereafter, cited as Harris Papers.)

71. Madge Phillips, "Sociological Considerations of the Female Participant," in *Women and Sport: A National Research Conference*, ed. Dorothy V. Harris, Penn State HPER Series no. 2 (University Park, Pa.: Pennsylvania State University Press, 1972), 187, 188.

72. Dorothy V. Harris, "What About Women in Sport?" *Pennsylvania Journal of Physical Education, Recreation, and Dance* 42 (September 1972): 5.

73. Leading sport scientists included Marlene Adrian, Anne Atwater, Barbara Drinkwater, Dorothy Harris, Emily Haymes, Sharon Plowman, Charlotte Sanborn, and Christine Wells.

74. Barbara L. Drinkwater, "Women and Exercise: Physiological Aspects," *ESSR* 12 (1984): 21.

75. Harris, "Little Girls?" 18, Harris Papers.

76. Dorothy V. Harris, "Overview: Is Biology Destiny?" in *The New Agenda: "A Blueprint for the Future of Women's Sports,"* Issue 1: Physiological Concerns (San Francisco: Women's Sports Foundation, 1985), 2: 2, 3.

77. Marlene Adrian, "Sex Differences in Biomechanics," in Harris, *Women and Sport*, 389–97; Anne E. Atwater, "Biomechanics and the Female Athlete," in *Sport Science Perspectives for Women*, ed. Jacqueline Puhl, C. Harmon Brown, and Robert O. Voy (Champaign, Ill.: Human Kinetics, 1985), 1–12; Barbara L. Drinkwater, "Physiological Responses of Women to Exercise," *ESSR* 1 (1973): 125–53; Dorothy V. Harris, "Conditioning for Stress in Sports," in *DGWS Research Reports: Women in Sports*, ed. Dorothy V. Harris (Washington, D.C.: AAHPER, 1973), 2:77–83; and Martha Yates, "Endurance Training for Women," in *NAGWS Research Reports*, ed. Marlene Adrian and Judith Brame, vol. 3 (Washington, D.C.: AAHPER, 1977), 3:5–13.

78. Adrian, "Sex Differences," 390 (height); and Christine L. Wells, "The Female Athlete: Myths and Superstitions Put to Rest," in *Toward an Understanding of Human Performance: Readings in Exercise Physiology for the Coach and Athlete*, ed. Edmund J. Burke (Ithaca, N.Y.: Mouvement Publications, 1978), 37.

79. Barbara L. Drinkwater, "Gender Differences in Heat Tolerance: Fact or Fiction?" in *Female Endurance Athletes*, ed. Barbara L. Drinkwater (Champaign, Ill.: Human Kinetics, 1986), 113–24; Barbara L. Drinkwater, "Maximal Oxygen Uptake of Females," in Harris, *Women and Sport*, 375–86; Nancy Oyster and Edna P. Wooten, "The Influence of

of Selected Anthropometric Measurements on the Ability of College Women to Perform the 35-Yard Dash," *Medicine and Science in Sports* 3 (1971): 130–34; and Christine L. Wells, "Sexual Differences in Heat Stress Response," *PSM* 5 (September 1977): 79–80, 83–84, 87–90.

80. Adrian, "Sex Differences," 392.

81. Bonnie J. Purdy, "Research Related to Women in Sport: Learning Aspects," in *DGWS Research Reports: Women in Sports*, ed. Dorothy V. Harris (Washington, D.C.: AAHPER, 1971), 1:97.

82. Melba B. Masse, Chair, Vermont DGWS, to Mary Rekstad, February 13, 1973; and Marlene Adrian, Chair, DGWS Research Committee, to Melba Masse, March 6, 1973, Box 23, Folder: Structures—Research Committee 1957–73, DGWS Papers (AC 3:6:1:6).

83. Joan Hult, "Competitive Athletics for Girls—We Must Act," *JOHPER* 45 (June 1974): 45–46.

84. *Philosophy and Standards for Girls and Women's Sport* (Washington, D.C.: DGWS, AAHPER, 1973), 17.

85. Hult, "Competitive Athletics," 46; and letter from Rachel E. Bryant, Consultant in Physical Education, DGWS, to Joyce E. Buckley, Secretary-Treasurer, Michigan DGWS, May 26, 1971, Box 25, Folder: "DGWS—Girls on Boys' Teams," Harris Papers.

86. DGWS, "Position Statement: Women on Men's Teams," Box 25, Folder: "DGWS—Girls on Boys' Teams," Harris Papers.

87. DGWS, *Philosophy and Standards* (1973), 17.

88. Linda Jean Carpenter and R. Vivian Acosta, *Title IX* (Champaign, Ill.: Human Kinetics, 2005), 42–47, 72–76 (quotation, 72).

89. Joan Hult, "Separate but Equal Athletics for Women," *JOHPER* 44 (June 1973): 57, 58.

90. Mary Jo Festle, *Playing Nice: Politics and Apologies in Women's Sports* (New York: Columbia University Press, 1996), 115–16, 122–25; and Ying Wushanley, *Playing Nice and Losing: The Struggle for Control of Women's Intercollegiate Athletics, 1960–2000* (Syracuse, N.Y.: Syracuse University Press, 2004), 62–69, 77–79. The AIAW later changed its position.

91. Examples from Linda Bunker, "What About Co-ed Competition?" in *Handbook for Youth Sports Coaches*, ed. Vern Seefeldt (Reston, Va.: AAHPERD, 1987), 342; Carole L. Mushier, *Team Sports for Girls and Women*, 2nd ed. (Princeton, N.J.: Princeton Book Company, 1983), 144; Sharon Plowman, "What is pseudo and what is scientific in the evidence concerning the capability of women?" in *The New Agenda*, Issue 1: Physiological Concerns, 2:15; and Kathryn M. Yandell and Waneen W. Spirduso, "Sex and Athletic Status as Factors in Reaction Latency and Movement Time," *RQ* 52 (1981): 495–504.

92. Bunker, "Co-ed Competition?" 347–48.

93. Dorothy V. Harris, "The Female Athlete: Strength, Endurance and Performance," in Burke, *Toward an Understanding*, 43.

94. Jerry R. Thomas, Amelia M. Lee, and Katherine T. Thomas, *Physical Education for Children: Concepts into Practice* (Champaign, Ill.: Human Kinetics, 1988), 7.

95. Marjorie Blaufarb, "Title IX: Implications for Campus Recreation," *JOPER* 51 (April 1980): 55–56; and Arlene A. Ignico, "Elementary Physical Education: Color It Androgynous," *JOPERD* 60 (February 1989): 23–24.

96. Ignico, "Elementary," 24; and Marie Weber, "Title IX in Action," *JOPER* 51 (May 1980): 20–21.

97. Harris, "Little Girls?" 10, Harris Papers.

98. Pat Griffin, "Coed Physical Education," *JOPERD* 55 (August 1984): 37.

99. Beverly Wilson, "The Battle Between the Sexes in Physical Education," *PE* 29 (October 1972): 139.

100. Judith Bischoff, "Equal Opportunity, Satisfaction and Success: An Exploratory Study on Coeducational Volleyball," *JTPE* 2 (Fall 1982): 3–12; Rosemary Selby, "What's Wrong (and Right)! With Coed Physical Education Classes: Secondary School Physical Educators' Views on Title IX Implementation," *PE* 34 (December 1977): 188–91; and Carol Lee Stamm, "Evaluation of Coeducational Physical Activity Classes," *JOPER* 50 (January 1979): 68–69.

101. Dawn E. Evans, in "Competitive Sports for Women—The Continuing Debate," *JOHPER* 45 (May 1974): 6.

102. Pamela Peridier, "What Should Women's Liberation Mean to You?" *JOHPER* 43 (January 1972): 32.

103. Fraser, "Equality, Difference, and Democracy," 101–2; Judith Lorber, *Gender Inequality: Feminist Theory and Politics*, 2nd ed. (Los Angeles: Roxbury, 2001), 33–34; and Weedon, *Feminism*, 14–16.

104. Weedon, *Feminism*, 104–7, and 99–130 in general.

105. Squires, *Gender in Political Theory*, 58.

106. Myra J. Hird, *Sex, Gender, and Science* (Houndmills, Eng.: Palgrave Macmillan, 2004), 5–6, 29–49; and van den Wijngaard, *Reinventing the Sexes*, 15–19.

107. Dorothy V. Harris, "Putting Myths and Misconceptions Behind Us!" (1988), 5, loose item, Box 32, Harris Papers.

108. Dorothy V. Harris, "Physical Sex Differences: A Matter of Degree," in Adrian and Brame, *NAGWS Research Reports*, 3:121–22; "Putting Myths," 4–6; and "Some Psychological Determinants of Women's Participation in Sport," in *Psychological Preparation of the Superior Sportsman* (Salford, Eng.: British Society of Sports Psychology, 1975), 45–47.

109. Harris, "Psychological Determinants," 46.

110. Wells, "Sexual Differences in Heat Stress Response," 90.

111. Dorothy V. Harris and Patricia Potter, "Special Considerations for the Female Athlete," 17, ca. 1985, Box 25, Folder: "Special Considerations," Harris Papers.

112. Harris, "Little Girls?" 19, Harris Papers.

113. Harris, "Female Aggression and Sport Involvement," in Harris, *DGWS Research Reports*, 2:49–54.

114. Cathy Small, "Requiem for an Issue," *JOHPER* 44 (January 1973): 27.

115. Dorothy V. Harris, "Femininity and Athleticism: Conflict or Consonant?" 12, speech, Immaculata College, November 11–12, 1976, Box 25, Folder: "Femininity and Athleticism," Harris Papers.

116. Cheska, "Women's Sports," 6.

117. For example, Jane Flax, "Postmodernism and Gender Relations in Feminist Theory," *Signs* 12 (1987): 621–43; and Linda Gordon, "On 'Difference,'" *Genders* 10 (1991): 91–111.

118. Phrases from Mary E. Duquin, "The Importance of Sport in Building Women's Potential," *JOPERD* 53 (March 1982): 20; and Cheska, "Women's Sports," 9.

119. Annelies Knoppers, "Equity for Excellence in Physical Education," *JOPERD* 59 (August 1988): 57.

120. Patricia S. Griffin, "'Gymnastics is a girl's thing': Student Participation and Interaction Patterns in a Middle School Gymnastics Unit," in *Teaching in Physical Education*, ed. Thomas J. Templin and Janice K. Olson, Big Ten Body of Knowledge Series, vol. 14 (Champaign, Ill.: Human Kinetics, 1983), 71, 84–85.

121. Harris, "Women in Society and Their Participation in Sport, I," *Olympic Review* 160 (1981): 91.

122. Harris, "Significant Issues of Women in Athletics in Higher Education: Psycho-Social Benefits of Participation," 6–7, handwritten notes, speech, Brown University, October 7, 1988, Box 39, Folder: "Women in Sport Administration," Harris Papers.

123. Kathy Davis, "Embody-ing Theory: Beyond Modernist and Postmodernist Readings of the Body," in *Embodied Practices: Feminist Perspectives on the Body*, ed. Kathy Davis (London: Sage, 1997), 1–8.

124. Lynda B. Ransdell and Christine L. Wells, "Sex Differences in Athletic Performance," *WSPAJ* 8 (1999): 76.

125. *Physical Activity and Health: A Report of the Surgeon General* (Atlanta, Ga.: U.S. Department of Health and Human Services, Centers for Disease Control and Prevention, National Center for Chronic Disease Prevention and Health Promotion; Washington, D.C.: President's Council on Physical Fitness and Sports, 1996), 6.

126. Online sources are http://www.healthypeople.gov and http://www.mypyramid.gov.

127. "Healthy People 2010: Physical Activity and Fitness," *PCPFS Research Digest*, Series 3, no. 13 (March 2001): 2.

128. Steven N. Blair and Jon C. Connelly, "How Much Physical Activity Should We Do? The Case for Moderate Amounts and Intensities of Physical Activity," *RQES* 67 (1996): 193–205; and Charles B. Corbin and Robert P. Pangrazi, "How Much Physical Activity Is Enough?" *JOPERD* 67 (April 1996): 33–37.

129. *Promoting Better Health for Young People Through Physical Activity and Sports: A Report to the President from the Secretary of Health and Human Services and the Secretary of Education* (Silver Spring, Md.: Centers for Disease Control and Prevention, National Center for Chronic Disease Prevention and Health Promotion, Division of Adolescent and School Health, 2000), 17.

130. U.S. Department of Health and Human Services, *Healthy People 2010*, 2nd ed. (Washington, D.C.: GPO, November 2000), vol. 2, Sec. 22: 4–5.

131. Carl J. Casperson, Mark A. Pereira, and Katy M. Curran, "Changes in Physical Activity Patterns in the United States, by Sex and Cross-Sectional Age," *MSSE* 32 (2000): 1601–9.

132. Comprehensive reports include President's Council on Physical Fitness and Sports, *Physical Activity and Sport in the Lives of Girls: Physical and Mental Health Dimensions from an Interdisciplinary Approach* (Washington, D.C.: The author, 1997); and Women's Sports Foundation, *Her Life Depends On It: Sport, Physical Activity and the Health and Well-Being of American Girls* (East Meadow, N. Y.: WSF, 2004).

133. George A. Langford and LaGary Carter, "Academic Excellence Must Include Physical Education," *PE* 60 (Late Winter 2003): 28.

134. Marilyn Strawbridge, "Current Activity Patterns of Women Intercollegiate Athletes of the Late 1960s and 1970s," *WSPAJ* 10 (2001): 55–72; and Doris L. Watson, Artur Poczwardowski, and Pat Eisenman, "After-School Physical Activity Programs for Adolescent Girls," *JOPERD* 71 (October 2000): 17.

135. National Association for Sport and Physical Education and American Heart Association, *2006 Shape of the Nation Report: Status of Physical Education in the USA* (Reston, Va.: NASPE, 2006), 8.

136. See "Issues" section in *JOPERD* 67 (October 1996): 6–7; 70 (January 1999): 11–12; and 75 (August 2004): 16–17. Advocates regard the "new PE" as girl-friendly; see Pangrazi et al., "Impact," 317–21.

137. Pat Griffin, "Equity in the Gym: What Are the Hurdles?" *CAHPER Journal* 55 (March–April 1989): 24.

138. Michael Sutliff, "Multicultural Education for Native American Students in Physical Education," *PE* 53 (Fall 1996): 160.

139. Fraser, "Equality, Difference, and Democracy," 101–3; Lorber, *Gender Inequality*, 16 (quotation), 147–62, 179–212; and Weedon, *Feminism*, 72–76, 99–130, 152–77.

140. Squires, *Gender in Political Theory*, 115, 139.

141. Fraser, "Equality, Difference, and Democracy," 101–3; Joan W. Scott, "Deconstructing Equality-Versus-Difference: Or, the Uses of Poststructuralist Theory for Feminism," *Feminist Studies* 14 (1988): 33–50; and Squires, *Gender in Political Theory*, 116–32.

142. Don Sabo and Janie Victoria Ward, "Wherefore Art Thou Feminisms? Feminist Activism, Academic Feminisms, and Women's Sports Advocacy," *Scholar and Feminist Online*, Issue 4.3 (Summer 2006), http://www.barnard.edu/sfonline.

143. My discussion focuses on curricular literature. Overviews are Joy T. DeSensi, "Understanding Multiculturalism and Valuing Diversity: A Theoretical Perspective," *Quest* 47 (1995): 34–43; and Carol C. Torrey and Madge Ashy, "Culturally Responsive Teaching in Physical Education," *PE* 54 (Fall 1997): 120–27.

144. Kay M. Williamson, "Is Your Inequity Showing? Ideas and Strategies for Creating a More Equitable Learning Environment," *JOPERD* 64 (October 1993): 15.

145. Quotations from Sandy Beveridge and Philip Scruggs, "TLC for Better PE: Girls and Elementary Physical Education," *JOPERD* 71 (October 2000): 23; and Gayle E. Hutchinson, "Gender-Fair Teaching in Physical Education," *JOPERD* 66 (January 1995): 45.

146. Quotations from Beveridge and Scruggs, "TLC," 24; and Amanda J. Daley and Joanne Buchanan, "Aerobic Dance and Physical Self-Perceptions in Female Adolescents: Some Implications for Physical Education," *RQES* 70 (1999): 198.

147. Williamson, "Inequity Showing?" 15.

148. Karen L. Butt and Markella L. Pahnos, "Why We Need a Multicultural Focus in Our Schools," *JOPERD* 66 (January 1995): 49.

149. Ibid., 48, 50.

150. Bonnie Mohnsen, *Teaching Middle School Physical Education* (Champaign, Ill.: Human Kinetics, 1997), 51.

151. Katherine Jamieson, "Latinas in Sport and Physical Activity," *JOPERD* 66 (September 1995): 42.

152. Phrase from Scott, "Deconstructing Equality-Versus-Difference," 48.

153. Robyn S. Lock, Leslie T. Minarik, and Joyce Omata, "Gender and the Problem of Diversity: Action Research in Physical Education," *Quest* 51 (1999): 403.

154. Laura Azzarito and Melinda A. Solmon, "A Reconceptualization of Physical Education: The Intersection of Gender/Race/Social Class," *Sport, Education and Society* 10 (2005): 41.

155. Lock, Minarik, and Omata, "Gender," 398–99, 400.

156. Catherine D. Ennis, "Creating a Culturally Relevant Curriculum for Disengaged Girls," *Sport, Education and Society* 4 (1999): 31–48 (quotations, 35, 36, 45).

157. Laura Azzarito and Catherine D. Ennis, "A Sense of Connection: Toward Social Constructivist Physical Education," *Sport, Education and Society* 8 (2003): 179–98 (quotations, 190, 191).

158. Ennis, "Creating," 33, 37.

159. Catherine D. Ennis, "Canaries in the Coal Mine: Responding to Disengaged Students Using Theme-Based Curricula," *Quest* 52 (2000): 125, 126–27.

160. Azzarito and Solmon, "Reconceptualization," 41–43; and Pat Griffin, "The Challenge to Live Up to Our Ideals: Appreciating Social Diversity and Achieving Social Justice in Schools," *JOPERD* 62 (August 1991): 58–61.

161. Celeste Ulrich, "Cherchez la Femme," 16, typescript of speech, n.d. (copy in Ulrich's private collection, Eugene, Ore.; photocopied by author, May 28, 1995).

162. Celeste Ulrich, "Journey Proud," 7, typescript of speech, n.d. (copy in Ulrich's private collection, Eugene, Ore.; photocopied by author, May 28, 1995).

Chapter 9

1. Angenette Parry, "The Athletic Girl and Motherhood," *Harper's Bazaar* 46 (August 1912): 380; and "Can Sports Make You Sterile?" *Harper's Bazaar* no. 3291 (February 1986): 214–15.

2. G. Bigelow Mullison, "Effects of Athletic Competition on Childbirth," *JAMA* 65 (1915): 2256–57; and Mona M. Shangold et al., "Evaluation and Management of Menstrual Dysfunction in Athletes," *JAMA* 263 (1990): 1665–69.

3. Elizabeth Halsey, "The College Curriculum in Physical Education for Women," *APER* 30 (1925): 495; and Meredith W. Burney and Barbara A. Brehm, "The Female Athlete Triad," *JOPERD* 69 (November–December 1998): 43–45.

4. Lynda Birke, *Feminism and the Biological Body* (New Brunswick, N.J.: Rutgers University Press, 2000), 85–111 (quotations, 91, 94); and Emily Martin, *The Woman in the Body: A Cultural Analysis of Reproduction* (Boston: Beacon, 1987), 32–53.

5. See Ineke Klinge, "Female Bodies and Brittle Bones: Medical Interventions in Osteoporosis," in *Embodied Practices: Feminist Perspectives on the Body*, ed. Kathy Davis (London: Sage, 1997), 59–72; and Nelly Oudshoorn, *Beyond the Natural Body: An Archeology of Sex Hormones* (London: Routledge, 1994).

6. Arthur H. Steinhaus et al., "The Role of Exercise in Physical Fitness," *JOHPE* 14 (June 1943): 300.

7. "Exercise and Fitness: A Statement on the Role of Exercise in Fitness by a Joint Committee of the American Medical Association and the American Association for Health, Physical Education, and Recreation," *JAMA* 188 (1964): 435, 436.

8. Emil Novak, *Textbook of Gynecology*, 3rd ed. (Baltimore, Md.: Williams and Wilkins, 1948), 116.

9. "Report of Committee on School Health: Competitive Athletics—A Statement of Policy," *Pediatrics* 18 (1956): 672–76.

10. Reviews included Gyula J. Erdelyi, "Women in Athletics," *Proceedings of the Second National Conference on the Medical Aspects of Sports* (Chicago: American Medical Association, 1961), 59–63; and David Ryde, "The Effects of Strenuous Exertion on Women," *Practitioner* 177 (July 1956): 73–77.

11. Ernst Jokl, "Some Clinical Data on Women's Athletics," *Journal of the Association for Physical and Mental Rehabilitation* 10 (March–April 1956): 49.

12. S. Leon Israel, *Diagnosis and Treatment of Menstrual Disorders and Sterility*, 4th ed. (New York: Paul B. Hoeber, 1959), 76–113, 217–22; and Robert W. Kistner, *Gynecology: Principles and Practice*, 1st ed. (Chicago: Year Book Medical Publishers, 1964), 187–88, 207–36.

13. Novak, *Textbook*, 2nd ed. (1944), 563.

14. John G. Gruhn and Ralph R. Kazer, *Hormonal Regulation of the Menstrual Cycle: The Evolution of Concepts* (New York: Plenum Medical Book, 1989), 67–94, 102–75.

15. Ibid., 160.

16. For example, John I. Brewer and Edwin J. DeCosta, *Textbook of Gynecology*, 4th ed. (Baltimore, Md.: Williams and Wilkins, 1967), 107.

17. Midwest Association of College Teachers of Physical Education for College Women, "Policies for Sports Days and Intramural Activities for College Women," *JOHPE* 13 (May 1942): 295.

18. Virginia Lee Horne, "Pool Regulations," in *Official Aquatic Guide, 1941–42* (New York: A. S. Barnes, 1941), 57; and Helen M. Petroskey, "Basketball and Health," in *Official Basketball and Officials Rating Guide for Women and Girls Containing Revised Rules, 1946–47* (New York: A. S. Barnes, 1946), 38.

19. Estelle Gilman, "The Exercise Program for the Correction of Dysmenorrhea," *JOHPE* 15 (September 1944): 377, 403–04; and Josephine W. Hubbell, "Specific and Non-Specific Exercises for the Relief of Dysmenorrhea," *RQ* 20 (1949): 378–86.

20. Grace Thwing, "Swimming During the Menstrual Period," *JOHPE* 14 (March 1943): 154; "Swimming and Diving Standards for Girls and Women," in *Official Aquatics, Winter Sports and Outing Activities Guide, 1949–1951* (Washington, D.C.: AAHPER, 1949), 40; and "Basketball Standards for Girls and Women," in *Official Basketball and Officials Rating Guide for Women and Girls Containing Revised Rules, 1948–49* (New York: A. S. Barnes, 1948), 41.

21. See *A.A.U. Study of Effect of Athletic Competition on Girls and Women* (New York: AAU, 1956; 2nd ed., 1959).

22. Martha E. Rogers, "Responses to Talks on Menstrual Health," *Nursing Outlook* 1 (1953): 272–74.

23. Frances A. Hellebrandt, "Physiology and the Physical Educator: Recent Advances in Applied Physiology and Their Implications for Physical Education," *RQ* 11 (October 1940): 22–23; and Christine White, "Report on Basketball Survey," in *Official Basketball Guide for Women and Girls Containing Revised Rules, 1940–41* (New York: A. S. Barnes, 1940), 16–17.

24. Letter from Rachel E. Bryant to Marjorie Phillips, December 2, 1958, new Box 23, Folder: Research Committee, 1957–73, Subseries 6: Structures, Papers of the NSWA/NSGWS/DGWS (AC 3:6:1), Archives, AAHPERD. Hereafter, collection cited as DGWS Papers (accession number and subseries).

25. Minnie Lynn, quoted in letter from Ruth V. Byler to Bernice Moss, August 14, 1957, Box 2, Folder: "Dr. Answers," 1957, DGWS Papers (AC 3:6:1:8 Publications).

26. Elizabeth M. Prange, "Report of the Research Committee, 1954," new Box 23, Folder: Research Committee, 1950–56, DGWS Papers (AC 3:6:1:6 Structures).

27. Marjorie Phillips, Katharine Fox, and Olive Young, "Sports Activity for Girls: A Report by the Research Committee of the Division of Girls and Women's Sports," *JOHPER* 30 (December 1959): 23–25, 54.

28. Letter from Mabel Locke to Marjorie Phillips, November 19, 1956, new Box 23, Folder: Research Committee, 1950–56, DGWS Papers (AC 3:6:1:6 Structures).

29. Lara Freidenfelds, *The Modern Period: Menstruation in Twentieth-Century America* (Baltimore, Md.: Johns Hopkins University Press, 2009), 88–94, 120–41; and Margot E. Kennard, "The Corporation in the Classroom: The Struggles over Meanings of Menstrual Education in Sponsored Films, 1947–1983" (Ph.D. diss., University of Wisconsin–Madison, 1989), 106–10.

30. Department of Hygiene and Physical Education, *Physical Education Bulletin, 1950–51*, 13; and *Bulletin, 1959–60*, 16, Box 1206, Folder: Bulletins, Records of the Physical Education Department, College Archives, Smith College, Northampton, Mass.

31. Angeline Watkins, compiler, "Opinions on the 1952–53 Girls Basketball Rules in Mississippi," 5, Box 1, Folder: Basketball Problem, 1953, DGWS Papers (AC 3:6:1:1 Executive Records); and Department of Physical Education for Women, "Procedures and Policies, Autumn 1955," 2, Box 15, Folder: 1946–1968 Departmental Regulations, Records of Women's Physical Education Department, Department of Special Collections, Green Library, Stanford University, Stanford, Calif.

32. Jewell Nolen, "Problems of Menstruation," *JOHPER* 36 (October 1965): 65.

33. Betty Foster McCue, "Why Exercise?" in *Physical Education Activities for Women*, ed. Betty Foster McCue (Toronto: Macmillan Company, 1969), 6–7.

34. Ibid., 7.

35. Marcia Barratt et al., *Foundations for Movement* (Dubuque, Iowa: Wm. C. Brown, 1964), 62.

36. Theresa W. Anderson, "Swimming and Exercise During Menstruation," *JOHPER* 36 (October 1965): 68.

37. Barratt et al., *Foundations*, 61–62.

38. Nolen, "Problems," 66.

39. Dorothy Kerth, "To a Young Swimming Instructor," in *Aquatics Guide, July 1961–July 1963, With Official Rules and Swimming and Diving Standards* (Washington, D.C.: DGWS/AAHPER, 1961), 32.

40. "Women and Competitive Sport," in *Proceedings of the First National Institute on Girls Sports Held November 4–9, 1963* (Washington, D.C.: AAHPER, 1965), 30.

41. See "Standards" in DGWS publications: *Basketball Guide, September 1962–September 1963*, 155; *Softball Guide, January 1964–January 1966*, 136; and *Track and Field Guide, January 1964–January 1966*, 121.

42. Committee on Standards of DGWS, *Philosophy and Standards for Girls and Women's Sports* (Washington, D.C.: DGWS/AAHPER, 1969), 18.

43. Ibid., 52–54.

44. "Report of the Research Committee of the Division for Girls and Women's Sports, December 1960," 2, new Box 23, Folder: Research Committee, 1957–73, DGWS Papers (AC 3:6:1:6 Structures).

45. From packet of research summaries, new Box 23, Folder: Research Committee, 1957–73, DGWS Papers (AC 3:6:1:6 Structures).

46. Jane A. Mott, *Conditioning and Basic Movement Concepts* (Dubuque, Iowa: Wm. C. Brown, 1968), 39.

47. Barratt et al., *Foundations*, 60–61.

48. Kimberly K. Yeager et al., "The Female Athlete Triad: Disordered Eating, Amenorrhea, Osteoporosis," *MSSE* 25 (1993): 775–77.

49. Carol L. Otis et al., "ACSM Position Stand: The Female Athlete Triad," *MSSE* 29, no. 5 (1997): v, and i–ix in general.

50. Elizabeth F. Yurth, "Female Athlete Triad," *Western Journal of Medicine* 162 (1995): 149.

51. *Science News* 133 (February 27, 1988): 137.

52. Edwin Dale et al., "Physical Fitness Profiles and Reproductive Physiology of the Female Distance Runner," *PSM* 7 (January 1979): 83–86, 89–91, 94–95; and Charlotte B. Feicht et al., "Secondary Amenorrhoea in Athletes," *Lancet* 2 (November 25, 1978): 1145–46.

53. Rose E. Frisch and Roger Revelle, "Height and Weight at Menarche and a Hypothesis of Critical Body Weights and Adolescent Events," *Science* 169 (1970): 397–99.

54. Rose E. Frisch and Janet W. McArthur, "Menstrual Cycles: Fatness as a Determinant of Minimum Weight for Height Necessary for Their Maintenance or Onset," *Science* 185 (1974): 949–51.

55. American College of Obstetricians and Gynecologists, *Précis: An Update in Obstetrics and Gynecology* (New York: McGraw-Hill, 1977), 145.

56. ACSM, "Opinion Statement on the Participation of the Female Athlete in Long-Distance Running," *MSSE* 11 (Winter 1979): ix–xi; and Richard W. Corbitt et al., "Female Athletics: Special Communication from the Committee on the Medical Aspects of Sports of the American Medical Association," *JAMA* 228 (1974): 1266–67.

57. For example, "Physical Activity During Menstruation and Pregnancy," *Physical Fitness Research Digest* Series 8 (July 1978): 1–25.

58. See Nadine Brozan, "Training Linked to Disruption of Female Reproductive Cycle," *New York Times*, April 17, 1978, C1, C10; and Deborah Larned-Romano and Jane Leavy, "Athletics and Fertility," *Ms. Magazine* 8 (October 1979): 38, 41.

59. For example, Donna Mae Miller, *Coaching the Female Athlete* (Philadelphia: Lea and Febiger, 1974), 33–35, 159–60.

60. Christine Wells, "The Female Athlete: Myths and Superstitions Put to Rest," in *Toward an Understanding of Human Performance: Readings in Exercise Physiology for the Coach and Athlete*, ed. Edmund J. Burke (Ithaca, N.Y.: Mouvement, 1978), 38.

61. Dorothy Harris, "The Female Athlete: Strength, Endurance and Performance," in Burke, *Toward an Understanding*, 42.

62. Quoted in J. F., "Secondary Amenorrhea Linked to Stress," *PSM* 6 (October 1978): 24.

63. Dorothy Harris, "Physical Sex Differences: Being Male and Being Female," in *The Study of Women: Enlarging Perspectives of Social Reality*, ed. Eloise C. Snyder (New York: Harper and Row, 1979), 189–90.

64. Tenley Albright, "Which Sports for Girls?" in *DGWS Research Reports: Women in Sports*, ed. Dorothy V. Harris (Washington, D.C.: AAHPER, 1971), 1:56.

65. Contemporary reviews included David C. Cumming, "The Reproductive Effects of Exercise and Training," *Current Problems in Obstetrics, Gynecology, and Fertility* 10 (June 1987): 225–85; and Charlotte F. Sanborn, "Menstrual Dysfunction in the Female Athlete," in *Scientific Foundations of Sports Medicine*, ed. Carol C. Teitz (Toronto: B. C. Decker, 1989), 117–34.

66. Jerilynn C. Prior and Yvette M. Vigna, "Ovulation Disturbances and Exercise Training," *Clinical Obstetrics and Gynecology* 34 (1991): 180–90.

67. Mary Jane De Souza, Joan Carles Arce, and Deborah A. Metzger, "Endocrine Basis of Exercise-Induced Amenorrhea," in *Women and Sport: Interdisciplinary Perspectives*, ed. D. Margaret Costa and Sharon R. Guthrie (Champaign, Ill.: Human Kinetics, 1994), 186, figure 13.1.

68. Christine M. Snow-Harter, "Bone Health and Prevention of Osteoporosis in Active and Athletic Women," *Clinics in Sports Medicine* 13 (1994): 389–404.

69. Terry Monahan, "Treating Athletic Amenorrhea: A Matter of Instinct?" *PSM* 15 (July 1987): 184.

70. Barbara L. Drinkwater, "Women: Menstrual Dysfunction, Premature Bone Loss, and Pregnancy," in *Future Directions in Exercise and Sport Science Research*, ed. James S. Skinner et al. (Champaign, Ill.: Human Kinetics, 1989), 251, 253.

71. Carol L. Otis and Roger Goldingay, "A Crucial Period," *Shape* 11 (March 1992): 51; and Aurelia Nattiv, with Lynda Lynch, "The Female Athlete Triad: Managing an Acute Risk to Long-Term Health," *PSM* 22 (January 1994): 67–68.

72. Robert W. Rebar, "Exercise and the Menstrual Cycle," in *Caring for the Exercising Woman*, ed. Ralph W. Hale, Current Topics in Obstetrics and Gynecology (New York: Elsevier Science, 1991), 69.

73. Charlotte Feicht Sanborn and Wiltz W. Wagner Jr., "Athletic Amenorrhea," in *Female Endurance Athletes*, ed. Barbara L. Drinkwater (Champaign, Ill.: Human Kinetics, 1986), 139.

74. Mary Jane De Souza and Deborah A. Metzger, "Reproductive Dysfunction in Amenorrheic Athletes and Anorexic Patients: A Review," *MSSE* 23 (1991): 995–1007.

75. Gruhn and Kazer, *Hormonal Regulation*, 102–63, 172–75. The hi-fi analogy appeared in Kenneth J. Ryan, Ross Berkowitz, and Robert L. Barbieri, *Kistner's Gynecology: Principles and Practice*, 5th ed. (Chicago: Year Book Medical, 1990), 18.

76. Arend Bonen, "Effect of Exercise and Training on Reproductive Hormones," *International Journal of Sports Medicine* 5 (1984): 195.

77. Otis et al., "ACSM Position Stand" (1997), v.

78. Anne B. Loucks, quoted in Frances Munnings, "Exercise and Estrogen in Women's Health: Getting a Clearer Picture," *PSM* 16 (May 1988): 152.

79. Jerilynn C. Prior, "Luteal Phase Defects and Anovulation: Adaptive Alterations Occurring with Conditioning Exercise," *Seminars in Reproductive Endocrinology* 3 (February 1985): 27.

80. See ACOG publications: "Women and Exercise," *Technical Bulletin*, No. 87 (September 1985); "Amenorrhea," *Technical Bulletin*, No. 128 (May 1989); "Women and Exercise," *Technical Bulletin*, No. 173 (October 1992); and *Précis III: An Update in Obstetrics and Gynecology* (1986), 69, 270–71, 285–86.

81. ACOG, *Exercise and Fitness: A Guide for Women*, ACOG Patient Education Pamphlet, AP045 (Washington, D.C.: ACOG, 1992).

82. Renie Rae Howard, "Rule Changes in Women's Tennis Target Medical Issues," *PSM* 23 (June 1995): 25–26; Andrew A. Skolnick, "Health Pros Want New Rules for Girl Athletes," *JAMA* 275 (1996): 22–24; and "Task Force on USA Gymnastics Response to the Female Athlete Triad," *Technique* 15 (October–November 1995): 18–21.

83. Jane E. Brody, "Effects of Exercise on Menstruation," *New York Times*, September 1, 1982, C6.

84. Aurelia Nattiv et al., "The Female Athlete Triad: The Inter-Relatedness of Disordered Eating, Amenorrhea, and Osteoporosis," *Clinics in Sports Medicine* 13 (1994): 407.

85. Mona M. Shangold and Gabe Mirkin, *The Complete Medicine Book for Women* (New York: Fireside, 1985), 111–24; and Linda Villarosa, ed., *Body & Soul: The Black Woman's Guide to Physical Health and Emotional Well-Being* (New York: HarperCollins, 1994), 156.

86. Felicia H. Stewart et al., *Understanding Your Body: Every Woman's Guide to a Lifetime of Health* (New York: Bantam, 1987), 577, 579–81.

87. Kathryn A. Cox, *The Good Housekeeping Illustrated Guide to Women's Health* (New York: Hearst, 1995), 56–57, 141, 179–80.

88. *U.S. News and World Report* 104 (March 7, 1988): 72; and *Mademoiselle* 93 (August 1987): 120.

89. Hunter Heath, "Athletic Women, Amenorrhea, and Skeletal Integrity," *Annals of Internal Medicine* 102 (1985): 258.

90. Ronald S. Laura and Christina Lee, "Amenorrhea: Your Cycle and Training—A Woman's Menstrual Status is More than a Matter of Body Fat," *Joe Weider's Muscle and Fitness* 54 (May 1993): 136.

91. Heath, "Athletic Women," 259.

92. My discussion draws on Iris M. Young, "Menstrual Meditations" in *On Female Body Experience: "Throwing Like a Girl" and Other Essays* (New York: Oxford University Press, 2005), 97–122 (quotations, 102, 109, 116).

93. Critique based on my review of dozens of North American and European scientific studies; and tables in the following sources: Sanborn, "Dysfunction," 119; Michelle P. Warren and Mona M. Shangold, *Sports Gynecology: Problems and Care of the Athletic Female* (Cambridge, Mass.: Blackwell Science, 1997), 6; and Christine L. Wells, *Women, Sport, and Performance*, 2nd ed. (Champaign, Ill.: Human Kinetics, 1991), 111–13, 117–18.

94. Arend Bonen, "Recreational Exercise Does Not Impair Menstrual Cycles: A Prospective Study," *International Journal of Sports Medicine* 13 (1992): 110–20; Loretta DiPietro and Nina S. Stachenfeld, "The Female Athlete Triad," *MSSE* 29 (1997): 1669–70; and Alan D. Rogol et al., "Durability of the Reproductive Axis in Eumenorrheic Women During 1 Year of Endurance Training," *Journal of Applied Physiology* 72 (1992): 1571–80.

95. Diane Wakat, in Issue 1: Physiological Concerns of Women in Sport, Topic C: "What are the reproductive and fertility concerns of athletic women?" in *The New Agenda: "A Blueprint for the Future of Women's Sports"* (San Francisco: Women's Sports Foundation, 1985), 28.

96. Joan Ullyot, "Amenorrhea: A Sensitive Subject," *Women's Sports* 3 (December 1981): 46.

97. Jerilynn C. Prior, "Endocrine 'Conditioning' with Endurance Training: A Preliminary Review," *Canadian Journal of Applied Sport Sciences* 7 (1982): 148.

98. Quotations from Wakat, "Reproductive," 28; and Joan Ullyot, "Periodic Concern," *Runner's World* 25 (August 1990): 24.

99. Wakat, "Reproductive," 28.

100. On the provocative hypothesis about cancer, see Rose E. Frisch, "Body Fat, Menarche, Fitness and Fertility," *Human Reproduction* 2 (1987): 521–33.

101. Mona M. Shangold, "Athletics Not Cause of Gynecological Concerns," *New Directions for Women* 10 (January–February 1981): 8.

102. Jerilynn C. Prior, Yvette M. Vigna, and Donald W. McKay, "Reproduction for the Athletic Woman: New Understandings of Physiology and Management," *Sports Medicine* 14, no. 3 (1992): 191.

103. Experts' summaries included Margaret A. Kolka and Lou A. Stephenson, "The Menstrual Cycle and the Female Athlete," *PE* 39 (October 1982): 136–41; and Gwen Hagenbuch Sasiene, "Secondary Amenorrhea Among Female Athletes: Current Understandings," *JOPERD* 54 (June 1983): 61–63.

104. N. Peggy Burke, "Nutrition for Women Athletes: Commonly Asked Questions," *JOPERD* 58 (March 1987): 42.

105. For example, Billie J. Lindsey and Kathleen F. Janz, "A Healthy Connection: Helping Physical Educators Address Eating Disorders," *JOPERD* 56 (November–December 1985): 41–44; and Virginia G. Overdorf, "Conditioning for Thinness," *JOPERD* 58 (April 1987): 62–65.

106. Sanborn, "Dysfunction," 128.

107. Feicht et al., "Secondary Amenorrhoea"; Barbara L. Drinkwater et al., "Bone Mineral Content of Amenorrheic and Eumenorrheic Athletes," *NEJM* 311 (1984): 277–81; and Barbara L. Drinkwater et al., "Bone Mineral Density After Resumption of Menses in Amenorrheic Athletes," *JAMA* 256 (1986): 380–82.

108. Quoted in Sanborn, "Dysfunction," 118.

109. Dorothy V. Harris and Patricia Potter, "Special Considerations for the Female Athlete," 10, typescript, 1982, Box 25, Folder: Special Considerations; and Harris, "The Effect of Exercise on Reproductive Health," 3, handwritten lecture notes, September 25, 1981, Box 38, Folder: Exercise and Reproductive Health, Papers of Dorothy V. Harris, Special Collections and University Archives, Penn State University, University Park, Pa.

110. Drinkwater, quoted in Terry Monahan, "Should Women Go Easy on Exercise?" *PSM* 12 (December 1986): 188, 190.

111. Christine L. Wells, "Menstruation, Pregnancy, and Menopause," in *Physical Activity and Well-Being*, ed. Vern Seefeldt (Reston, Va.: AAHPERD, 1986), 212.

112. Stephen R. Wall and David C. Cumming, "Effects of Physical Activity on Reproductive Function and Development in Males," *Seminars in Reproductive Endocrinology* 3 (February 1985): 65, 68.

113. Sharon Ann Plowman, "Maturation and Exercise Training in Children," *Pediatric Exercise Science* 1 (1989): 304.

114. Wall and Cumming, "Effects of Physical Activity," 65.

115. Michelle P. Warren, "Effects of Undernutrition on Reproductive Function in the Human," *Endocrine Reviews* 4 (1983): 363, 368.

116. Reviews include Katherine A. Beals and Nanna L. Meyer, "Female Athlete Triad Update," *Clinics in Sports Medicine* 26 (2007): 69–89; and Leanne M. Redman and Anne B. Loucks, "Menstrual Disorders in Athletes," *Sports Medicine* 35 (2005): 747–55.

117. Anne B. Loucks, "Energy Availability, Not Body Fatness, Regulates Reproductive Function in Women," *ESSR* 31 (2003): 146.

118. Mary Jane De Souza and Nancy I. Williams, "Beyond Hypoestrogenism in Amenorrheic Athletes: Energy Deficiency As a Contributing Factor for Bone Loss," *Current Sports Medicine Reports* 4 (2005): 40.

119. Anne B. Loucks, "Prevailing View," in "Contrasting Perspectives in Exercise Science and Sports Medicine: The Female Athlete Triad—Do Female Athletes Need to Take Special Care to Avoid Low Energy Availability?" *MSSE* 38 (2006): 1694.

120. Christine A. Dueck et al., "Treatment of Athletic Amenorrhea with a Diet and Training Intervention Program," *International Journal of Sport Nutrition* 6 (1996): 35.

121. Cathy L. Zanker and Carlton B. Cooke, "Energy Balance, Bone Turnover, and Skeletal Health in Physically Active Individuals," *MSSE* 36 (2004): 1379.

122. Alan D. Rogol, "Delayed Puberty in Girls and Primary and Secondary Amenorrhea," in *The Child and Adolescent Athlete*, ed. Oded Bar-Or, vol. 6 of *The Encyclopaedia of Sports Medicine* (Cambridge, Mass.: Blackwell Science, 1996), 313–16; and Warren and Shangold, *Sports Gynecology*, 5–7, 35–37.

123. Aurelia Nattiv et al., "ACSM Position Stand: The Female Athlete Triad," *MSSE* 39 (2007): 1871.

124. Constance Marie Lebrun, "The Female Athlete Triad: What's a Doctor to Do?" *Current Sports Medicine Reports* 6 (2007): 397–404; and Paula E. Papanek, "The Female Athlete Triad: An Emerging Role for Physical Therapy," *Journal of Orthopedic and Sports Physical Therapy* 33 (2003): 594–614.

125. See American Academy of Pediatrics, Committee on Sports Medicine and Fitness, "Medical Concerns in the Female Athlete: Policy Statement," *Pediatrics* 106 (2000): 610–13; Melinda M. Manore, Susan I. Barr, and Gail E. Butterfield, "Position of the American Dietetic Association, Dieticians of Canada, and the American College of Sports Medicine: Nutrition and Athletic Performance," *Journal of the American Dietetic Association* 100 (2000): 1544–46; Nattiv et al., "ACSM Position Stand" (2007), 1867–69; "What is the Female Athlete Triad?" Female Athlete Triad Coalition, http://www.femaleathletetriad.org/faq.html (accessed December 9, 2007); and "Female Athlete Issues for the Team Physician: A Consensus Statement," *MSSE* 35 (2003): 1789–90.

126. *NCAA Coaches Handbook: Managing the Female Athlete Triad*, 3, 19, 31, http://princeton.edu/uhs/pdfs/NCAA%20Managing%20the%20Female%20Athlete%20Triad.pdf (accessed December 15, 2007); "IOC Consensus Statement on the Female Athlete Triad, November 9, 2005," http://www.olympic.org/uk/organisation/commissions/medical/full_story_uk.asp?id=1540 (accessed December 14, 2007); International Olympic Committee (IOC) Medical Commission Working Group Women in Sport, *Position Stand on the Female Athlete Triad*, 2006, http://multimedia.olympic.org/pdf/en_report_917.pdf (accessed December 14, 2007); and Women's Sports Foundation, "The Female Athlete Triad," http://womenssportsfoundation.org/binary-data/WSF_ARTICLE/pdf_file/721.pdf (accessed January 3, 2008).

127. For example, Lola Ramos and Gregory L. Welch, "The Female Triad," *American Fitness* 22 (May–June 2004): 56–63.

128. Carol L. Otis and Roger Goldingay, *The Athletic Woman's Survival Guide* (Champaign, Ill.: Human Kinetics, 2000), 113; and "What is the Female Athlete Triad?" FAT Coalition website.

129. Monica L. Rencken, Charles H. Chesnut III, and Barbara L. Drinkwater, "Bone Density at Multiple Skeletal Sites in Amenorrheic Athletes," *JAMA* 276 (July 17, 1996): 238–40.

130. Katherine A. Beals, Rebecca A. Brey, and Julianna B. Gonyou, "Understanding the Female Athlete Triad: Eating Disorders, Amenorrhea, and Osteoporosis," *Journal of School Health* 69 (1999): 337.

131. Nattiv et al., "ACSM Position Stand" (2007), 1870.

132. Otis and Goldingay, *Survival Guide*, 1.

133. Lebrun, "Triad," 397.

134. Nattiv et al., "ACSM Position Stand" (2007), 1868.

135. Otis and Goldingay, *Survival Guide*, 126.

136. "The Health Effects and Benefits of Physical Activity in Women," *Women's Health Issues* 8 (March–April 1998): 78.

137. Angela D. Smith, "The Female Athlete Triad: Causes, Diagnosis, and Treatment," *PSM* 24 (July 1996): 68.

138. JoAnn E. Manson and I-Min Lee, "Exercise for Women—How Much Pain for Optimal Gain?" *NEJM* 334 (1996): 1325–27.

139. Karen J. Carlson, Stephanie A. Eisenstat, and Terra Ziporyn, *The Harvard Guide to Women's Health* (Cambridge, Mass.: Harvard University Press, 1996), 33; and Cox, *Good Housekeeping*, 141, 179–80.

140. Michelle P. Warren and Shanmugan Shantha, "The Female Athlete," *Baillière's Clinical Endocrinology and Metabolism* 14 (2000): 48.

141. Otis and Goldingay, *Survival Guide*, 124.

142. Zanker and Cooke, "Energy Balance," 1375, 1376.

143. For example, "Research Works: Can Adequate Caloric Intake Prevent 'Exercise-Induced' Amenorrhea?" *JOPERD* 67 (February 1996): 15; and Katherine A. Beals and Sarah E. Warner, "The Female Athlete Triad," in *Ensuring the Health of Active and Athletic Girls and Women*, ed. Lynda Ransdell and Linda Petlichkoff (Reston, Va.: NAGWS, 2005), 215–16, 218, 220.

144. Burney and Brehm, "Triad," 43.

145. Katherine A. Beals, "Subclinical Eating Disorders in Female Athletes," *JOPERD* 71 (September 2000): 23–29.

146. Burney and Brehm, "Triad," 45; and Jane Shimon, "In the Shadow of Obesity: The Female Triad," *JOPERD* 77 (August 2006): 54.

147. For example, Deborah H. Rhea, "Physical Activity and Body Image of Female Adolescents: Moving Toward the 21st Century," *JOPERD* 69 (May–June 1998): 27–31; Karen M. Skemp-Arlt, "Body Image Dissatisfaction and Eating Disturbances Among Children and Adolescents: Prevalence, Risk Factors, and Prevention Strategies," *JOPERD* 77 (January 2006): 45–51; and Sarah E. Warner and Janet M. Shaw, "Estrogen, Physical Activity, and Bone Health," *JOPERD* 71 (August 2000): 19–23, 27–28.

Conclusion

1. See Jepkorir Rose Chepyator-Thomson, JeongAe You, and Brent Hardin, "Issues and Perspectives on Gender in Physical Education," *WSPAJ* 9 (2000): 99–121; Alison Dewar, "Oppression and Privilege in Physical Education: Struggles in the Negotiation of Gender in a University Programme," in *Physical Education, Curriculum and Culture: Critical Issues in the Contemporary Crisis*, ed. David Kirk and Richard Tinning (London: Falmer, 1991), 67–100; Anne Flintoff, "Gender, Physical Education and Initial Teacher Education," in *Equality, Education and Physical Education*, ed. John Evans (London: Falmer, 1993), 184–204; and Susan Wilkinson, Kay M. Williamson, and Ruth Rozdilsky, "Gender and Fitness Standards," *WSPAJ* 5 (1996): 1–25.

2. Judith Lorber, "Believing Is Seeing: Biology as Ideology," *Gender & Society* 7 (1993): 568–71.

3. David Kirk and Richard Tinning, "Embodied Self-Identity, Healthy Lifestyles and School Physical Education," *Sociology of Health & Illness* 16 (1994): 606.

4. Sandra Lee Bartky, "Foucault, Femininity, and the Modernization of Patriarchal Power," in *Feminism and Foucault: Reflections on Resistance*, ed. Irene Diamond and Lee Quinby (Boston: Northeastern University Press, 1988), 61–86; and Michel Foucault, "Body/Power," in *Power/Knowledge: Selected Interviews and Other Writings, 1972–1977*, ed. Colin Gordon (New York: Pantheon, 1980), 55–62.

5. Allan M. Brandt and Paul Rozin, eds., *Morality and Health* (New York: Routledge, 1997); and Bryan S. Turner, *The Body and Society: Explorations in Social Theory*, 2nd ed. (London: Sage, 1996), 159–96.

6. John Evans and Brian Davies, "Introduction," in Evans, *Equality, Education and Physical Education*, 3–5; and David Kirk, "Physical Education, Discourse, and Ideology: Bringing the Hidden Curriculum Into View," *Quest* 44 (1992): 35–56.

7. Phrase from Arthur W. Frank, "Bringing Bodies Back In: A Decade Review," *Theory, Culture & Society* 7 (1990): 131.

8. Although histories of the profession's research bloc consider intellectual context, my analysis of the relationships between instructional physical education and science is distinctive.

9. Frances E. Willard, *How I Learned to Ride the Bicycle: Reflections of an Influential 19th Century Woman*, ed. Carol O'Hare, introduction by Edith Mayo (Sunnyvale, Calif.: Fair Oaks, 1991), 45.

10. Ibid., 31, 33, 46.

11. Emily Martin, *The Woman in the Body: A Cultural Analysis of Reproduction* (Boston: Beacon, 1987), 194–95.

12. Robyn Wiegman and Lynda Zwinger, "Tonya's Bad Boot, or, Go Figure," in *Women on Ice: Feminist Essays on the Tonya Harding/Nancy Kerrigan Spectacle*, ed. Cynthia Baughman (New York: Routledge, 1995), 105.

13. See Jepkorir Rose Chepyator-Thomson and Catherine D. Ennis, "Reproduction and Resistance to the Culture of Femininity and Masculinity in Secondary School Physical Education," *RQES* 68 (1997): 89–99; President's Council on Physical Fitness and Sports, *Physical Activity and Sport in the Lives of Girls: Physical and Mental Health Dimensions from an Interdisciplinary Approach* (Washington, D.C.: President's Council, 1997); and Women's Sports Foundation, *Her Life Depends On It: Sport, Physical Activity and the Health and Well-Being of American Girls* (East Meadow, N.Y.: WSF, 2004).

14. Willard, *How I Learned*, 27, 41–42, 49–50, 61.

15. For example, Nate McCaughtry, "Learning to Read Gender Relations in Schooling: Implications of Personal History and Teaching Context on Identifying Disempowerment for Girls," *RQES* 75 (2004): 400–412.

16. See Laura Azzarito and Melinda A. Solmon, "A Reconceptualization of Physical Education: The Intersection of Gender/Race/Social Class," *Sport, Education and Society* 10 (2005): 25–47; Mary Jo Kane, "Resistance/Transformation of the Oppositional Binary: Exposing Sport as a Continuum," *Journal of Sport and Social Issues* 19 (1995): 191–218; and Inez Rovegno and David Kirk, "Articulations and Silences in Socially Critical Work on Physical Education: Toward a Broader Agenda," *Quest* 47 (1995): 447–74.

17. Evans and Davies, "Introduction," in Evans, *Equality, Education and Physical Education*, 21.

{ SELECT BIBLIOGRAPHY }

The entries under manuscript collections, oral histories, and primary journals are inclusive. The listings of government documents and primary books and articles emphasize works by American physical educators or items especially pertinent to them. The sections on secondary sources feature scholarship that informed individual chapters and my overall analysis. The endnotes provide a more comprehensive record of this book's extensive research base.

Manuscript Collections

Agnes Scott College, Decatur, Ga. McCain Library. Special Collections and Archives.
    Kate McKemie Papers.
    Physical Education Department File.
American Alliance for Health, Physical Education, Recreation and Dance, Reston, Va.
    Archives. (Now housed at Babson Library, Springfield College, Springfield, Mass.)
    Papers of the American Academy of Physical Education.
    Papers of Blanche Trilling.
    Papers of the Division of Girls and Women's Sports (1957–74), Coll. AC 4:6:5.
    Papers of Mabel Lee.
    Papers of the National Section on Women's Athletics (1932–53), National Section for
        Girls and Women's Sports (1953–57), and Division of Girls and Women's Sports
        (1957–74), Coll. AC 3:6:1.
    Papers of the Women's Athletic Section (1898–1932) and National Section on Women's
        Athletics (1932–53), Coll. AC 2:6:7.
    Papers of the Women's Division of the National Amateur Athletic Federation.
Brown University, Providence, R.I. John Hay Library. University Archives.
    Records of the Department of Physical Education of Pembroke College.
Bryn Mawr College, Bryn Mawr, Pa. Mariam Coffin Canaday Library. Special Collections
    and College Archives.
    Papers of Constance M. K. Applebee.
    Papers of M. Carey Thomas.
    Records of the Physical Education Department.
Charles Sumner School Museum and Archives, Washington, D.C. Research Library and
    Archives.
    Minutes of the Board of Education, District of Columbia Public Schools.
Duke University, Durham, N.C. William R. Perkins Library. Rare Book, Manuscript, and
    Special Collections Library.
    Papers of the Grout Family.

Duke University, Durham, N.C. William R. Perkins Library. University Archives.
    Papers of Alice Mary Baldwin.
    Papers of Julia R. Grout.
    Papers of William Hane Wannamaker.
    Papers of William Preston Few.
    Records of the Women's Department of Health and Physical Education.
Hampton University, Hampton, Va. Hampton University Museum. University Archives.
    Faculty Files.
    Faculty information cards.
    Papers of Hollis Burke Frissell.
    Records of the College of Education: Division of Physical Education, Coll. 19/11.
Howard University, Washington, D.C. Moorland-Spingarn Research Center. University
    Archives.
    Annual Reports of the College of Liberal Arts.
    Howardiana Vertical Files.
Howard University, Washington, D.C. Moorland-Spingarn Research Center. Manuscript
    Division.
    Papers of Cato Adams.
    Papers of Charlotte Moton Hubbard.
    Papers of Edwin Bancroft Henderson.
    Papers of Maryrose Reeves Allen.
Lawrence University, Appleton, Wisc. Seeley G. Mudd Library. University Archives.
    Archives of Milwaukee-Downer College: Papers of Althea Heimbach.
Oberlin College, Oberlin, Ohio. Mudd Center. College Archives.
    Alumni and Development Records: Faculty Files.
    Oberlin Files.
    Papers of the Office of the Secretary: Administrative Records of Departments and
        Offices—Annual Reports Received.
    Records of the Physical Education Department: Physical Education for Women (Coll.
        9/6), including Papers of Gertrude Moulton.
Ohio State University, Columbus, Ohio. Library Book Depository. University Archives.
    Papers of the Division of Student Services: Athletic Department, including Records
        of the Director's Office (9/e-1) and Records of Women's Recreational and Intra-
        mural Sports (9/e-5a).
    Records of Women's Athletics (9/e-5a, Acc. 124/89).
    Records of the College of Education: School of Health, Physical Education, and Recrea-
        tion (unprocessed Acc. 89/89 and 36/84).
Pennsylvania State University, University Park, Pa. Paterno Library. Eberly Family Special
    Collections Library. University Archives.
    Papers of Dorothy V. Harris.
Radcliffe Institute, Harvard University, Cambridge, Mass. Radcliffe College Archives.
    Papers of the Office of the President: LeBaron Russell Briggs and Ada L. Comstock.
    Papers of the Physical Education Department, including Records of the Athletic
        Association.
    Records of the Alumnae Association: Class Collections.
    Records of the Radcliffe College Governing Board.

Smith College, Northampton, Mass. Neilson Library. College Archives.
  General Faculty Files—Individuals (Series 42): Dorothy S. Ainsworth, Senda Berenson,
    Florence Gilman, Florence Meredith, and Anna Mann Richardson.
  Papers of Dorothy S. Ainsworth (Coll. 3A).
  Presidential Papers (Series 32): Herbert John Davis and William H. Neilson.
  Records of College Departments (Series 52): Papers of the Physical Education
    Department (processed and unprocessed).
  Records of Students—Athletics and Activities (Series 80): Papers of the Athletic
    Association.
Spelman College, Atlanta, Ga. Cosby Academic Center. College Archives.
  Personnel Records.
Stanford University, Stanford, Calif. Stanford University Libraries. Department of Special
  Collections and University Archives.
  Faculty Biographical Files.
  Papers of Clelia Duel Mosher.
  Papers of Luell Weed Guthrie.
  Papers of President Ray Lyman Wilbur.
  Records of the Department of Physical Education for Women.
  Records of the Women's Athletic Association/Women's Recreation Association.
Tulane University, New Orleans, La. Howard-Tilton Memorial Library. University
  Archives.
  Newcomb College Scrapbooks.
  University Faculty Files.
Tuskegee University, Tuskegee, Ala. Hollis Burke Frissell Library. University Archives.
  Papers of Nell Cecilia Jackson.
  Papers of Robert Russa Moton.
  Papers of Robert Stewart Darnaby.
  Papers of Ross C. Owen.
University of California at Berkeley, Berkeley, Calif. The Bancroft Library.
  Papers of Anna S. Espenschade.
  Papers of the Women's Athletic Association.
  Papers of the Women's Division of the National Amateur Athletic Federation.
University of California at Berkeley, Berkeley, Calif. Hearst Gymnasium Historical
  Collections.
  Papers of Winifred Van Hagen.
University of Illinois at Urbana-Champaign, Urbana, Ill. Main Library. University Archives.
  Records of the College of Applied Life Studies: Physical Education for Women
    Department, including Papers of Jennette E. Carpenter Lincoln, Papers of Laura
    J. Huelster, and Papers of Louise Freer.
University of Michigan, Ann Arbor, Mich. Bentley Historical Library.
  Papers of Eliza Maria Mosher.
  Papers of Margaret Bell.
  Papers of Marie D. Hartwig.
  Papers of the Department of Physical Education for Women.
  Papers of President Clarence Cook Little.
  Records of the Women's Athletic Association, 1905–62.

University of Minnesota, Minneapolis, Minn. Elmer L. Andersen Library. University Archives.

    Alumnae Association of the Physical Education Association: Misc. documents.

    Papers of Anne Maud Butner.

    Papers of Gertrude M. Baker.

    Papers of the President's Office, 1911–45.

    Records of the College of Education, 1917–50 (Coll. AQ1.1).

    Tape-recorded interview, Gertrude M. Baker, May 24, 1968.

    Women's Athletic Association: Misc. documents.

University of Nebraska at Lincoln, Lincoln, Neb. UNL Libraries. Archives and Special Collections.

    Papers of the Board of Regents.

    Papers of the Office of the Chancellor: Samuel Avery; E. A. Burnett; C. S. Boucher; R. G. Gustavson; John K. Selleck; Clifford Hardin; and D. B. Varner.

    Records of the Teachers College: Department of Physical Education for Women (Coll. 23/18).

University of North Carolina at Greensboro, Greensboro, N.C. Walter Clinton Jackson Library. Special Collections and University Archives.

    Papers of Chancellor Julius Isaac Foust.

    Papers of Chancellor Walter Clinton Jackson.

    Papers of the National Association for Physical Education of College Women.

    Papers of the Southern Association for Physical Education of College Women.

    Records of the School of Health, Physical Education, Recreation, and Dance, including Papers of Mary Channing Coleman.

    Records of Student Organizations: Recreation Association.

University of Wisconsin, Madison, Wisc. Steenbock Memorial Library. Steenbock Archives.

    Papers of the School of Education: Department of Women's Physical Education (Acc. 82/50), including Files of Blanche Trilling.

    Papers of the School of Education: Department of Women's Physical Education (Acc. 16/82).

    Papers of the School of Education: Department of Women's Physical Education (Coll. 13/5).

University of Wisconsin, Madison, Wisc. Memorial Library. University Archives.

    Papers of the Chancellors of the University.

Wellesley College, Wellesley, Mass. Margaret Clapp Library. College Archives.

    Papers of Amy Morris Homans (Coll. 3P).

    Papers of the Department of Hygiene and Physical Education (Coll. 3L), including Student Records.

    Records of the Alumnae Association: Hygiene and Physical Education Section— Biographical Data.

Oral Histories (Interviews conducted by the author)

Beavers, Irene. By telephone. Tuskegee, Ala. May 27, 1996.

Benson, Rita. Northampton, Mass. March 1, 1996.

Bookhout, Elizabeth C. Tape recording. Durham, N.C. May 7, 1992.

Broer, Marion R. Tape recording. Irvine, Calif. August 7, 1993.

Bryan, Margaret (Peg). Lewisburg, Pa. Various dates, 1995–2005.

Espenschade, Anna S. Tape recording, Laguna Hills, Calif. August 9, 1993.

Hooten, Henry. Tape recording. Tuskegee, Ala. July 28, 1994.

Jewett, Ann E. Tape recording. Athens, Ga. July 29, 1994.

Levinson, Ruth Diamond. Tape recording. Lincoln, Neb. November 11, 1991.

Manuel, Kay. Tape recording. Decatur, Ga. August 3, 1994.

Maver, Jane. West Lafayette, Ind. June 29, 1994.

McKemie, Kate. Tape recording. Decatur, Ga. August 3, 1994.

Phillips, Madge M. Tape recording. Knoxville, Tenn. August 6, 1994.

Russell, Helen. Northampton, Mass. March 1, 1996.

Schellberg, Ruth. Tape recording. Mankato, Minn. November 18, 1991.

Sherman, Helen. Tape recording. Wayland, Mass. August 6, 1992.

Shrader, Ray Anne. West Lafayette, Ind. June 29, 1994.

Simon, Marguerite. Tape recording. Atlanta, Ga. May 28, 1996.

Ulrich, Celeste. Tape recording. Eugene, Ore. May 28, 1995.

Van Cleve, Whitney. Tape recording. Tuskegee, Ala. July 28, 1994.

Wilson, Ruth M. Tape recording. Irvine, Calif. August 7, 1993.

Yost, Mary. Tape recording. Columbus, Ohio. July 7, 1994.

Primary Journals and Serials

American Physical Education Review (1896–1929)

Exercise and Sport Sciences Reviews (1973–current)

Journal of Health and Physical Education (1930–48)

Journal of Health, Physical Education, and Recreation (1949–75)

Journal of Physical Education and Recreation (1976–80)

Journal of Physical Education, Recreation and Dance (1981–current)

Journal of Teaching in Physical Education (1981–current)

Medicine and Science in Sports (1969–79)

Medicine and Science in Sports and Exercise (1980–current)

Mind and Body (1894–1936)

Official Sports Guides for Women and Girls (1901–85, covering various sports. Publisher: Spalding's American Sports Publishing Company, 1901–38; A. S. Barnes and Company, 1938–49; AAHPER, 1949–85)

PCPFS Research Digest (1993–current; preceded by *Physical Fitness Research Digest* and *Physical Activity and Fitness Research Digest*)

The Physical Educator (1940–current)

The Physician and Sportsmedicine (1973–current)

Proceedings of the American Association for the Advancement of Physical Education (1885–95)

Proceedings of the Annual Meeting of the American Student Health Association (1919–64)

Quest (1963–current)

Research Quarterly (1930–79)

Research Quarterly for Exercise and Sport (1980–current)

Women in Sport and Physical Activity Journal (1992–current)

Government Documents

Boykin, James C. "Physical Training." In *Report of the [U.S.] Commissioner of Education for the Year 1891–92*, 1:580–94. Washington, D.C.: Government Printing Office, 1894.

Brammell, P. Roy. *Intramural and Interscholastic Athletics*. National Survey of Secondary Education Monograph no. 27, Office of Education Bulletin, 1932, no. 17. Washington, D.C.: Government Printing Office, 1933.

Caliver, Ambrose. "Education of Negro Teachers." In *National Survey of the Education of Teachers*, U.S. Office of Education Bulletin, 1933, no. 10, vol. 4. Washington, D.C.: Government Printing Office, 1933; repr., Westport, Conn.: Greenwood Press, 1970.

Jones, Thomas Jesse. *Negro Education: A Study of the Private and Higher Schools for Colored People in the United States*. Bureau of Education Bulletin, 1916, no. 39. Washington, D.C.: Government Printing Office, 1917.

Klein, Arthur J. *Survey of Negro Colleges and Universities*. Bureau of Education Bulletin, 1928, no. 7. Washington, D.C.: Government Printing Office, 1929; repr., New York: Negro Universities Press, 1969.

Physical Activity and Health: A Report of the Surgeon General. Atlanta: U.S. Department of Health and Human Services, Centers for Disease Control and Prevention, National Center for Chronic Disease Prevention and Health Promotion; Washington, D.C.: President's Council on Physical Fitness and Sports, 1996.

Promoting Better Health for Young People Through Physical Activity and Sports: A Report to the President from the Secretary of Health and Human Services and the Secretary of Education. Silver Spring, Md.: Centers for Disease Control and Prevention, National Center for Chronic Disease Prevention and Health Promotion, Division of Adolescent and School Health, 2000.

Ready, Marie M. *Physical Education in American Colleges and Universities*. Bureau of Education Bulletin, 1927, no. 14. Washington, D.C.: Government Printing Office, 1927.

———. *Physical Education in City Public Schools*. Bureau of Education Physical Education Series, no. 10. Washington, D.C.: Government Printing Office, 1929.

Rogers, James Frederick. *State-Wide Trends in School Hygiene and Physical Education*. Office of Education Pamphlet no. 5, rev. Washington, D.C.: Government Printing Office, 1934.

Storey, Thomas A., and Willard S. Small. *Recent State Legislation for Physical Education*. Bureau of Education Bulletin, 1918, no. 40. Washington, D.C.: Government Printing Office, 1919.

Storey, Thomas A., Willard S. Small, and Elon G. Salisbury. *Recent State Legislation for Physical Education*. Bureau of Education Bulletin, 1922, no. 1. Washington, D.C.: Government Printing Office, 1922.

U.S. Department of Health and Human Services, Office of Disease Prevention and Health Promotion. *Healthy People 2010*. http://www.healthypeople.gov.

Primary Works

Adrian, Marlene, and Judith Brame, eds. *NAGWS Research Reports*. Vol. 3. Washington, D.C.: AAHPER, 1977.

Ainsworth, Dorothy S. "Recreational Trends in Physical Education at Smith College." *Smith Alumnae Quarterly* 27 (May 1936): 255–57.

American Academy of Pediatrics, Committee on Sports Medicine. "Medical Concerns in the Female Athlete: Policy Statement." *Pediatrics* 106 (2000): 610–13.

American College of Obstetricians and Gynecologists. "Amenorrhea." *Technical Bulletin*, No. 128 (May 1989).

———. *Exercise and Fitness: A Guide for Women*. ACOG Patient Education Pamphlet, AP045. Washington, D.C.: ACOG, 1992.

———. "Women and Exercise." *Technical Bulletin*, No. 87 (September 1985).

———. "Women and Exercise." *Technical Bulletin*, No. 173 (October 1992).

Andrews, Gladys, Jeannette Saurborn, and Elsa Schneider. *Physical Education for Today's Boys and Girls*. Boston: Allyn and Bacon, 1960.

Åstrand, P.-O., et al. "Girl Swimmers with Special Reference to Respiratory and Circulatory Adaptation and Gynaecological and Psychiatric Aspects." *Acta Paediatrica Scandinavica* suppl. 147 (1963): 1–75.

Azzarito, Laura, and Melinda A. Solmon. "A Reconceptualization of Physical Education: The Intersection of Gender/Race/Social Class." *Sport, Education and Society* 10 (2005): 25–47.

Baker, Gertrude M. "Survey of the Administration of Physical Education in Public Schools in the United States." *Research Quarterly* 33 (1962): 632–36.

———. "A Survey of Administrative Relationships of Departments of Physical Education in Colleges and Universities." *Research Quarterly* 13 (1942): 217–28.

Baker, Gertrude M., Elsie Annis, and Jean Bontz. "Supervision of Physical Education in the Elementary School. Part 1: The Supervisor's Viewpoint." *Research Quarterly* 23 (1952): 379–90.

———. "Supervision of Physical Education in the Elementary School. Part 2: The Classroom Teacher's Viewpoint." *Research Quarterly* 25 (1954): 379–86.

Barratt, Marcia, et al. *Foundations for Movement*. Dubuque, Iowa: Wm. C. Brown, 1964.

Beals, Katherine A., and Nanna L. Meyer. "Female Athlete Triad Update." *Clinics in Sports Medicine* 26 (2007): 69–89.

Bell, Margaret. *The Doctor Answers Some Practical Questions on Menstruation*. Washington, D.C.: National Section on Women's Athletics, AAHPER, 1937; rev. ed., 1952; rev. ed., 1955.

Bell, Margaret, and Eloise Parsons. "Dysmenorrhea in College Women." *Medical Woman's Journal* 38 (February 1931): 31–35.

Bilhuber, Gertrude. "The Effect of Functional Periodicity on the Motor Ability of Women in Sports." D.P.H. diss., University of Michigan, 1926.

Bocker, Dorothy, ed. *Basket Ball for Women: A Guide for Player, Coach and Official*. New York: Thos. E. Wilson, 1920.

Bouchard, Claude, Roy J. Shephard, and Thomas Stephens, eds. *Physical Activity, Fitness, and Health: Consensus Statement*. Champaign, Ill.: Human Kinetics, 1993.

Bowen, W. P. "The Preparation of Teachers of Physical Education." *American Physical Education Review* 19 (1914): 421–25.

Bowers, Ethel. *Recreation for Girls and Women*. New York: A. S. Barnes, 1934.

Cheska, Alyce T. "Women's Sports—The Unlikely Myth of Equality." In *The Female Athlete: A Socio-Psychological and Kinanthropometric Approach*, edited by Jan Borms, Marcel Hebbelinck, and Antonio Venerando, 1–11. Medicine and Sport Series, vol. 15. Basel and New York: Karger, 1981.

Coleman, Mary Channing. "Games and Athletics in the School Program." *North Carolina Parent-Teacher Bulletin* 8 (1930): 107–8, 111.

Coops, Helen Leslie. *High School Standards in Girls Athletics in the State of Ohio.* New York: Teachers College, Columbia University, 1933.

Cumming, David C. "The Reproductive Effects of Exercise and Training." *Current Problems in Obstetrics, Gynecology, and Fertility* 10 (June 1987): 225–85.

DeSensi, Joy T. "Understanding Multiculturalism and Valuing Diversity: A Theoretical Perspective." *Quest* 47 (1995): 34–43.

De Souza, Mary Jane, and Nancy I. Williams. "Physiological Aspects and Clinical Sequelae of Energy Deficiency and Hypoestrogenism in Exercising Women." *Human Reproduction Update* 10 (2004): 433–48.

DiPietro, Loretta, and Nina S. Stachenfeld. "The Female Athlete Triad." *Medicine and Science in Sports and Exercise* 29 (1997): 1669–71.

Division of Girls and Women's Sports. *Philosophy and Standards for Girls and Women's Sports.* Washington, D.C.: DGWS/AAHPER, 1969; rev. ed., 1970; rev. ed., 1973.

———. *Policies and Procedures for Competition in Girls and Women's Sports.* Washington, D.C.: DGWS/AAHPER, 1958; rev. ed., 1961.

Drinkwater, Barbara L. "Athletic Amenorrhea: A Review." *American Academy of Physical Education Papers* 17 (1983): 120–31.

———, ed. *Female Endurance Athletes.* Champaign, Ill.: Human Kinetics, 1986.

———. "Women and Exercise: Physiological Aspects." *Exercise and Sport Sciences Reviews* 12 (1984): 21–51.

Drinkwater, Barbara L., et al. "Bone Mineral Content of Amenorrheic and Eumenorrheic Athletes." *New England Journal of Medicine* 311 (1984): 277–81.

Dudley, Gertrude, and Frances A. Kellor. *Athletic Games in the Education of Women.* New York: Henry Holt, 1909.

Elliott, Ruth. *The Organization of Professional Training in Physical Education in State Universities.* Contributions to Education, No. 268. New York: Bureau of Publications, Teachers College, Columbia University, 1927.

Ennis, Catherine D. "Creating a Culturally Relevant Curriculum for Disengaged Girls." *Sport, Education and Society* 4 (1999): 31–48.

Ennis, Catherine D., et al. "Creating a Sense of Family in Urban Schools Using the 'Sport for Peace' Curriculum." *Research Quarterly for Exercise and Sport* 70 (1999): 273–85.

Erdelyi, Gyula J. "Effects of Exercise on the Menstrual Cycle." *Physician and Sportsmedicine* 4 (March 1976): 79–81.

———. "Women in Athletics." In *Proceedings of the Second National Conference on the Medical Aspects of Sports*, 59–63. Chicago: American Medical Association, 1961.

Espenschade, Anna S. "Development of Motor Coordination in Boys and Girls." *Research Quarterly* 18 (1947): 30–44.

———. "Women and Competitive Sport." In *Proceedings of the First National Institute on Girls Sports*, 28–32. Washington, D.C.: AAHPER, 1965.

Espenschade, Anna S., and Helen M. Eckert. *Motor Development.* Columbus, Ohio: Charles E. Merrill, 1967.

Evans, Melvin I. "The Vanishing Americans." *Journal of Health, Physical Education, and Recreation* 44 (October 1973): 55–57.

"Exercise and Fitness: A Statement on the Role of Exercise in Fitness by a Joint Committee of the American Medical Association and the American Association for Health, Physical Education, and Recreation." *Journal of Health, Physical Education, and Recreation* 35 (May 1964): 42–44, 82.

"The Female Athlete Triad—Do Female Athletes Need to Take Special Care to Avoid Low Energy Availability? Contrasting Perspectives in Exercise Science and Sports Medicine" (Anne B. Loucks, and Nina S. Stachenfeld and Loretta DiPietro). *Medicine and Science in Sports and Exercise* 38 (2006): 1694–1700.

"Female Athletics: A Special Communication from the Committee on the Medical Aspects of Sports of the American Medical Association." *Journal of Physical Education and Recreation* 46 (January 1975): 45–46.

Folsom, Mrs. Richard S. "Report of the National Women's Sport Committee, A.A.U." *Mind and Body* 39 (1933): 300–302.

Frisch, Rose E. *Female Fertility and the Body Fat Connection.* Chicago: University of Chicago Press, 2002.

Frost, Lorraine. "Dysmenorrhea and Exercise." *Physiotherapy Review* 12 (1932): 251–54.

Frymir, Alice W. *Basket Ball for Women: How to Coach and Play the Game.* New York: A. S. Barnes, 1930.

———. *Track and Field for Women.* New York: A. S. Barnes, 1930.

Gendel, Evalyn S. "Women and the Medical Aspects of Sports." *Journal of School Health* 37 (1967): 427–31.

Griffin, Pat. "The Challenge to Live Up to Our Ideals: Appreciating Social Diversity and Achieving Social Justice in Schools." *Journal of Physical Education, Recreation, and Dance* 62 (August 1991): 58–61.

Hanna, Delphine. "Present Status of Physical Training in Normal Schools." *American Physical Education Review* 8 (1903): 293–97.

Harber, Vicki J. "Energy Balance and Reproductive Function in Active Women." *Canadian Journal of Applied Physiology* 29 (2004): 48–58.

Harmon, Kimberly G., and Rosemary Agostini, eds. "The Athletic Woman." *Clinics in Sports Medicine* 19 (April 2000): xiii–380.

Harris, Dorothy V., ed. *DGWS Research Reports: Women in Sports.* Vol. 1. Washington, D.C.: AAHPER, 1971.

———, ed. *DGWS Research Reports: Women in Sports.* Vol. 2. Washington, D.C.: AAHPER, 1973.

———. "Monthly Mystery." *womenSports* 4 (September 1977): 49.

———. "Physical Sex Differences: A Matter of Degree." In *NAGWS Research Reports,* edited by Marlene Adrian and Judith Brame, 117–24. Washington, D.C.: AAHPER, 1977.

———, ed. *Women and Sport: A National Research Conference.* Penn State HPER Series no. 2. University Park, Pa.: Pennsylvania State University, 1972.

Hawley, Gertrude. *An Anatomical Analysis of Sports.* New York: A. S. Barnes, 1940.

Heimbach, Althea. "Women's Physical Education in Milwaukee." *Historical Messenger* 25 (June 1969): 63–67.

Henderson, Edwin Bancroft. "An Experiment in Elementary School Athletics." *Journal of Health, Physical Education, and Recreation* 22 (June 1951): 21–22.

———. *The Negro in Sports.* 2nd ed. Washington, D.C.: Associated Publishers, 1949.

———. "Negro Women in Sports." *Negro History Bulletin* 15 (December 1951): 55.

———. "Progress and Problems in Health and Physical Education Among Colored Americans." *Journal of Health and Physical Education* 6 (June 1935): 9, 55.

———. "Tolerance." *Journal of Health and Physical Education* 17 (February 1946): 76.

Hoferek, Mary J. "At the Crossroad: Merger or ———?" *Quest* 32 (1980): 95–102.

Huelster, Laura J. "The Role of Sports in the Culture of Girls." In *Proceedings of the Second National Institute on Girls Sports*, 119–23. Washington, D.C.: AAHPER, 1966.

Hult, Joan. "Competitive Athletics for Girls—We Must Act." *Journal of Health, Physical Education, and Recreation* 45 (June 1974): 45–46.

———. "Separate but Equal Athletics for Women." *Journal of Health, Physical Education, and Recreation* 44 (June 1973): 57–58.

Ireland, Mary Lloyd, and Aurelia Nattiv, eds. *The Female Athlete*. Philadelphia: W. B. Saunders, 2003.

Jackson, Nell C. "Contribution of Track and Field to the Development of Girls and Women." In *Proceedings of the First National Institute on Girls Sports*, 93–94. Washington, D.C.: AAHPER, 1965.

Johnson, Georgia Borg. *Organization of the Required Physical Education for Women in State Universities*. Contributions to Education, no. 253. New York: Bureau of Publications, Teachers College, Columbia University, 1927.

Jokl, Ernst. "Some Clinical Data on Women's Athletics." *Journal of the Association for Physical and Mental Rehabilitation* 10 (March–April 1956): 48–49.

Kidwell, Kathro, and Dorothy Simpson. "A Study and Investigation of the Health of Women Teachers of Physical Education." *American Physical Education Review* 34 (1929): 83–91.

Leavitt, Norma M., and Margaret M. Duncan. "The Status of Intramural Programs for Women." *Research Quarterly* 8 (March 1937): 68–79.

Lee, Mabel. "The Case For and Against Intercollegiate Athletics for Women and the Situation as It Stands To-Day." *American Physical Education Review* 29 (1924): 13–19.

———. "The Case For and Against Intercollegiate Athletics for Women and the Situation Since 1923." *Research Quarterly* 2 (May 1931): 93–127.

———. *The Conduct of Physical Education: Its Organization and Administration for Girls and Women*. New York: A. S. Barnes, 1937.

———. "A Consideration of the Fundamental Differences between Boys and Girls as They Affect the Girls' Program of Physical Education." *Education* 53 (1933): 467–71.

———. *Memories Beyond Bloomers (1924–1954)*. Washington, D.C.: American Alliance for Health, Physical Education, and Recreation, 1978.

———. *Memories of a Bloomer Girl (1894–1924)*. Washington, D.C.: American Alliance for Health, Physical Education, and Recreation, 1977.

Lock, Robyn S., Leslie T. Minarik, and Joyce Omata. "Gender and the Problem of Diversity: Action Research in Physical Education." *Quest* 51 (1999): 393–407.

Marshall, Violet B. "The Status of Physical Education for Women in Colleges and Universities." *Research Quarterly* 7 (October 1936): 3–13.

McCue, Betty Foster. "Why Exercise?" In *Physical Education Activities for Women*, ed. Betty Foster McCue, 3–10. Toronto: Macmillan Company, 1969.

McCurdy, J. H. *Report of the Committee on the Curriculum of the 139 Institutions Preparing Teachers of Physical Education in the United States, 1929*. Springfield, Mass.: American Physical Education Association, 1929.

McKinstry, Helen. "The Hygiene of Menstruation." *Mary Hemenway Alumnae Association Bulletin* (1916–17): 15–27.

Meaker, Samuel R. "Menstrual Disorders in Adolescent Girls and Young Women." *Journal of Health and Physical Education* 12 (January 1941): 12–15, 62–63.

Meyer, Margaret H., and Marguerite M. Schwarz. *Team Sports for Girls and Women.* 4th ed. Philadelphia: W. B. Saunders, 1965.

Miller, Donna Mae. *Coaching the Female Athlete.* Philadelphia: Lea and Febiger, 1974.

Miller, Donna Mae, and Katherine L. Ley. *Individual and Team Sports for Women.* New York: Prentice Hall, 1955.

Mohnsen, Bonnie S., ed. *Concepts and Principles of Physical Education: What Every Student Needs to Know.* Reston, Va.: NASPE, 2003.

Moore, Roy B. "An Analytical Study of Sex Differences as They Affect the Program of Physical Education." *Research Quarterly* 12 (1941): 587–608.

Mosher, Clelia Duel. "Functional Periodicity in Women and Some of the Modifying Factors." *American Physical Education Review* 16 (1911): 494–95.

———. "A Physiologic Treatment of Congestive Dysmenorrhea and Kindred Disorders Associated with the Menstrual Function." *Journal of the American Medical Association* 62 (1914): 1297–1301.

National Association for Sport and Physical Education. *Physical Education for Lifelong Fitness: The Physical Best Teacher's Guide.* 2nd ed. Champaign, Ill.: Human Kinetics, 2005.

National Association for Sport and Physical Education and American Heart Association. *2006 Shape of the Nation Report: Status of Physical Education in the USA.* http://www.aahperd.org/naspe/ShapeOfTheNation/ (accessed February 15, 2008).

National Association of State Boards of Education. *Healthy Schools: State-Level School Health Policies.* http://www.nasbe.org/HealthySchools/States/State_Policy.asp (accessed September 21, 2006).

National Section for Girls and Women's Sports. *Standards in Sports for Girls and Women: Guiding Principles in the Organization and Administration of Sports Programs.* Washington, D.C.: NSGWS/AAHPER, 1953.

National Section on Women's Athletics. *Standards in Athletics for Girls and Women: Guiding Principles in the Organization and Administration of Athletic Programs.* Washington, D.C.: NSWA/APEA, 1937; rev. ed., NSWA/AAHPER, 1948.

Nattiv, Aurelia, et al. "ACSM Position Stand: The Female Athlete Triad." *Medicine and Science in Sports and Exercise* 39 (2007): 1867–82.

Nattiv, Aurelia, Rosemary Agostini, Barbara Drinkwater, and Kimberly K. Yeager. "The Female Athlete Triad: The Inter-Relatedness of Disordered Eating, Amenorrhea, and Osteoporosis." *Clinics in Sports Medicine* 13 (1994): 405–18.

Neal, Patsy. *Basketball Techniques for Women.* New York: Ronald Press, 1966.

———. *Coaching Methods for Women.* Reading, Mass.: Addison-Wesley, 1969.

Nilges, Lynda M. "I Thought Only Fairy Tales Had Supernatural Power: A Radical Feminist Analysis of Title IX in Physical Education." *Journal of Teaching in Physical Education* 17 (January 1998): 172–94.

Norris, J. Anna. "Dangers in Basket Ball: Popular Sport Should be Made Safe for Girls." *Child Health* 5 (1924): 512–14.

Otis, Carol L., and Roger Goldingay. *The Athletic Woman's Survival Guide.* Champaign, Ill.: Human Kinetics, 2000.

Otis, Carol L., et al. "ACSM Position Stand: The Female Athlete Triad." *Medicine and Science in Sports and Exercise* 29, n. 5 (1997): i–ix.

Pate, Russell R., et al. "Physical Activity and Public Health: A Recommendation from the Centers for Disease Control and Prevention and the American College of Sports Medicine." *Journal of the American Medical Association* 273 (1995): 402–7.

Paterson, Ann, ed. *Team Sports for Girls.* New York: Ronald Press, 1958.

Perrin, Ethel. "The Confessions of a Once Strict Formalist." *Journal of Health and Physical Education* 9 (1938): 533–36, 589–90.

———. "Outdoor Recreation as a Factor in Child Welfare." *Playground* 18 (July 1924): 240–42, 246, 266.

Phillips, Marjorie. "Compensation Practices and Extracurricular Responsibilities of Women High School Physical Education Teachers." *Research Quarterly* 28 (1957): 379–94.

Phillips, Marjorie, Katharine Fox, and Olive Young. "Recommendations from Women Doctors and Gynecologists about Sports Activity for Girls: A Report by the Research Committee of the Division of Girls and Women's Sports." *Journal of Health, Physical Education, and Recreation* 30 (December 1959): 23–25, 54.

"Pioneer Women in Physical Education." *Research Quarterly* 12, suppl. (October 1941): 615–703.

Plowman, Sharon. "Physiological Characteristics of Female Athletes." *Research Quarterly* 45 (1974): 349–62.

Popma, Anne, ed. *The Female Athlete: Proceedings of a National Conference about Women in Sports and Recreation.* Burnaby, British Columbia: Institute for Human Performance, Simon Fraser University, 1980.

President's Council on Physical Fitness and Sports. *Physical Activity and Sport in the Lives of Girls: Physical and Mental Health Dimensions from an Interdisciplinary Approach.* Washington, D.C.: The Council, 1997.

Proceedings of the First National Institute on Girls Sports. Washington, D.C.: AAHPER, 1965.

Proceedings of the Second National Institute on Girls Sports. Washington, D.C.: AAHPER, 1966.

Proceedings of the Third National Institute on Girls Sports. Washington, D.C.: AAHPER, 1966.

Puhl, Jacqueline, and C. Harmon Brown, eds. *The Menstrual Cycle and Physical Activity.* Champaign, Ill.: Human Kinetics, 1986.

Puhl, Jacqueline, C. Harmon Brown, and Robert O. Voy, eds. *Sport Science Perspectives for Women.* Champaign, Ill.: Human Kinetics, 1988.

Ransdell, Lynda, and Linda Petlichkoff, eds. *Ensuring the Health of Active and Athletic Girls and Women.* Reston, Va.: National Association for Girls and Women in Sport, 2005.

Ransdell, Lynda B., and Christine L. Wells. "Sex Differences in Athletic Performance." *Women in Sport and Physical Activity Journal* 8 (Spring 1999): 55–81.

Redman, Leanne M., and Anne B. Loucks. "Menstrual Disorders in Athletes." *Sports Medicine* 35 (2005): 747–55.

Sabo, Donald F., Kathleen Elizabeth Miller, Merrill J. Melnick, and Leslie Heywood. *Her Life Depends On It: Sport, Physical Activity and the Health and Well-Being of American Girls.* East Meadow, N.Y.: Women's Sports Foundation, 2004.

Sanborn, Charlotte Feicht. "Menstrual Dysfunction in the Female Athlete." In *Scientific Foundations of Sports Medicine*, edited by Carol C. Teitz, 117–34. Toronto: B. C. Decker, 1989.

Savage, Howard J., et al. *American College Athletics*. New York: Carnegie Foundation for the Advancement of Teaching, 1929.

Schoedler, Lillian. "Girls' Athletics—Wise and Otherwise." *Child Welfare Magazine* 20 (1926): 591–95.

Scott, M. Gladys. "Competition for Women in American Colleges and Universities." *Research Quarterly* 16 (1945): 49–71.

Scott, M. Phebe, and Virginia R. Crafts. *Track and Field for Girls and Women*. New York: Appleton-Century-Crofts, 1964.

Smeal, Georgia, Belinda Carpenter, and Gordon Tait. "Ideals and Realities: Articulating Feminist Perspectives in Physical Education." *Quest* 46 (1994): 410–24.

Smith, Helen Norman, and Helen Leslie Coops. *Physical and Health Education: Principles and Procedures*. New York: American Book, 1938.

Somers, Florence. *Principles of Women's Athletics*. New York: A. S. Barnes, 1930.

Stoneroad, Rebecca. "How Far Should Physical Training Be Educational and How Far Recreative in Grammar Schools?" *Addresses and Proceedings of the National Education Association*, 1905, 768–72.

———. "Physical Education of Girls During Childhood and Pubescent Period, or Upper-Grammar and Lower-High-School Age." *Addresses and Proceedings of the National Education Association*, 1910, 936–41.

———. "Public School Conditions, Problems and Methods from the Standpoint of Physical Education." *American Physical Education Review* 4 (1899): 42–49.

Sumption, Dorothy. *Sports for Women*. New York: Prentice-Hall, 1940.

Thomas, Jerry R., and Katherine T. Thomas. "Gender Differences Across Age in Motor Performance: A Meta-Analysis." *Psychological Bulletin* 98 (1985): 260–82.

Thomas, Jerry R., Amelia M. Lee, and Katherine T. Thomas. *Physical Education for Children: Concepts into Practice*. Champaign, Ill.: Human Kinetics, 1988.

Toogood, Ruth. "A Survey of Recreational Interests and Pursuits of College Women." *Research Quarterly* 10 (October 1939): 90–100.

Torrey, Carol C., and Madge Ashy. "Culturally Responsive Teaching in Physical Education." *Physical Educator* 54 (Fall 1997): 120–27.

Trilling, Blanche M. "The Playtime of a Million Girls or an Olympic Victory—Which?" *Nation's Schools* 4 (August 1929): 51–54.

Ullyot, Joan. "Amenorrhea: A Sensitive Subject." *Women's Sports* 3 (December 1981): 46.

Vannier, Maryhelen, and Mildred Foster. *Teaching Physical Education in Elementary Schools*. Philadelphia: W. B. Saunders, 1968.

Vannier, Maryhelen, and Hally Beth Poindexter. *Physical Activities for College Women*. 2nd ed. Philadelphia: W. B. Saunders, 1969.

Warren, Michelle P., and Mona M. Shangold. *Sports Gynecology: Problems and Care of the Athletic Female*. Cambridge, Mass.: Blackwell Science, 1997.

Wayman, Agnes R. *Education through Physical Education: Its Organization and Administration for Girls and Women*. 2nd ed. Philadelphia: Lea and Febiger, 1928.

———. *A Modern Philosophy of Physical Education, with Special Implications for Girls and Women and for the College Freshman Program*. Philadelphia: W. B. Saunders, 1938.

Wells, Christine L. "The Female Athlete: Myths and Superstitions Put to Rest." In *Toward an Understanding of Human Performance: Readings in Exercise Physiology for the Coach and Athlete*, edited by Edmund J. Burke, 37–40. Ithaca, N.Y.: Mouvement Publications, 1978.

———. "Menstruation, Pregnancy, and Menopause." In *Physical Activity and Well-Being*, edited by Vern Seefeldt, 212–34. Reston, Va.: AAHPERD, 1986.

———. *Women, Sport, and Performance: A Physiological Perspective*. 2nd ed. Champaign, Ill.: Human Kinetics, 1991.

Wells, Christine L., and Sharon A. Plowman. "Sexual Differences in Athletic Performance: Biological or Behavioral?" *Physician and Sportsmedicine* 11 (August 1983): 52–56, 59–63.

Williams, Charles H. "'Darkest Africa' at 'A Century of Progress.'" *Southern Workman* 62 (November 1933): 429–37.

———. "The Hampton Institute Creative Dance Group." *Dance Observer* 4 (1937): 97–98.

———. "Recreation in the Lives of Young People." *Southern Workman* 46 (February 1917): 95–100.

Williamson, Kay M. "Is Your Inequity Showing? Ideas and Strategies for Creating a More Equitable Learning Environment." *Journal of Physical Education, Recreation, and Dance* 64 (October 1993): 15–23.

Women's Division of the National Amateur Athletic Federation, comp. *Women and Athletics*. New York: A. S. Barnes, 1930.

Secondary Works: Articles, Books, and Book Chapters

Abney, Robertha. "African American Women in Sport." *Journal of Physical Education, Recreation, and Dance* 70 (April 1999): 35–38.

Abney, Robertha, and Dorothy Richey. "Barriers Encountered by Black Female Athletic Administrators and Coaches." *Journal of Physical Education, Recreation, and Dance* 62 (August 1991): 19–21.

Acosta, R. Vivian, and Linda Jean Carpenter. "As the Years Go By—Coaching Opportunities in the 1990s." *Journal of Physical Education, Recreation, and Dance* 63 (March 1992): 36–41.

———. "Women in Athletics: A Status Report." *Journal of Physical Education, Recreation, and Dance* 56 (August 1985): 30–34.

———. "Women in Intercollegiate Sport: A Longitudinal, National Study—Twenty-Seven-Year Update, 1977–2004." *Women in Sport and Physical Activity Journal* 13 (2004): 62–89.

Ainsworth, Dorothy S. *The History of Physical Education in Colleges for Women*. New York: A. S. Barnes, 1930.

Anderson, Eric, and Alfred A. Moss Jr. *Dangerous Donations: Northern Philanthropy and Southern Black Education, 1902–1930*. Columbia: University of Missouri Press, 1999.

Anderson, James D. *The Education of Blacks in the South, 1860–1935*. Chapel Hill: University of North Carolina Press, 1988.

———. "The Hampton Model of Normal School Industrial Education, 1868–1900." In *New Perspectives on Black Educational History*, edited by Vincent P. Franklin and James D. Anderson, 61–96. Boston: G. K. Hall, 1978.

Angus, David L., and Jeffrey E. Mirel. *The Failed Promise of the American High School, 1890–1995*. New York: Teachers College Press, 1999.

Bacchi, Carol Lee. *Same Difference: Feminism and Sexual Difference*. Sydney: Allen and Unwin, 1990.

Bain, Linda L. "A Critical Analysis of the Hidden Curriculum in Physical Education." In *Physical Education, Curriculum and Culture: Critical Issues in the Contemporary Crisis*, edited by David Kirk and Richard Tinning, 23–42. London: Falmer Press, 1990.

Banner, Lois W. *American Beauty: A Social History through Two Centuries of the American Idea, Ideal, and Image of the Beautiful Woman*. New York: Alfred A. Knopf, 1983.

Barnes, Barbara A., Susan G. Zieff, and David I. Anderson. "Racial Difference and Social Meanings: Research on 'Black' and 'White' Infants' Motor Development, c. 1931–1992." *Quest* 51 (1999): 328–45.

Barney, Robert Knight. "A Historical Reinterpretation of the Forces Underlying the First State Legislation for Physical Education in the Public Schools of the U.S." *Research Quarterly* 44 (1973): 346–60.

Bartky, Sandra Lee. "Foucault, Femininity, and the Modernization of Patriarchal Power." In *Feminism and Foucault: Reflections on Resistance*, edited by Irene Diamond and Lee Quinby, 61–86. Boston: Northeastern University Press, 1988.

Bederman, Gail. *Manliness and Civilization: A Cultural History of Gender and Race in the United States, 1880–1917*. Chicago: University of Chicago Press, 1995.

Bennett, Bruce L. "This Is Our Heritage: 1960–1985." *Research Quarterly for Exercise and Sport*, Centennial Issue (April 1985): 102–20.

Bennett, Michael, and Vanessa D. Dickerson, eds. *Recovering the Black Female Body: Self-Representations by African American Women*. New Brunswick, N.J.: Rutgers University Press, 2000.

Beran, Janice A. "Daughters of the Middle Border: Iowa Women in Sport and Physical Activity, 1850–1910." *Iowa State Journal of Research* 62 (November 1987): 161–81.

———. "Playing to the Right Drummer: Girls' Basketball in Iowa, 1892–1927." *Research Quarterly for Exercise and Sport*, Centennial Issue (April 1985): 78–85.

Berryman, Jack W., and Roberta J. Park, eds. *Sport and Exercise Science: Essays in the History of Sports Medicine*. Urbana: University of Illinois Press, 1992.

Betts, Edith, and Hazel Peterson. "Dorothy Sears Ainsworth: Pioneer in International Relations." *Journal of Physical Education, Recreation, and Dance* 56 (May–June 1985): 63–65, 67.

Birke, Lynda. *Feminism and the Biological Body*. New Brunswick, N.J.: Rutgers University Press, 2000.

Birrell, Susan. "Racial Relations Theories and Sport: Suggestions for a More Critical Analysis." *Sociology of Sport Journal* 6 (1989): 212–27.

———. "Women of Color, Critical Autobiography, and Sport." In *Sport, Men, and the Gender Order: Critical Feminist Perspectives*, edited by Michael A. Messner and Donald F. Sabo, 185–99. Champaign, Ill.: Human Kinetics, 1990.

Bloom, John. *To Show What an Indian Can Do: Sports at Native American Boarding Schools*. Minneapolis: University of Minnesota Press, 2000.

Bolden, Frank P. "In Memoriam: Edwin Bancroft Henderson." *Journal of Physical Education and Recreation* 48 (May 1977): 6–7.

Bordo, Susan R. "The Body and the Reproduction of Femininity: A Feminist Appropriation of Foucault." In *Gender/Body/Knowledge: Feminist Reconstructions of Being and Knowing*, edited by Alison M. Jaggar and Susan R. Bordo, 13–33. New Brunswick, N.J.: Rutgers University Press, 1989.

Borish, Linda J. "'Athletic Activities of Various Kinds': Physical Health and Sport Programs for Jewish American Women." *Journal of Sport History* 26 (1999): 240–70.

———. "'An Interest in Physical Well-Being Among the Feminine Membership': Sporting Activities for Women at Young Men's and Young Women's Hebrew Associations." *American Jewish History* 87 (1999): 61–93.

Brandt, Allan M. "Behavior, Disease, and Health in the Twentieth-Century United States: The Moral Valence of Individual Risk." In *Morality and Health: Interdisciplinary Perspectives*, edited by Allan M. Brandt and Paul Rozin, 53–77. New York: Routledge, 1997.

Bredemeier, Brenda Jo Light, et al. "Changers and the Changed: Moral Aspects of Coming Out in Physical Education." *Quest* 51 (1999): 418–31.

Brooks, George A., ed. *Perspectives on the Academic Discipline of Physical Education: A Tribute to G. Lawrence Rarick*. Champaign, Ill.: Human Kinetics, 1981.

Brown, Elsa Barkley. "'What Has Happened Here': The Politics of Difference in Women's History and Feminist Politics." *Feminist Studies* 18 (1992): 295–312.

Brown, Victoria Bissell. "The Fear of Feminization: Los Angeles High Schools in the Progressive Era." *Feminist Studies* 16 (1990): 493–518.

Brumberg, Joan Jacobs. *The Body Project: An Intimate History of American Girls*. New York: Random House, 1997.

———. "'Something Happens to Girls': Menarche and the Emergence of the Modern American Hygienic Imperative." *Journal of the History of Sexuality* 4 (1993): 99–127.

Burgeson, Charlene R., et al. "Physical Education and Activity: Results from the School Health Policies and Programs Study 2000." *Journal of Physical Education, Recreation, and Dance* 74 (January 2003): 20–36.

Burt, Ramsay. "The Trouble with the Male Dancer . . ." In *The Male Dancer: Bodies, Spectacle, Sexualities*, 10–30. London: Routledge, 1995.

Cadden, Joan. *Meanings of Sex Difference in the Middle Ages: Medicine, Science, and Culture*. Cambridge: Cambridge University Press, 1993.

Cahn, Susan K. *Coming on Strong: Gender and Sexuality in Twentieth-Century Women's Sport*. New York: Free Press, 1994.

———. "Crushes, Competition, and Closets: The Emergence of Homophobia in Women's Physical Education." In *Women, Sport, and Culture*, edited by Susan Birrell and Cheryl L. Cole, 327–39. Champaign, Ill.: Human Kinetics, 1994.

Canaday, Margot. *The Straight State: Sexuality and Citizenship in Twentieth-Century America*. Princeton, N.J.: Princeton University Press, 2009.

Carlson, Shirley J. "Black Ideals of Womanhood in the Late Victorian Era." *Journal of Negro History* 77 (Spring 1992): 61–73.

Carlson, Teresa B. "We Hate Gym: Student Alienation from Physical Education." *Journal of Teaching in Physical Education* 14 (1995): 467–77.

Carpenter, Linda Jean, and R. Vivian Acosta. *Title IX*. Champaign, Ill.: Human Kinetics, 2005.

Carrington, Bruce, and Oliver Leaman. "Equal Opportunities and Physical Education." In *Physical Education, Sport and Schooling: Studies in the Sociology of Physical Education*, edited by John Evans, 215–26. London: Falmer Press, 1986.

Casperson, Carl J., Mark A. Pereira, and Katy M. Curran. "Changes in Physical Activity Patterns in the United States, by Sex and Cross-Sectional Age." *Medicine and Science in Sports and Exercise* 32 (2000): 1601–9.

Cavallo, Dominick. *Muscles and Morals: Organized Playgrounds and Urban Reform, 1880–1920*. Philadelphia: University of Pennsylvania Press, 1981.

Cayleff, Susan E. *Babe: The Life and Legend of Babe Didrikson Zaharias*. Urbana: University of Illinois Press, 1995.

Chambers, Ted. *The History of Athletics and Physical Education at Howard University*. New York: Vantage Press, 1986.

Chepyator-Thomson, Jepkorir Rose, JeongAe You, and Brent Hardin. "Issues and Perspectives on Gender in Physical Education." *Women in Sport and Physical Activity Journal* 9 (September 2000): 99–121.

Clarke, Gill. "Playing a Part: The Lives of Lesbian Physical Education Teachers." In *Researching Women and Sport*, edited by Gill Clarke and Barbara Humberstone, 36–49. Houndmills: Macmillan, 1997.

Clifford, Geraldine Jonçich, ed. *Lone Voyagers: Academic Women in Coeducational Universities, 1870–1937*. New York: Feminist Press, 1989.

Cole, Cheryl L. "Resisting the Canon: Feminist Cultural Studies, Sport, and Technologies of the Body." *Journal of Sport and Social Issues* 17 (1993): 77–97.

Connell, R. W. *Masculinities*. 2nd ed. Berkeley: University of California Press, 2005.

Cooke, Paul. "The Cost of Segregated Public Schools in the District of Columbia." *Journal of Negro Education* 18 (1949): 95–103.

Corbett, Doris, and William Johnson. "The African-American Female in Collegiate Sport: Sexism and Racism." In *Racism in College Athletics: The African-American Athlete's Experience*, edited by Dana D. Brooks and Ronald C. Althouse, 179–204. Morgantown, W. Va.: Fitness Information Technology, 1993.

Cordts, Harold John, and John H. Shaw. "Status of the Physical Education Required or Instructional Programs in Four-Year Colleges and Universities." *Research Quarterly* 31 (1960): 409–19.

Costa, D. Margaret, and Sharon R. Guthrie, eds. *Women and Sport: Interdisciplinary Perspectives*. Champaign, Ill.: Human Kinetics, 1994.

Cott, Nancy F. "Feminist Theory and Feminist Movements: The Past Before Us." In *What Is Feminism? A Re-Examination*, edited by Juliet Mitchell and Ann Oakley, 49–62. New York: Pantheon, 1986.

———. *The Grounding of Modern Feminism*. New Haven, Conn.: Yale University Press, 1987.

Cottrell, Debbie M. "The Sargent School for Physical Education." *Journal of Physical Education, Recreation, and Dance* 65 (March 1994): 32–37.

Coursey, Leon N. "Anita J. Turner: Early Black Female Physical Educator." *Journal of Health, Physical Education, and Recreation* 45 (March 1974): 71–72.

———. "Pioneer Black Physical Educators: Contributions of Anita J. Turner and Edwin B. Henderson." *Journal of Physical Education and Recreation* 51 (May 1980): 54–56.

Craig, Maxine Leeds. *Ain't I a Beauty Queen? Black Women, Beauty, and the Politics of Race*. New York: Oxford University Press, 2002.

Cranz, Galen. "Women in Urban Parks." *Signs* 5, no. 3 suppl. (1980): S79–S95.

Crase, Darrell, and Michael H. Hamrick. "Gender and Race/Ethnicity Differentials Among Physical Education Doctorates." *Physical Educator* 51 (Fall 1994): 162–68.

Crase, Darrell, and Hollie Walker Jr. "The Black Physical Educator—An Endangered Species." *Journal of Physical Education, Recreation, and Dance* 59 (October 1988): 65–69.

Crase, Darrell, et al. "Perspectives on Physical Education in Traditionally Black Institutions." *Journal of Physical Education, Recreation, and Dance* 62 (September 1991): 28–32, 75.

Cravens, Hamilton. *The Triumph of Evolution: The Heredity-Environment Controversy, 1900–1941*. Baltimore, Md.: Johns Hopkins University Press, 1988.

Crawford, Robert. "Individual Responsibility and Health Politics in the 1970s." In *Health Care in America: Essays in Social History*, edited by Susan Reverby and David Rosner, 247–68. Philadelphia: Temple University Press, 1979.

Crespo, Carlos J. "Physical Activity in Minority Populations: Overcoming a Public Health Challenge." *PCPFS Research Digest*, Series 6, no. 2 (June 2005): 1–8.

Cuban, Larry. *How Scholars Trumped Teachers: Change Without Reform in University Curriculum, Teaching, and Research, 1890–1990*. New York: Teachers College, Columbia University, 1999.

Dabney, Lillian G. *The History of Schools for Negroes in the District of Columbia, 1807–1947*. Washington, D.C.: Catholic University of America Press, 1949.

Davis, Kathryn L. "Teaching for Gender Equity in Physical Education: A Review of the Literature." *Women in Sport and Physical Activity Journal* 12 (September 2003): 55–81.

Davis, Kathy. "Embody-ing Theory: Beyond Modernist and Postmodernist Readings of the Body." In *Embodied Practices: Feminist Perspectives on the Body*, edited by Kathy Davis, 1–23. London: Sage, 1997.

Degler, Carl N. *In Search of Human Nature: The Decline and Revival of Darwinism in American Social Thought*. New York: Oxford University Press, 1991.

Delaney, Janice, Mary Jane Lupton, and Emily Toth. *The Curse: A Cultural History of Menstruation*. Rev. ed. Urbana: University of Illinois Press, 1988.

DeLuzio, Crista. *Female Adolescence in American Scientific Thought, 1830–1930*. Baltimore, Md.: Johns Hopkins University Press, 2007.

D'Emilio, John. *Sexual Politics, Sexual Communities: The Making of a Homosexual Minority in the United States, 1940–1970*. 2nd ed. Chicago: University of Chicago Press, 1998.

D'Emilio, John, and Estelle B. Freedman. *Intimate Matters: A History of Sexuality in America*. New York: Harper and Row, 1988.

DeFrantz, Thomas. "Simmering Passivity: The Black Male Body in Concert Dance." In *Moving History/Dancing Cultures: A Dance History Reader*, edited by Ann Dils and Ann Cooper Albright, 342–49. Middletown, Conn.: Wesleyan University Press, 2001.

Dewar, Alison. "The Social Construction of Gender in Physical Education." *Women's Studies International Forum* 10 (1987): 453–65.

Dosch, Nancy Cole. "'The Sacrifice of Maidens' or Healthy Sportswomen? The Medical Debate Over Women's Basketball." In *A Century of Women's Basketball: From Frailty to Final Four*, edited by Joan S. Hult and Marianna Trekell, 125–36. Reston, Va.: AAH-PERD, 1991.

Drewry, Henry N., and Humphrey Doermann. *Stand and Prosper: Private Black Colleges and Their Students.* Princeton, N.J.: Princeton University Press, 2001.

Dyreson, Mark. *Making the American Team: Sport, Culture, and the Olympic Experience.* Urbana: University of Illinois Press, 1998.

Dyson, Walter. *Howard University: The Capstone of Negro Education—A History, 1867–1940.* Washington, D.C.: Graduate School, Howard University, 1941.

Eisen, George. "Sport, Recreation and Gender: Jewish Immigrant Women in Turn-of-the-Century America (1880–1920)." *Journal of Sport History* 18 (1991): 103–20.

Elliott, Orrin Leslie. *Stanford University: The First Twenty-Five Years.* 1937. Repr., New York: Arno, 1977.

Ellis, A. W. "The Status of Health and Physical Education for Women in Negro Colleges and Universities." *Research Quarterly* 10 (May 1939): 135–41.

Evans, John, ed. *Equality, Education and Physical Education.* London: Falmer Press, 1993.

Evans, John, and Brian Davies. "Introduction." In *Equality, Education and Physical Education,* edited by John Evans, 1–9. London: Falmer Press, 1993.

Evans, John, Brian Davies, and Jan Wright, eds. *Body Knowledge and Control: Studies in the Sociology of Physical Education and Health.* London: Routledge, 2004.

Evans, John, and Trefor Williams. "Moving Up and Getting Out: The Classed and Gendered Career Opportunities of Physical Education Teachers." In *Socialization into Physical Education: Learning to Teach,* edited by Thomas J. Templin and Paul G. Schempp, 235–49. Indianapolis: Benchmark, 1989.

Faderman, Lillian. *Odd Girls and Twilight Lovers: A History of Lesbian Life in Twentieth-Century America.* New York: Penguin Books, 1992.

Farrell-Beck, Jane, and Laura Klosterman Kidd. "The Roles of Health Professionals in the Development and Dissemination of Women's Sanitary Products, 1880–1940." *Journal of the History of Medicine and Allied Sciences* 51 (1996): 325–52.

Fass, Paula S. *The Damned and the Beautiful: American Youth in the 1920s.* New York: Oxford University Press, 1977.

———. *Outside In: Minorities and the Transformation of American Education.* New York: Oxford University Press, 1989.

Faucette, F. Nell, et al. "'I'd Rather Chew on Aluminum Foil': Overcoming Classroom Teachers' Resistance to Teaching Physical Education." *Journal of Teaching in Physical Education* 21 (2002): 287–308.

Fausto-Sterling, Anne. "Gender, Race, and Nation: The Comparative Anatomy of 'Hottentot' Women in Europe, 1815–1817." In *Deviant Bodies: Critical Perspectives on Difference in Science and Popular Culture,* edited by Jennifer Terry and Jacqueline Urla, 19–48. Bloomington: Indiana University Press, 1995.

———. *Myths of Gender: Biological Theories About Women and Men.* Rev. ed. New York: Basic Books, 1992.

———. *Sexing the Body: Gender Politics and the Construction of Sexuality.* New York: Basic Books, 2000.

Festle, Mary Jo. *Playing Nice: Politics and Apologies in Women's Sports.* New York: Columbia University Press, 1996.

Filene, Peter G. *Him/Her/Self: Gender Identities in Modern America*. 3rd ed. Baltimore, Md.: Johns Hopkins University Press, 1998.

"Final Rites for Miss Anita Turner, Phys. Ed. Director." *Washington Tribune*, February 15, 1941.

Flax, Jane. "Postmodernism and Gender Relations in Feminist Theory." *Signs* 12 (1987): 621–43.

Fletcher, Sheila. *Women First: The Female Tradition in English Physical Education, 1880–1980*. London: Athlone Press, 1984.

Foucault, Michel. *Power/Knowledge: Selected Interviews and Other Writings, 1972–1977*. Edited by Colin Gordon. New York: Pantheon, 1980.

Frank, Arthur W. "Bringing Bodies Back In: A Decade Review." *Theory, Culture & Society* 7 (1990): 131–62.

Fraser, Nancy. "Equality, Difference, and Democracy: Recent Feminist Debates in the United States." In *Feminism and the New Democracy: Re-siting the Political*, edited by Jodi Dean, 98–109. Thousand Oaks, Calif.: Sage, 1997.

Freidenfelds, Lara. *The Modern Period: Menstruation in Twentieth-Century America*. Baltimore, Md.: Johns Hopkins University Press, 2009.

Fultz, Michael. "Teacher Training and African American Education in the South, 1900–1940." *Journal of Negro Education* 64 (1995): 196–210.

Gaines, Stanley O. Jr. "Sexuality and Race." In *The African American Experience: An Historiographical and Bibliographical Guide*, edited by Arvarh E. Strickland and Robert E. Weems Jr., 315–35. Westport, Conn.: Greenwood Press, 2001.

Gatewood, Willard B. *Aristocrats of Color: The Black Elite, 1880–1920*. Bloomington: Indiana University Press, 1990.

Gems, Gerald R. "Sport and the Americanization of Ethnic Women in Chicago." In *Ethnicity and Sport in North American History and Culture*, edited by George Eisen and David K. Wiggins, 177–200. Westport, Conn.: Greenwood Press, 1994.

George, Judith Jenkins. "Women's Riflery Teams: A Collegiate Anomaly of the Post World War I Period." *Canadian Journal of the History of Sport* 23 (1992): 32–45.

Gerber, Ellen W. "The Controlled Development of Collegiate Sport for Women, 1923–1936." *Journal of Sport History* 2 (1975): 1–28.

———. *Innovators and Institutions in Physical Education*. Philadelphia: Lea and Febiger, 1971.

Giddings, Paula. *When and Where I Enter: The Impact of Black Women on Race and Sex in America*. 2nd ed. New York: William Morrow, 1996.

Gilman, Sander L. *Difference and Pathology: Stereotypes of Sexuality, Race, and Madness*. Ithaca, N.Y.: Cornell University Press, 1985.

Gissendanner, Cindy Himes. "African-American Women and Competitive Sport, 1920–1960." In *Women, Sport, and Culture*, edited by Susan Birrell and Cheryl L. Cole, 81–92. Champaign, Ill.: Human Kinetics, 1994.

———. "African American Women Olympians: The Impact of Race, Gender, and Class Ideologies, 1932–1968." *Research Quarterly for Exercise and Sport* 67 (1996): 172–82.

Goodson, Martia Graham, ed. *Chronicles of Faith: The Autobiography of Frederick D. Patterson*. Tuscaloosa: University of Alabama Press, 1991.

Gordon, Lynn D. *Gender and Higher Education in the Progressive Era*. New Haven, Conn.: Yale University Press, 1990.

Gordon, Tuula. "Citizenship, Difference and Marginality in Schools: Spatial and Embodied Aspects of Gender Construction." In *Equity in the Classroom: Towards Effective Pedagogy for Girls and Boys*, edited by Patricia F. Murphy and Caroline V. Gipps, 34–45. London: Falmer Press, 1996.

Gossett, Thomas F. *Race: The History of an Idea in America*. New York: Schocken Books, 1965.

Gotfrit, Leslie. "Women Dancing Back: Disruption and the Politics of Pleasure." In *Postmodernism, Feminism, and Cultural Politics: Redrawing Educational Boundaries*, edited by Henry A. Giroux, 174–95. Albany: State University of New York Press, 1991.

Gray, Miriam, ed. *A Century of Growth: The Historical Development of Physical Education for Women in Selected Colleges of Six Midwestern States*. Ann Arbor, Mich.: Edwards Brothers, 1951.

Green, Constance McLaughlin. *The Secret City: A History of Race Relations in the Nation's Capital*. Princeton, N.J.: Princeton University Press, 1967.

———. *Washington: Capital City, 1879–1950*. Princeton, N.J.: Princeton University Press, 1963.

———. *Washington: Village and Capital, 1800–1878*. Princeton, N.J.: Princeton University Press, 1962.

Green, Harvey. *Fit for America: Health, Fitness, Sport, and American Society*. New York: Pantheon, 1986.

Greendorfer, Susan L., and Laurna Rubinson. "Homophobia and Heterosexism in Women's Sport and Physical Education." *Women in Sport and Physical Activity Journal* 6 (Fall 1997): 189–212.

Griego, Elizabeth. "The Making of a 'Misfit': Clelia Duel Mosher, 1863–1940." In *Lone Voyagers: Academic Women in Coeducational Institutions, 1870–1937*, edited by Geraldine Jonçich Clifford, 149–82. New York: The Feminist Press, 1989.

Grieve, Andrew. "State Legal Requirements for Physical Education." *Journal of Health, Physical Education, and Recreation* 42 (April 1971): 19–23.

Griffin, Patricia S. "Boys' Participation Styles in a Middle School Physical Education Team Sports Unit." *Journal of Teaching in Physical Education* 4, no. 2 (1985): 100–110.

———. "Changing the Game: Homophobia, Sexism, and Lesbians in Sport." *Quest* 44 (1992): 251–65.

———. "Girls' Participation Patterns in a Middle School Team Sports Unit." *Journal of Teaching in Physical Education* 4, no. 1 (1984): 30–38.

———. *Strong Women, Deep Closets: Lesbians and Homophobia in Sport*. Champaign, Ill.: Human Kinetics, 1998.

Grosz, Elizabeth. "Notes Towards a Corporeal Feminism." *Australian Feminist Studies* 5 (1987): 1–16.

Grover, Kathryn, ed. *Fitness in American Culture: Images of Health, Sport and the Body, 1830–1940*. Amherst: University of Massachusetts Press; Rochester, N.Y.: Margaret Woodbury Strong Museum, 1989.

Gruhn, John G., and Ralph R. Kazer. *Hormonal Regulation of the Menstrual Cycle: The Evolution of Concepts*. New York: Plenum Medical Book Company, 1989.

Grundy, Pamela. *Learning to Win: Sports, Education, and Social Change in Twentieth-Century North Carolina*. Chapel Hill: University of North Carolina Press, 2001.

Guy-Sheftall, Beverly. "Black Women and Higher Education: Spelman and Bennett Colleges Revisited." *Journal of Negro Education* 51 (1982): 278–87.

———. *Daughters of Sorrow: Attitudes Toward Black Women, 1880–1920.* Black Women in United States History, vol. 11. Brooklyn, N.Y.: Carlson, 1990.

Guterl, Matthew Pratt. *The Color of Race in America, 1900–1940.* Cambridge, Mass.: Harvard University Press, 2001.

Hale, Grace Elizabeth. *Making Whiteness: The Culture of Segregation in the South, 1890–1940.* New York: Pantheon, 1998.

Hall, M. Ann. *Feminism and Sporting Bodies: Essays on Theory and Practice.* Champaign, Ill.: Human Kinetics, 1996.

———. "How Should We Theorize Gender in the Context of Sport?" In *Sport, Men, and the Gender Order: Critical Feminist Perspectives*, edited by Michael A. Messner and Donald F. Sabo, 223–39. Champaign, Ill.: Human Kinetics, 1990.

———. "Knowledge and Gender: Epistemological Questions in the Social Analysis of Sport." *Sociology of Sport Journal* 2 (1985): 25–42.

Hammonds, Evelynn. "Black (W)holes and the Geometry of Black Female Sexuality." *differences: A Journal of Feminist Cultural Studies* 6 (1994): 127–45.

Hammonds, Evelynn, and Rebecca M. Herzig, eds. *The Nature of Difference: Sciences of Race in the United States from Jefferson to Genomics.* Cambridge, Mass.: MIT Press, 2009.

Hannaford, Ivan. *Race: The History of an Idea in the West.* Washington, D.C.: Woodrow Wilson Center, 1996.

Hardy, Stephen. "'Adopted by All the Leading Clubs': Sporting Goods and the Shaping of Leisure, 1800–1900." In *Sport in America: From Wicked Amusement to National Obsession*, edited by David K. Wiggins, 133–50. Champaign, Ill.: Human Kinetics, 1995.

———. "'Parks for the People': Reforming the Boston Park System, 1870–1915." *Journal of Sport History* 7 (1980): 5–24.

Hargreaves, Jennifer A. "Gender on the Sports Agenda." *International Review for the Sociology of Sport* 25 (1990): 287–307.

———. *Sporting Females: Critical Issues in the History and Sociology of Women's Sports.* London: Routledge, 1994.

Harley, Sharon. "Beyond the Classroom: The Organizational Lives of Black Female Educators in the District of Columbia, 1890–1930." *Journal of Negro Education* 51 (1982): 254–65.

Harlow, Siobán D. "Function and Dysfunction: A Historical Critique of the Literature on Menstruation and Work." In *Culture, Society, and Menstruation*, edited by Virginia E. Olesen and Nancy Fugate Woods, 39–50. Washington, D.C.: Hemisphere, 1986.

Harris, Mary B., and Joy Griffin. "Stereotypes and Personal Beliefs about Women Physical Education Teachers." *Women in Sport and Physical Activity Journal* 6 (1997): 49–58.

Henderson, James H. M., and Betty F. Henderson. *Molder of Men: Portrait of a 'Grand Old Man'—Edwin Bancroft Henderson.* Washington, D.C.: Vantage, 1985.

Hensley, Larry D. "Current Status of Basic Instruction Programs in Physical Education at American Colleges and Universities." *Journal of Physical Education, Recreation, and Dance* 71 (November–December 2000): 30–36.

Herndl, Diane Price. "The Invisible (Invalid) Woman: African-American Women, Illness, and Nineteenth-Century Narrative." *Women's Studies* 24 (1995): 553–72.

Higginbotham, Evelyn Brooks. "African-American Women's History and the Metalanguage of Race." *Signs* 17 (1992): 251–74.

———. "Beyond the Sound of Silence: Afro-American Women in History." *Gender & History* 1 (1989): 50–67.

———. "Rethinking the Subject of African American Women's History." In *New Viewpoints in Women's History: Working Papers from the Schlesinger Library 50th Anniversary Conference, March 4–5, 1994,* edited by Susan Ware, 64–70. Cambridge, Mass.: Schlesinger Library, Radcliffe College, 1994.

———. *Righteous Discontent: The Women's Movement in the Black Baptist Church, 1880–1920.* Cambridge, Mass.: Harvard University Press, 1993.

Hill, Ruth Edmonds, ed. *The Black Women Oral History Project.* 10 vols. Westport, Conn.: Meckler, 1990.

Himes, Cindy. "From Equity to Equality: Women's Athletics at Brown." In *The Search for Equity: Women at Brown University, 1891–1991,* edited by Polly Welts Kaufman, 121–54. Hanover, N.H.: University Press of New England, 1991.

Hine, Darlene Clark. "Rape and the Inner Lives of Black Women in the Middle West: Preliminary Thoughts on the Culture of Dissemblance." *Signs* 14 (1989): 912–20.

Hine, Darlene Clark, and Kathleen Thompson. *A Shining Thread of Hope: The History of Black Women in America.* New York: Broadway Books, 1998.

Hird, Myra J. *Sex, Gender, and Science.* Houndmills, Basingstoke, Hampshire, U.K.: Palgrave Macmillan, 2004.

Hoberman, John. *Darwin's Athletes: How Sport Has Damaged Black America and Preserved the Myth of Race.* Boston: Houghton Mifflin, 1997.

hooks, bell. *Ain't I a Woman: Black Women and Feminism.* Boston: South End Press, 1981.

Horowitz, Helen Lefkowitz. *Alma Mater: Design and Experience in the Women's Colleges from Their Nineteenth-Century Beginnings to the 1930s.* 2nd ed. Amherst: University of Massachusetts Press, 1993.

———. *Campus Life: Undergraduate Cultures from the End of the Eighteenth Century to the Present.* New York: Alfred A. Knopf, 1987.

———. *The Power and Passion of M. Carey Thomas.* New York: Alfred A. Knopf, 1994.

Houchins, Joseph R. "The Negro in Professional Occupations in the United States." *Journal of Negro Education* 22 (1953): 405–15.

Howell, Reet, ed. *Her Story in Sport: A Historical Anthology of Women in Sport.* West Point, N.Y.: Leisure Press, 1982.

Hughes, William Hardin, and Frederick D. Patterson, eds. *Robert Russa Moton of Hampton and Tuskegee.* Chapel Hill: University of North Carolina Press, 1956.

Hult, Joan S. "The Governance of Athletics for Girls and Women: Leadership by Women Physical Educators, 1899–1949." *Research Quarterly for Exercise and Sport,* Centennial Issue (April 1985): 64–77.

———. "The Philosophical Conflicts in Men's and Women's Collegiate Athletics." *Quest* 32 (1980): 77–94.

———. "Women's Struggle for Governance in U.S. Amateur Athletics." *International Review for the Sociology of Sport* 24 (1989): 249–63.

Hult, Joan S., and Marianna Trekell, eds. *A Century of Women's Basketball: From Frailty to Final Four.* Reston, Va.: AAHPERD, 1991.

Humbert, M. Louise. "On the Sidelines: The Experiences of Young Women in Physical Education Classes." *Avanté* 1 (1995): 58–77.

"In Memoriam [Dorothy S. Ainsworth]." *Journal of Physical Education and Recreation* 48 (February 1977): 44–45.

Inglis, Sue, Karen E. Danylchuk, and Donna L. Pastore. "Multiple Realities of Women's Work Experiences in Coaching and Athletic Management." *Women in Sport and Physical Activity Journal* 9 (Fall 2000): 1–26.

"Interview with Jessie Harriet (Scott) Abbott." In *Black Women Oral History Project*, edited by Ruth Edmonds Hill, 1:1–137. Westport, Conn.: Meckler, 1991.

Jordanova, Ludmilla. *Sexual Visions: Images of Gender in Science and Medicine between the Eighteenth and Twentieth Centuries*. Madison: University of Wisconsin Press, 1989.

Kadzielski, Mark A. "'As a Flower Needs Sunshine': The Origins of Organized Children's Recreation in Philadelphia, 1886–1911." *Journal of Sport History* 4 (Fall 1977): 169–88.

Kahan, David. "Islam and Physical Activity: Implications for American Sport and Physical Educators." *Journal of Physical Education, Recreation, and Dance* 74 (March 2003): 48–54.

Kane, Mary Jo. "Resistance/Transformation of the Oppositional Binary: Exposing Sport as a Continuum." *Journal of Sport and Social Issues* 19 (1995): 191–218.

Kasson, John F. *Houdini, Tarzan, and the Perfect Man: The White Male Body and the Challenge of Modernity in America*. New York: Hill and Wang, 2001.

Kieckhefer, Grace Norton. "The History of Milwaukee-Downer College, 1851–1951." *Milwaukee-Downer College Bulletin* series 33, no. 2 (November 1950).

Kilson, Marion. "Black Women in the Professions, 1890–1970." *Monthly Labor Review* 100 (May 1977): 38–41.

Kirby, John B. *Black Americans in the Roosevelt Era: Liberalism and Race*. Knoxville: University of Tennessee Press, 1980.

Kirk, David. *Defining Physical Education: The Social Construction of a School Subject in Postwar Britain*. London: Falmer, 1992.

———. "Physical Education, Discourse, and Ideology: Bringing the Hidden Curriculum Into View." *Quest* 44 (1992): 35–56.

———. "Schooling Bodies in New Times: The Reform of School Physical Education in High Modernity." In *Critical Postmodernism in Human Movement, Physical Education, and Sport*, edited by Juan-Miguel Fernández-Balboa, 39–63. Albany: State University of New York Press, 1997.

———. *Schooling Bodies: School Practice and Public Discourse, 1880–1950*. London: Leicester University Press, 1998.

Kirk, David, and Richard Tinning. "Embodied Self-Identity, Healthy Lifestyles and School Physical Education." *Sociology of Health & Illness* 16 (1994): 600–625.

Kirk, Robert H. "The Posture of Predominantly Negro College and University Health and Physical Education Faculties." *Journal of Health, Physical Education, and Recreation* 40 (February 1969): 83–84, 86.

Klinge, Ineke. "Female Bodies and Brittle Bones: Medical Interventions in Osteoporosis." In *Embodied Practices: Feminist Perspectives on the Body*, edited by Kathy Davis, 59–72. London: Sage, 1997.

Krane, Vikki, and Heather Barber. "Identity Tensions in Lesbian Intercollegiate Coaches." *Research Quarterly for Exercise and Sport* 76 (2005): 67–81.

Ladd, Wayne M., and Angela Lumpkin, eds. *Sport in American Education: History and Perspective*. Washington, D.C.: AAHPERD, 1979.

Ladd-Taylor, Molly. "Women's Health and Public Policy." In *Women, Health, and Medicine in America: A Historical Handbook*, edited by Rima D. Apple, 391–410. New York: Garland, 1990.

Lapchick, Richard. "The 2005 Racial and Gender Report Card: College Sports." http://www.bus.ucf.edu/sport/public/downloads/2005_Racial_Gender_Report_Card_Colleges.pdf (accessed January 11, 2007).

Laqueur, Thomas. *Making Sex: Body and Gender from the Greeks to Freud*. Cambridge, Mass.: Harvard University Press, 1990.

Lasch-Quinn, Elisabeth. *Black Neighbors: Race and the Limits of Reform in the American Settlement House Movement, 1890–1945*. Chapel Hill: University of North Carolina Press, 1993.

Lears, T. J. Jackson. "From Salvation to Self-Realization: Advertising and the Therapeutic Roots of the Consumer Culture, 1880–1930." In *The Culture of Consumption: Critical Essays in American History, 1880–1980*, edited by Richard Wightman Fox and T. J. Jackson Lears, 1–38. New York: Pantheon Books, 1983.

Lee, Mabel. *A History of Physical Education and Sports in the U.S.A.* New York: John Wiley and Sons, 1983.

Lee, Mabel, and Bruce L. Bennett. "This is Our Heritage." *Journal of Health, Physical Education, and Recreation* 31 (April 1960): 25–33, 38–47, 52–58, 62–73, 76–85.

Lenskyj, Helen. *Out of Bounds: Women, Sport and Sexuality*. Toronto: Women's Press, 1986.

———. *Out on the Field: Gender, Sport and Sexualities*. Toronto: Women's Press, 2003.

———. "Power and Play: Gender and Sexuality Issues in Sport and Physical Activity." *International Review for the Sociology of Sport* 25 (1990): 235–43.

———. "Women, Sport, and Sexualities: Breaking the Silences." In *Sport and Gender in Canada*, edited by Philip White and Kevin Young, 170–81. Ontario: Oxford University Press, 1999.

Levine, David O. *The American College and the Culture of Aspiration, 1915–1940*. Ithaca, N.Y.: Cornell University Press, 1986.

Levine, Peter. "'Our Crowd' at Play: The Elite Jewish Country Club in the 1920s." In *Sports and the American Jew*, edited by Steven A. Riess, 160–84. Syracuse, N.Y.: Syracuse University Press, 1998.

Lewis, Guy M. "Adoption of the Sports Program, 1906–39: The Role of Accommodation in the Transformation of Physical Education." *Quest* 12 (1969): 34–46.

Liberti, Rita M. "'We Were Ladies, We Just Played Basketball Like Boys': African American Womanhood and Competitive Basketball at Bennett College, 1928–1942." *Journal of Sport History* 26 (1999): 567–84.

———. "Women's Sport History and Black Feminist Theory." *Womanist Theory and Research* 3.2/4.1 (2001/2002): 45–50.

Little, Monroe H. "The Extra-Curricular Activities of Black College Students, 1868–1940." *Journal of Negro History* 65 (1980): 135–48.

Lockhart, Aileene S., and Betty Spears, eds. *Chronicle of American Physical Education: Selected Readings, 1855–1930*. Dubuque, Iowa: William C. Brown, 1972.

Logan, Rayford W. *Howard University: The First Hundred Years, 1867–1967*. New York: New York University Press, 1969.

Long, Howard H. "The Support and Control of Public Education in the District of Columbia." *Journal of Negro Education* 7 (1938): 390–99.

Lorber, Judith. "Believing Is Seeing: Biology as Ideology." *Gender & Society* 7 (1993): 568–81.

———. *Gender Inequality: Feminist Theories and Politics*. 2nd ed. Los Angeles: Roxbury, 2001.

Lord, Alexandra. "'The Great Arcana of the Deity': Menstruation and Menstrual Disorders in Eighteenth-Century British Medical Thought." *Bulletin of the History of Medicine* 73 (1999): 38–63.

Lowe, Margaret A. *Looking Good: College Women and Body Image, 1875–1930*. Baltimore, Md.: Johns Hopkins University Press, 2003.

Lowen, Rebecca S. *Creating the Cold War University: The Transformation of Stanford*. Berkeley: University of California Press, 1997.

Lowry, Richard. "Participation in High School Physical Education—United States, 1991–2003." *Journal of School Health* 75 (February 2005): 47–49.

Lowry, Richard, et al. "Recent Trends In Participation in Physical Education Among US High School Students." *Journal of School Health* 71 (April 2001): 145–52.

Loy, John W., David L. Andrews, and Robert E. Rinehart. "The Body in Culture and Sport." *Sport Science Review* 2 (1993): 69–91.

Lumpkin, Angela, and Jane Jenkins. "Basic Instruction Programs: A Brief History." *Journal of Physical Education, Recreation, and Dance* 64 (August 1993): 32–36.

Lydon, Mary C. "Secondary School Programs: Diversity in Practice." In *Women in Sport: Issues and Controversies*, edited by Greta L. Cohen, 95–103. Thousand Oaks, Calif.: Sage, 1993.

Macdonald, Doune. "The 'Professional' Work of Experienced Physical Education Teachers." *Research Quarterly for Exercise and Sport* 70 (1999): 41–54.

———. "The Role of Proletarianization in Physical Education Teacher Attrition." *Research Quarterly for Exercise and Sport* 66 (1995): 129–41.

Macdonald, Doune, and David Kirk. "Private Lives, Public Lives: Surveillance, Identity and Self in the Work of Beginning Physical Education Teachers." *Sport, Education and Society* 1 (1996): 59–75.

MacKinnon, Catherine. *Feminism Unmodified: Discourses on Life and Law*. Cambridge, Mass.: Harvard University Press, 1987.

Mangan, J. A., and Roberta J. Park, eds. *From 'Fair Sex' to Feminism: Sport and the Socialization of Women in the Industrial and Post-Industrial Eras*. London: Frank Cass, 1987.

Manley, Robert N. *Frontier University (1869–1919)*. Vol. 1, *Centennial History of the University of Nebraska*. Lincoln: University of Nebraska Press, 1969.

"Margaret Bell, 1888–1969." *Journal of Health, Physical Education, and Recreation* 40 (April 1969): 88.

Markula, Pirkko, and Richard Pringle. *Foucault, Sport and Exercise: Power, Knowledge and Transforming the Self*. New York: Routledge, 2006.

Martin, Emily. *The Woman in the Body: A Cultural Analysis of Reproduction*. Boston: Beacon Press, 1987.

Martin, Karin A. "Becoming a Gendered Body: Practices of Preschools." *American Sociological Review* 63 (1998): 494–511.

Massengale, John D., and Richard A. Swanson, eds. *The History of Exercise and Sport Science*. Champaign, Ill.: Human Kinetics, 1997.

Maynard, Mary. "'Race,' Gender and the Concept of 'Difference' in Feminist Thought." In *The Dynamics of 'Race' and Gender: Some Feminist Interventions*, edited by Haleh Afshar and Mary Maynard, 9–25. London: Taylor and Francis, 1994.

McCallister, Sarah G., Elaine M. Blinde, and Jessie M. Phillips. "Prospects for Change in a New Millennium: Gender Beliefs of Young Girls in Sport and Physical Activity." *Women in Sport and Physical Activity Journal* 12 (2003): 83–109.

McLaren, Peter L. "Schooling the Postmodern Body: Critical Pedagogy and the Politics of Enfleshment." In *Postmodernism, Feminism, and Cultural Politics: Redrawing Educational Boundaries*, edited by Henry A. Giroux, 144–73. Albany: State University of New York Press, 1991.

McPherson, James M. *The Abolitionist Legacy: From Reconstruction to the NAACP*. 2nd ed. Princeton, N.J.: Princeton University Press, 1995.

———. "White Liberals and Black Power in Negro Education, 1865–1915." *American Historical Review* 75 (1970): 1357–86.

Messner, Michael A. "Sports and Male Domination: The Female Athlete as Contested Ideological Terrain." *Sociology of Sport Journal* 5 (1988): 197–211.

Meyerowitz, Joanne, ed. *Not June Cleaver: Women and Gender in Postwar America, 1945–1960*. Philadelphia: Temple University Press, 1994.

Mihesuah, Devon A. *Cultivating the Rosebuds: The Education of Women at the Cherokee Female Seminary, 1851–1909*. Urbana: University of Illinois Press, 1993.

Miller, Glenn A., Linus J. Dowell, and Robert H. Pender. "Physical Activity Programs in Colleges and Universities: A Status Report." *Journal of Physical Education, Recreation, and Dance* 60 (August 1989): 20–23.

Miller, Patrick B. "The Anatomy of Scientific Racism: Racialist Responses to Black Athletic Achievement." *Journal of Sport History* 25 (1998): 119–51.

———. "To 'Bring the Race along Rapidly': Sport, Student Culture, and Educational Mission at Historically Black Colleges during the Interwar Years." *History of Education Quarterly* 35 (1995): 111–33.

Miller, Patrick B., and David K. Wiggins, eds. *Sport and the Color Line: Black Athletes and Race Relations in Twentieth-Century America*. New York: Routledge, 2004.

Minow, Martha. *Making All the Difference: Inclusion, Exclusion, and American Law*. Ithaca, N.Y.: Cornell University Press, 1990.

Mirel, Jeffrey. "From Student Control to Institutional Control of High School Athletics: Three Michigan Cities, 1883–1905." *Journal of Social History* 16 (1982): 83–100.

Mitchell, J. Pearce. *Stanford University, 1916–1941*. Stanford, Calif.: Stanford University Press, 1958.

Moore, Jacqueline M. *Leading the Race: The Transformation of the Black Elite in the Nation's Capital, 1880–1920*. Charlottesville: University Press of Virginia, 1999.

Morantz-Sanchez, Regina Markell. *Sympathy and Science: Women Physicians in American Medicine*. New York: Oxford University Press, 1985.

More, Ellen S. *Restoring the Balance: Women Physicians and the Profession of Medicine, 1850–1995*. Cambridge, Mass.: Harvard University Press, 1999.

Morrow, James R. "2004 C. H. McCloy Research Lecture: Are American Children and Youth Fit? It's Time We Learned." *Research Quarterly for Exercise and Sport* 76 (2005): 377–88.

Morrow, Ronald G., and Diane L. Gill. "Perceptions of Homophobia and Heterosexism in Physical Education." *Research Quarterly for Exercise and Sport* 74 (2003): 205–14.

Morton, Mary A. "The Education of Negroes in the District of Columbia." *Journal of Negro Education* 16 (1947): 325–39.

Mrozek, Donald J. "The 'Amazon' and the American 'Lady': Sexual Fears of Women as Athletes." In *From 'Fair Sex' to Feminism: Sport and the Socialization of Women in the Industrial and Post-Industrial Eras*, edited by J. A. Mangan and Roberta J. Park, 282–98. London: Frank Cass, 1987.

———. *Sport and American Mentality, 1880–1910*. Knoxville: University of Tennessee Press, 1983.

Mumford, Arnett W. "The Present Status of Health and Physical Education Programs in Negro Senior Colleges." *Research Quarterly* 19 (1948): 190–97.

National Coalition for Women and Girls in Education. "Title IX at 30: Report Card on Gender Equity (June 2002)." http://iweb.aahperd.org/nagws/pdf_files/title930.pdf (accessed October 9, 2006).

Neverdon-Morton, Cynthia. *Afro-American Women of the South and the Advancement of the Race, 1895–1925*. Knoxville: University of Tennessee Press, 1989.

Nicholson, Linda. "Interpreting Gender." *Signs* 20 (1994): 79–105.

"Normal Schools: Exploring Our Heritage." *Journal of Physical Education, Recreation, and Dance* 65 (March 1994): 25–56.

Olafson, Lori. "'I Hate Phys. Ed.': Adolescent Girls Talk About Physical Education." *Physical Educator* 59 (Spring 2002): 67–74.

O'Sullivan, Mary. "Failing Gym is Like Failing Lunch or Recess: Two Beginning Teachers' Struggle for Legitimacy." *Journal of Teaching in Physical Education* 8 (April 1989): 227–42.

O'Sullivan, Mary, Kim Bush, and Margaret Gehring. "Gender Equity and Physical Education: A USA Perspective." In *Gender and Physical Education: Contemporary Issues and Future Directions*, edited by Dawn Penney, 163–89. London: Routledge, 2002.

Oudshoorn, Nelly. *Beyond the Natural Body: An Archeology of Sex Hormones*. London: Routledge, 1994.

Owen, Janet. *Sports in Women's Colleges*. New York: New York Herald-Tribune, 1932.

Oxendine, Joseph B. "100 Years of Basic Instruction." *Journal of Physical Education, Recreation, and Dance* 56 (September 1985): 32–36.

———. "Status of Required Physical Education Programs in Colleges and Universities." *Journal of Health, Physical Education, and Recreation* 40 (January 1969): 32–35.

Park, Roberta J. "1989 C. H. McCloy Research Lecture: Health, Exercise, and the Biomedical Impulse, 1870–1914." *Research Quarterly for Exercise and Sport* 61 (1990): 126–40.

———. "The Contributions of Women to Exercise Science and Sports Medicine, 1870–1994." *Women in Sport and Physical Activity Journal* 3 (Spring 1995): 41–69.

———. "The Emergence of the Academic Discipline of Physical Education in the United States." In *Perspectives on the Academic Discipline of Physical Education: A Tribute to*

G. Lawrence Rarick, edited by George A. Brooks, 20–45. Champaign, Ill.: Human Kinetics, 1981.

———. "For Pleasure? Or Profit? Or Personal Health? College Gymnasia as Contested Terrain." In *Sites of Sport: Space, Place, Experience*, edited by Patricia Vertinsky and John Bale, 177–204. London: Routledge, 2004.

———. "Healthy, Moral, and Strong: Educational Views of Exercise and Athletics in Nineteenth-Century America." In *Fitness in American Culture: Images of Health, Sport, and the Body, 1830–1940*, edited by Kathryn Grover, 123–68. Amherst: University of Massachusetts Press; Rochester, N.Y.: Margaret Woodbury Strong Museum, 1989.

———. "High-Protein Diets, 'Damaged Hearts,' and Rowing Men: Antecedents of Modern Sports Medicine and Exercise Science, 1867–1928." *Exercise and Sport Sciences Reviews* 25 (1997): 137–69.

———. "History and Structure of the Department of Physical Education at the University of California, with Special Reference to Women's Sports." In *Her Story in Sport: A Historical Anthology of Women in Sport*, edited by Reet Howell, 405–16. West Point, N.Y.: Leisure Press, 1982.

———. *Measurement of Physical Fitness: A Historical Perspective*. Office of Disease Prevention and Health Promotion Monograph Series. Washington, D.C.: U.S. Department of Health and Human Services, Public Health Service, [1989].

———. "Physiologists, Physicians, and Physical Educators: Nineteenth-Century Biology and Exercise, *Hygienic* and *Educative*." In *Sport and Exercise Science: Essays in the History of Sports Medicine*, edited by Jack W. Berryman and Roberta J. Park, 137–81. Urbana: University of Illinois Press, 1992.

———. "The *Research Quarterly* and Its Antecedents." *Research Quarterly for Exercise and Sport* 51 (1980): 1–22.

———. "Science, Service, and the Professionalization of Physical Education: 1885–1905." *Research Quarterly for Exercise and Sport* Centennial Issue (April 1985): 7–20.

———. "The Second 100 Years: Or, Can Physical Education Become the Renaissance Field of the 21st Century?" *Quest* 41 (1989): 1–27.

———. "Sport and Recreation Among Chinese American Communities of the Pacific Coast From Time of Arrival to the 'Quiet Decade' of the 1950s." *Journal of Sport History* 27 (2000): 445–80.

Park, Roberta J., and Joan S. Hult. "Women as Leaders in Physical Education and School-Based Sports, 1865 to the 1930s." *Journal of Physical Education, Recreation, and Dance* 64 (March 1993): 35–40.

Pate, Russell R. "Recent Statements and Initiatives on Physical Activity and Health." *Quest* 47 (1995): 304–10.

Pate, Russell R., et al. "School Physical Education." *Journal of School Health* 65 (October 1995): 312–18.

Peiss, Kathy. *Cheap Amusements: Working Women and Leisure in Turn-of-the-Century New York*. Philadelphia: Temple University Press, 1986.

———. *Hope in a Jar: The Making of America's Beauty Culture*. New York: Henry Holt and Company, 1998.

Perkins, Linda M. "The African American Female Elite: The Early History of African American Women in the Seven Sister Colleges, 1880–1960." *Harvard Educational Review* 67 (Winter 1997): 718–56.

————. "The History of Blacks in Teaching: Growth and Decline Within the Profession." In *American Teachers: Histories of a Profession at Work*, edited by Donald Warren, 344–69. New York: Macmillan, 1989.

Perpener, John O., III. *African-American Concert Dance: The Harlem Renaissance and Beyond*. Urbana: University of Illinois Press, 2001.

Peterson, Carla L. "Foreword: Eccentric Bodies." In *Recovering the Black Female Body: Self-Representations by African American Women*, edited by Michael Bennett and Vanessa D. Dickerson, ix–xvi. New Brunswick, N.J.: Rutgers University Press, 2000.

Peterson, Hazel C. *Dorothy S. Ainsworth: Her Life, Professional Career and Contributions to Physical Education*. Rev. ed. Moscow: University of Idaho Press, 1975.

Pfister, Gertrud. "The Medical Discourse on Female Physical Culture in Germany in the 19th and Early 20th Centuries." *Journal of Sport History* 17 (1990): 183–98.

Pfister, Gertrud, and Dagmar Reese. "Gender, Body Culture, and Body Politics in National Socialism." *Sport Science Review* 4 (1995): 91–121.

Pierro, Armstead A. "A History of Professional Preparation in Physical Education in Selected Negro Colleges and Universities to 1958." In *A History of Physical Education and Sport in the United States and Canada: Selected Topics*, edited by Earle F. Zeigler, 255–71. Champaign, Ill.: Stipes, 1975.

Plank, David N., and Rick Ginsberg, eds. *Southern Cities, Southern Schools: Public Education in the Urban South*. Westport, Conn.: Greenwood Press, 1990.

Pope, S. W. *Patriotic Games: Sporting Traditions in the American Imagination, 1876–1926*. New York: Oxford University Press, 1997.

Prescott, Heather Munro. *Student Bodies: The Influence of Student Health Services in American Society and Medicine*. Ann Arbor: University of Michigan Press, 2007.

Preston, Emmett D. Jr. "The Development of Negro Education in the District of Columbia." *Journal of Negro Education* 9 (1940): 595–603.

————. "The Development of Negro Education in the District of Columbia, 1800–1860." *Journal of Negro Education* 12 (1943): 189–98.

Read, Florence Matilda. *The Story of Spelman College*. Princeton, N.J.: Princeton University Press, 1961.

Remley, Mary L. "Amy Homans and the Boston Normal School of Gymnastics." *Journal of Physical Education, Recreation, and Dance* 65 (March 1994): 47–49, 52.

Ritterhouse, Jennifer. *Growing Up Jim Crow: How Black and White Southern Children Learned Race*. Chapel Hill: University of North Carolina Press, 2006.

Rosenberg, Rosalind. *Beyond Separate Spheres: Intellectual Roots of Modern Feminism*. New Haven, Conn.: Yale University Press, 1982.

————. *Divided Lives: American Women in the Twentieth Century*. New York: Hill and Wang, 1992.

Rosenzweig, Roy. "Middle-Class Parks and Working-Class Play: The Struggle over Recreational Space in Worcester, Massachusetts, 1870–1910." *Radical History Review* 21 (Fall 1979): 31–46.

Rossiter, Margaret W. *Women Scientists in America: Struggles and Strategies to 1940*. Baltimore, Md.: Johns Hopkins University Press, 1982.

Rotundo, E. Anthony. *American Manhood: Transformations in Masculinity from the Revolution to the Modern Era*. New York: Basic Books, 1993.

Rovegno, Inez, and David Kirk. "Articulations and Silences in Socially Critical Work on Physical Education: Toward a Broader Agenda." *Quest* 47 (1995): 447–74.

Russett, Cynthia Eagle. *Sexual Science: The Victorian Construction of Womanhood.* Cambridge, Mass.: Harvard University Press, 1989.

Ryan, Mary P. *Mysteries of Sex: Tracing Women and Men through American History.* Chapel Hill: University of North Carolina Press, 2006.

Sabo, Don, and Janie Victoria Ward. "Wherefore Art Thou Feminisms? Feminist Activism, Academic Feminisms, and Women's Sports Advocacy." *Scholar and Feminist Online*, Issue 4.3 (Summer 2006). http://www.barnard.edu/sfonline/sport/sabo_ward_01.htm

Sawyer, R. McLaran. *The Modern University, 1920–1969.* Vol. 2, *Centennial History of the University of Nebraska.* Lincoln, Neb.: Centennial Press, 1973.

Schiebinger, Londa. *The Mind Has No Sex? Women in the Origins of Modern Science.* Cambridge, Mass.: Harvard University Press, 1989.

———. *Nature's Body: Gender in the Making of Modern Science.* Boston: Beacon Press, 1993.

Scott, Joan W. "Deconstructing Equality-Versus-Difference: Or, the Uses of Poststructuralist Theory for Feminism." *Feminist Studies* 14 (1988): 33–50.

Scott, Patricia Bell. "Schoolin' 'Respectable' Ladies of Color: Issues in the History of Black Women's Higher Education." *Journal of the National Association of Women's Deans, Administrators, and Counselors* 43 (Winter 1979–80): 22–28.

Scraton, Sheila. "Gender and Physical Education: Ideologies of the Physical and the Politics of Sexuality." In *Changing Policies, Changing Teachers: New Directions for Schooling?* edited by Stephen Walker and Len Barton, 169–89. Milton Keynes, U.K.: Open University, 1987.

———. "Reconceptualizing Race, Gender and Sport: The Contribution of Black Feminism." In *"Race," Sport and British Society*, edited by Ben Carrington and Ian McDonald, 170–87. London: Routledge, 2001.

———. *Shaping Up to Womanhood: Gender and Girls' Physical Education.* Buckingham, U.K.: Open University, 1992.

Scraton, Sheila, and Anne Flintoff. "Sport Feminism: The Contribution of Feminist Thought to Our Understandings of Gender and Sport." In *Gender and Sport: A Reader*, edited by Sheila Scraton and Anne Flintoff, 30–46. London: Routledge, 2002.

Sedgwick, Eve Kosofsky. "Gender Criticism." In *Redrawing the Boundaries: The Transformation of English and American Literary Studies*, edited by Stephen Greenblatt and Giles Gunn, 271–302. New York: Modern Language Association of America, 1992.

Shapin, Steven. *The Scientific Revolution.* Chicago: University of Chicago Press, 1996.

Shaw, Stephanie J. *What a Woman Ought to Be and to Do: Black Professional Women Workers During the Jim Crow Era.* Chicago: University of Chicago Press, 1996.

Shilling, Chris. "Educating the Body: Physical Capital and the Production of Social Inequalities." *Sociology* 25 (1991): 653–72.

Sicherman, Barbara, and Carol Hurd Green, eds. *Notable American Women: The Modern Period.* Cambridge, Mass.: Belknap Press of Harvard University Press, 1980.

Silver, Catherine Bodard. *Black Teachers in Urban Schools: The Case of Washington, D.C.* New York: Praeger, 1973.

Sitkoff, Harvard. *A New Deal For Blacks: The Emergence of Civil Rights as a National Issue—The Depression Decade.* New York: Oxford University Press, 1978.

Smith, Roger. *The Norton History of the Human Sciences*. New York: W. W. Norton and Company, 1997.

Smith, Yevonne R. "Issues and Strategies for Working with Multicultural Athletes." *Journal of Physical Education, Recreation, and Dance* 62 (March 1991): 39–44.

———. "Recruitment and Retention of African American and Other Multicultural Physical Educators." *Journal of Physical Education, Recreation, and Dance* 64 (March 1993): 66–70.

———. "Women of Color in Society and Sport." *Quest* 44 (1992): 228–50.

Smith-Rosenberg, Carroll. "Puberty to Menopause: The Cycle of Femininity in Nineteenth-Century America." *Feminist Studies* 1 (Winter/Spring 1973): 58–72.

Smith-Rosenberg, Carroll, and Charles Rosenberg. "The Female Animal: Medical and Biological Views of Woman and Her Role in Nineteenth-Century America." *Journal of American History* 60 (1973): 332–56.

Solomon, Barbara Miller. *In the Company of Educated Women: A History of Women and Higher Education in America*. New Haven, Conn.: Yale University Press, 1985.

Somerville, Siobhan B. *Queering the Color Line: Race and the Invention of Homosexuality in American Culture*. Durham, N.C.: Duke University Press, 2000.

Sparkes, Andrew C. "Self, Silence and Invisibility as a Beginning Teacher: A Life History of Lesbian Experience." *British Journal of Sociology of Education* 15 (1994): 93–118.

Sparkes, Andrew C., and Arto Tiihonen. "Silent Voices in a Marginal World: The Life-Story of a Lesbian Physical Education Teacher." In *On the Fringes of Sport*, edited by Leena Laine, 40–47. St. Augustine, Germany: Academia Verlag, 1993.

Sparkes, Andrew C., Thomas J. Templin, and Paul G. Schempp. "Exploring Dimensions of Marginality: Reflecting on the Life Histories of Physical Education Teachers." *Journal of Teaching in Physical Education* 12 (July 1993): 386–98.

Spears, Betty. *Leading the Way: Amy Morris Homans and the Beginnings of Professional Education for Women*. Contributions in Women's Studies, no. 64. New York: Greenwood Press, 1986.

———. "Success, Women, and Physical Education." In *Women as Leaders in Physical Education and Sports*, edited by M. Gladys Scott and Mary J. Hoferek, 5–19. Iowa City: University of Iowa Press, 1979.

Spivey, Donald. *Schooling for the New Slavery: Black Industrial Education, 1868–1915*. Contributions in Afro-American and African Studies, no. 38. Westport, Conn.: Greenwood Press, 1978.

Spring, Joel H. "Mass Culture and School Sports." *History of Education Quarterly* 14 (1974): 483–99.

Squires, Judith. *Gender in Political Theory*. Malden, Mass.: Polity Press, 2000.

Squires, Sarah L., and Andrew C. Sparkes. "Circles of Silence: Sexual Identity in Physical Education and Sport." *Sport, Education and Society* 1 (1996): 77–101.

Stepan, Nancy Leys. "Race and Gender: The Role of Analogy in Science." In *The "Racial" Economy of Science: Toward a Democratic Future*, edited by Sandra Harding, 359–76. Bloomington: Indiana University Press, 1993.

Stern, Alexandra Minna, and Howard Markel, eds. *Formative Years: Children's Health in the United States, 1880–2000*. Ann Arbor: University of Michigan Press, 2002.

Stier, William F. Jr., and Jerome Quarterman. "Characteristics of Physical Education Faculty in Historically Black Colleges and Universities (HBCUs)." *Physical Educator* 49 (Spring 1992): 73–80.

Stier, William F., Jerome Quarterman, and Mark Martin Stier. "The Status of Physical Education Performance Classes Within Historically Black Colleges and Universities." *Journal of Physical Education, Recreation, and Dance* 64 (May–June 1993): 87–92.

Stroot, Sandra A., et al. "Contextual Hoops and Hurdles: Workplace Conditions in Secondary Physical Education." *Journal of Teaching in Physical Education* 13 (July 1994): 342–60.

Swanson, Richard A., and Betty M. Spears. *History of Sport and Physical Education in the United States.* 4th ed. Madison, Wisc.: Brown and Benchmark, 1995.

Sykes, Heather. "Constr(i)(u)cting Lesbian Identities in Physical Education: Feminist and Poststructural Approaches to Researching Sexuality." *Quest* 48 (1996): 459–69.

Tannehill, Deborah, and Dorothy Zakrajsek. "Student Attitudes Towards Physical Education: A Multicultural Study." *Journal of Teaching in Physical Education* 13 (1993): 78–84.

Tannehill, Deborah, et al. "Attitudes Toward Physical Education: Their Impact on How Physical Education Teachers Make Sense of Their Work." *Journal of Teaching in Physical Education* 13 (1994): 406–20.

Terry, Jennifer. *An American Obsession: Science, Medicine, and Homosexuality in Modern Society.* Chicago: University of Chicago Press, 1999.

Terry, Jennifer, and Jacqueline Urla, eds. *Deviant Bodies: Critical Perspectives on Difference in Science and Popular Culture.* Bloomington: Indiana University Press, 1995.

Thaxton, Nolan A. "Tuskegee Institute: Pioneer in Women's Track & Field." *Physical Educator* 29 (May 1972): 77–79.

Theberge, Nancy. "Reflections on the Body in the Sociology of Sport." *Quest* 43 (1991): 123–34.

Thelin, John R. *A History of American Higher Education.* Baltimore, Md.: Johns Hopkins University Press, 2004.

Theriot, Nancy. "Towards a New Sporting Ideal: The Women's Division of the National Amateur Athletic Federation." *Frontiers* 3, no. 1 (1978): 1–7.

Todd, Jan. *Physical Culture and the Body Beautiful: Purposive Exercise in the Lives of American Women, 1800–1870.* Macon, Ga.: Mercer University Press, 1998.

Tomko, Linda J. *Dancing Class: Gender, Ethnicity, and Social Divides in American Dance, 1890–1920.* Bloomington: Indiana University Press, 1999.

Townes, Ross E. "Professional Physical Education in Selected Negro Colleges." *Journal of Negro Education* 20 (1951): 174–80.

Trimble, R. Thomas, and Larry D. Hensley. "Basic Instruction Programs At Four-Year Colleges and Universities. Parts 1 and 2." *Journal of Physical Education, Recreation, and Dance* 61 (August 1990): 64–73.

Tuana, Nancy. "The Weaker Seed: The Sexist Bias of Reproductive Theory." In *Feminism and Science*, edited by Nancy Tuana, 147–71. Bloomington: Indiana University Press, 1989.

Turner, Bryan S. *The Body and Society: Explorations in Social Theory.* 2nd ed. London: Sage, 1996.

Twin, Stephanie. "Ethel Perrin." In *Notable American Women: The Modern Period*, edited by Barbara Sicherman and Carol Hurd Green, 539–41. Cambridge, Mass.: Belknap Press of Harvard University Press, 1980.

Tyack, David B. *The One Best System: A History of American Urban Education.* Cambridge, Mass.: Harvard University Press, 1974.

Tyack, David B., and Elisabeth Hansot. *Learning Together: A History of Coeducation in American Public Schools*. New Haven, Conn.: Yale University Press; New York: Russell Sage Foundation, 1990.

Urban, Wayne, and Jennings Wagoner Jr. *American Education: A History*. New York: McGraw-Hill, 1996.

Valdiserri, Ronald O. "Menstruation and Medical Theory: An Historical Overview." *Journal of the American Medical Women's Association* 38 (May–June 1983): 66–70.

Verbrugge, Martha H. *Able-Bodied Womanhood: Personal Health and Social Change in Nineteenth-Century Boston*. New York: Oxford University Press, 1988.

———. "Clelia Duel Mosher." In *American National Biography*, edited by John A. Garraty and Mark C. Carnes, 15:976–78. New York: Oxford University Press, 1999.

———. "Climbing Toward Health: School-Based Physical Education and the Emergence of Physical Activity as a Public Health Priority in the United States, 1920–2005." Paper presented at conference on "Public Health and the State: Yesterday, Today, and Tomorrow," Columbia University, New York, October 2005.

———. "Gender, Science & Fitness: Perspectives on Women's Exercise in the United States in the 20th Century." *Health and History* 4 (2002): 52–72.

———. "Gym Periods and Monthly Periods: Concepts of Menstruation in American Physical Education, 1900–1940." In *Body Talk: Rhetoric, Technology, Reproduction*, edited by Mary M. Lay, Laura J. Gurak, Clare Gravon, and Cynthia Myntti, 67–97. Madison: University of Wisconsin Press, 2000.

———. "The Institutional Politics of Women's Sports in American Colleges, 1920–1940." Paper presented at the annual meeting of the North American Society for Sport History, Auburn, Ala., May 1996.

———. "Knowledge and Power: Health and Physical Education for Women in America." In *Women, Health, and Medicine in America: A Historical Handbook*, edited by Rima D. Apple, 369–90. New York: Garland, 1990.

———. "Recreating the Body: Women's Physical Education and the Science of Sex Differences in America, 1900–1940." *Bulletin of the History of Medicine* 71 (1997): 273–304.

———. "Recreation and Racial Politics in the Young Women's Christian Association of the United States, 1920s–1950s." *International Journal of the History of Sport* 27 (2010): 1191–1218.

Vertinsky, Patricia A. "Embodying Normalcy: Anthropometry and the Long Arm of William H. Sheldon's Somatotyping Project." *Journal of Sport History* 29 (2002): 95–133.

———. *The Eternally Wounded Woman: Women, Doctors, and Exercise in the Late Nineteenth Century*. Urbana: University of Illinois Press, 1994.

———. "Reclaiming Space, Revisioning the Body: The Quest for Gender-Sensitive Physical Education." *Quest* 44 (1992): 373–96.

———. "Science, Social Science, and the 'Hunger for Wonders' in Physical Education: Moving Toward a Future Healthy Society." In *New Possibilities, New Paradigms?* American Academy of Physical Education Papers, no. 24, 70–88. Champaign, Ill.: Human Kinetics, 1991.

Vertinsky, Patricia A., and Gwendolyn Captain. "More Myth than History: American Culture and Representations of the Black Female's Athletic Ability." *Journal of Sport History* 25 (1998): 532–61.

Walden, Janelle. "Sports." In *The Contributions of Black Women to America*, edited by Marianna W. Davis, 1:493–589. Columbia, S.C.: Kenday Press, 1982.

Warren, Donald, ed. *American Teachers: Histories of a Profession at Work*. New York: Macmillan, 1989.

Weatherford, Allen Ericson II. "Professional Health, Physical Education, and Recreation Education in Negro Colleges, 1948–1949." *Journal of Negro Education* 22 (1953): 527–33.

Weedon, Chris. *Feminism, Theory and the Politics of Difference*. Oxford: Blackwell, 1999.

Weiss, Beverly J. "An African American Teacher in Washington, D.C.: Marion P. Shadd (1856–1943)." In *Lives of Women Public School Teachers: Scenes from Educational History*, edited by Madelyn Holmes and Beverly J. Weiss, 191–218. New York: Garland, 1995.

Welch, Paula D. *History of American Physical Education and Sport*. 3rd ed. Springfield, Ill.: Charles C. Thomas, 2004.

Wellman, Susan, and Elaine Blinde. "Homophobia in Women's Intercollegiate Basketball: Views of Women Coaches Regarding Coaching Careers and Recruitment of Athletes." *Women in Sport and Physical Activity Journal* 6 (Fall 1997): 63–82.

Weston, Arthur. *The Making of American Physical Education*. New York: Appleton-Century-Crofts, 1962.

Whitson, David. "Sport in the Social Construction of Masculinity." In *Sport, Men, and the Gender Order: Critical Feminist Perspectives*, ed. Michael A. Messner and Donald F. Sabo, 19–29. Champaign, Ill.: Human Kinetics, 1990.

Whorton, James C. *Crusaders for Fitness: The History of American Health Reformers*. Princeton, N.J.: Princeton University Press, 1982.

———. *Inner Hygiene: Constipation and the Pursuit of Health in Modern Society*. New York: Oxford University Press, 2000.

Wiggins, David K. "Edwin Bancroft Henderson, African American Athletes, and the Writing of Sport History." In *Glory Bound: Black Athletes in a White America*, 221–40. Syracuse, N.Y.: Syracuse University Press, 1997.

———. "Edwin Bancroft Henderson: Physical Educator, Civil Rights Activist, and Chronicler of African American Athletes." *Research Quarterly for Exercise and Sport* 70 (1999): 91–112.

———. "'Great Speed But Little Stamina': The Historical Debate Over Black Athletic Superiority." *Journal of Sport History* 16 (1989): 158–85.

———. "The Notion of Double-Consciousness and the Involvement of Black Athletes in American Sport." In *Glory Bound: Black Athletes in a White America*, 200–220. Syracuse, N.Y.: Syracuse University Press, 1997.

Wijngaard, Marianne van den. *Reinventing the Sexes: The Biomedical Construction of Femininity and Masculinity*. Bloomington: Indiana University Press, 1997.

Wilkinson, Susan, Kay M. Williamson, and Ruth Rozdilsky. "Gender and Fitness Standards." *Women in Sport and Physical Activity Journal* 5 (1996): 1–25.

Wiltse, Jeff. *Contested Waters: A Social History of Swimming Pools in America*. Chapel Hill: University of North Carolina Press, 2007.

Wolters, Raymond. *The New Negro on Campus: Black College Rebellions of the 1920s*. Princeton, N.J.: Princeton University Press, 1975.

Women's Sports and Fitness Facts & Statistics (updated 3/26/09). http://www.womenss-portsfoundation.org/~/media/Files/PDFs%20and%20other%20files%20by%20Topic/Issues/Coaching/C/WSF%20FACTS%20March%202009.pdf (accessed January 30, 2010).

Woods, Sherry E. "Describing the Experience of Lesbian Physical Educators: A Phenomenological Study." In *Research in Physical Education and Sport: Exploring Alternative Visions*, edited by Andrew C. Sparkes, 90–117. London: Falmer Press, 1992.

Woods, Sherry E., and Karen M. Harbeck. "Living in Two Worlds: The Identity Management Strategies Used by Lesbian Physical Educators." In *Coming Out of the Classroom Closet: Gay and Lesbian Students, Teachers, and Curricula*, edited by Karen M. Harbeck, 141–66. New York: Haworth, 1992.

Wrynn, Alison M. "A Fine Balance: Margaret Bell, Physician and Physical Educator." *Research Quarterly for Exercise and Sport* 76 (2005): 149–65.

Wushanley, Ying. *Playing Nice and Losing: The Struggle for Control of Women's Intercollegiate Athletics, 1960–2000*. Syracuse, N.Y.: Syracuse University Press, 2004.

Young, Elizabeth Barber. *A Study of the Curricula of Seven Selected Women's Colleges of the Southern States*. Contributions to Education, no. 511. New York: Bureau of Publications, Teachers College, Columbia University, 1932; repr. ed., 1972.

Young, Iris M. *On Female Body Experience: "Throwing Like a Girl" and Other Essays*. New York: Oxford University Press, 2005.

Young, Lola. "Racializing Femininity." In *Women's Bodies: Discipline and Transgression*, edited by Jane Arthurs and Jean Grimshaw, 67–90. London: Cassell, 1999.

Zakrajsek, Dorothy, and Deborah Tannehill. "Parents Look at Physical Education: A Cross Cultural Perspective." *Future Focus* 8, no. 3 (1993): 16–20.

Zeigler, Earle F. "Historical Perspective on Contrasting Philosophies of Professional Preparation for Physical Education." *Canadian Journal of History of Sport and Physical Education* 6 (1975): 23–42.

———, ed. *A History of Physical Education and Sport in the United States and Canada: Selected Topics*. Champaign, Ill.: Stipes, 1975.

Zieff, Susan G. "The American 'Alliance' of Health and Physical Education: Scholastic Programs and Professional Organizations, 1920–1950." *Research Quarterly for Exercise and Sport* 77 (2006): 437–50.

———. "From Badminton to the Bolero: Sport and Recreation in San Francisco's Chinatown, 1895–1950." *Journal of Sport History* 27 (2000): 1–29.

Unpublished Theses and Dissertations

Abney, Robertha. "The Effects of Role Models and Mentors on Career Patterns of Black Women Coaches and Athletic Administrators in Historically Black and Historically White Institutions of Higher Education." Ph.D. diss., University of Iowa, 1988.

Alexander, Alpha. "Status of Minority Women in the Association of Intercollegiate Athletics for Women." M.Ed. thesis, Temple University, 1978.

Brandford, Pat A. "Training and Opportunities for Negro Women in Physical Education." M.A. thesis, State University of Iowa, 1939.

Brockmeyer, Gretchen Ann. "A Survey of Basic Instruction Physical Education Programs for Women in Selected Colleges and Universities." M.S. thesis, Springfield College, 1966.

Burr, John Harold. "A Survey of Physical Education in Negro Colleges and Universities." M.Ed. thesis, International Young Men's Christian Association College, 1931.

Carkin, Janice W. "A Study of Five Women in the Field of Physical Education Who Have Been Recipients of the Gulick Award Up to 1950." Ed.D. diss., Stanford University, 1952.

Chepko, Steveda. "The Impact of Mabel Lee, Ethel Perrin and Agnes Wayman on Women's Intercollegiate Athletics between 1920 and 1935." Ed.D. diss., Temple University, 1987.

Cottrell, Debora Lynn. "Women's Minds, Women's Bodies: The Influence of the Sargent School for Physical Education." Ph.D. diss., University of Texas at Austin, 1993.

Coursey, Leon N. "The Life of Edwin Bancroft Henderson and His Professional Contributions to Physical Education." Ph.D. diss., Ohio State University, 1971.

Dosch, Nancy Cole. "Exploring Alternatives: The Use of Exercise as a Medical Therapeutic in Mid-Nineteenth Century America, 1830–1870." Ph.D. diss., University of Maryland, 1993.

Duval, Earl Henry Jr. "An Historical Analysis of the Central Intercollegiate Athletic Association and Its Influence on the Development of Black Intercollegiate Athletics: 1912–1984." Ph.D. diss., Kent State University, 1985.

Godfrey, Jessie. "The Organization and Administration of Women's Athletic and Recreation Associations." M.S. thesis, Wellesley College, 1951.

Gormley, Helen. "A Study of the Factors Which Influence the Success of Women Majors in Physical Education." M.S. thesis, University of Wisconsin, 1937.

Gormley, Katherine Frances. "A Study of Interests and Personality Traits of Women Students Majoring in Physical Education." M.A. thesis, University of California at Berkeley, 1939.

Haddock, Frances C. "A Study of Physical Education for Women in Accredited Negro Colleges and Universities." Special Study Project, Hygiene 323: Graduate Seminar, Department of Hygiene and Physical Education, Wellesley College, May 1938.

Handorf, William George. "An Historical Study of the Superintendency of Dr. Frank W. Ballou in the Public School System of the District of Columbia." Ed.D. diss., American University, 1962.

Himes, Cindy L. *The Female Athlete in American Society: 1860–1940*. Ann Arbor: University Microfilms International, 1986; Ph.D. diss., University of Pennsylvania, 1986.

Hodgdon, Paula D. "An Investigation of Interscholastic and Intercollegiate Activities for Girls and Women from 1917–1970." Ph.D. diss., Springfield College, 1973.

Jacobs, Mary G. "An Evaluation of the Physical Education Service Program for Women in Certain Selected Colleges." Ed.D. diss., New York University, 1957.

Kennard, Margot E. "The Corporation in the Classroom: The Struggles over Meanings of Menstrual Education in Sponsored Films, 1947–1983." Ph.D. diss., University of Wisconsin at Madison, 1989.

Leyhe, Naomi Laura. "Attitudes of the Women Members of the American Association for Health, Physical Education, and Recreation Toward Competition in Sports for Girls and Women." D.P.E. diss., Indiana University, 1955.

Liberti, Rita M. "'We Were Ladies, We Just Played Basketball Like Boys': A Study of Women's Basketball at Historically Black Colleges and Universities in North Carolina, 1925–1945." Ph.D. diss., University of Iowa, 1998.

Lisberger, Sylvia Virginia. "Federal and State Legislation Regarding Physical Education in the United States From 1935 to 1945." M.S. thesis, Stanford University, 1946.

Lupcho, Paula Rogers. "The Professionalization of American Physical Education, 1885–1930." Ph.D. diss., University of California, Berkeley, 1986.

Lynn, Minnie L. "An Historical Analysis of the Professional Career of Delphine Hanna." M.S. thesis, Pennsylvania State University, 1937.

Mitchell, Florence Nightingale. "A Survey of Physical Education Personnel for Women in Negro Colleges and Universities." M.Ed. thesis, Springfield College, 1958.

Murphy, Margaret Dianne. "The Involvement of Blacks in Women's Athletics in Member Institutions of the Association of Intercollegiate Athletics for Women." Ph.D. diss., Florida State University, 1980.

Neilson, Herman Newman. "An Evaluation of the Physical Education of Negro Professional Schools." M.Ed. thesis, International Young Men's Christian Association College, 1936.

O'Hanlon, Timothy P. "Interscholastic Athletics, 1900–1940: Shaping Citizens for Unequal Roles in the Modern Industrial State." Ph.D. diss., University of Illinois, Urbana-Champaign, 1979.

Peterson, Hazel Clara. "Dorothy S. Ainsworth: Her Life, Professional Career and Contributions to Physical Education." Ph.D. diss., Ohio State University, 1975.

Phillips, Madge Marie. "Biographies of Selected Women Leaders in Physical Education in the United States." Ph.D. diss., University of Iowa, 1960.

Pierro, Armstead A. "A History of Professional Preparation for Physical Education in Some Selected Negro Colleges and Universities, 1924–1958." Ph.D. diss., University of Michigan, 1962.

Pullum, Fred Douglas. "Professional Preparation in Physical Education at Historically Black Institutions in Georgia." Ed.D. diss., University of Georgia, 1974.

Riffe, Terri Dean. "A History of Women's Sports at the University of Arizona." Ph.D. diss., University of Arizona, 1986.

Robinson, William Hannibal. "The History of Hampton Institute, 1868–1949." Ph.D. diss., New York University, 1954.

Roe, Donald L. "The Struggle for Quality Education: The Desegregation of the District of Columbia Public School System, 1947–1962." Ph.D. diss., Howard University, 1994.

Smith, Nina Jo Woolley. "'Out of Adversity, We Survived': Oral Histories of Seven Black Women Physical Educators." M.A. thesis, San Francisco State University, 1992.

St. Clair, Stephen Isaac. "The Play Day/Sport Day Movement in Selected Colleges of the South." Ed.D. diss., University of North Carolina at Greensboro, 1984.

Szady, Sheryl Marie. "The History of Intercollegiate Athletics for Women at the University of Michigan." Ed.D. diss., University of Michigan, 1987.

Thaxton, Nolan A. "A Documentary Analysis of Competitive Track and Field for Women at Tennessee State A&I University and Tuskegee Institute." Ph.D. diss., Springfield College, 1970.

Thompson, William Dove. "The Development of Physical Education in the District of Columbia Public Schools." Ed.D. diss., New York University, 1941.

Townes, Ross Emile. "A Study of Professional Education in Physical Education In Selected Negro Colleges." D.P.E. diss., Indiana University, 1950.

Trekell, Marianna. "Gertrude Evelyn Moulton, M.D.: Her Life and Professional Career in Health and Physical Education." Ph.D. diss., Ohio State University, 1962.

Twin, Stephanie Lee. "Jock and Jill: Aspects of Women's Sports History in America, 1870–1940." Ph.D. diss., Rutgers University, 1978.

Umstead, Elizabeth Claire. "Mary Channing Coleman: Her Life and Contributions to Health, Physical Education and Recreation, 1883–1947." Ed.D. diss., University of North Carolina at Chapel Hill, 1967.

Vostral, Sharra L. "Conspicuous Menstruation: The History of Menstruation and Menstrual Hygiene Products in America, 1870–1960." Ph.D. diss., Washington University, 2000.

Waterman, Emma Fuller. "The Physiologic and Anatomic Basis for the Selection and Limitation of Women's Motor Activities." M.A. thesis, Department of Hygiene and Physical Education, Wellesley College, 1925.

Weatherford, Allen Ericson II. "Professional Health Education, Physical Education, and Recreation in Negro Colleges and Universities in the United States." Ph.D., Pennsylvania State College, 1948.

Wilke, Phyllis Kay. "The History of Physical Education for Women at the University of Nebraska from the Early Beginnings to 1952." M.Ed. thesis, University of Nebraska, 1973.

Williams, Linda Darnette. "An Analysis of American Sportswomen in Two Negro Newspapers: The 'Pittsburgh Courier,' 1924–1948 and the 'Chicago Defender,' 1932–1948." Ph.D. diss., Ohio State University, 1987.

Wrynn, Alison M. "The Contributions of Women Researchers to the Development of a Science of Physical Education in the United States." Ph.D. diss., University of California, Berkeley, 1996.

Zeigler, Earle F. "A History of Professional Preparation for Physical Education in the United States, 1861–1948." Ph.D. diss., Yale University, 1951.

Zieff, Susan G. "The Medicalization of Higher Education: Women Physicians and Physical Training, 1870–1920." Ph.D. diss., University of California, Berkeley, 1994.

Zimmerli, Elizabeth K. "A History of Physical Education for Women at Stanford University and a Survey of the Department of Physical Education for Women in 1943–1944." Ed.D. diss., Stanford University, 1945.

{ INDEX }

Abbott, Cleveland L., 136–37, 139, 142
Abbott, Jessie H. (Scott), 19, 136, 138, 142
abbreviations, 259–60
academic settings, gym teachers, 28–29, 30, 181, 188–89, 191–93
administrative structure and power
colleges and universities, 38–41, 183–84, 191–92, 194–95
Howard University (Allen), 94–96
menstrual rules, 74–75
University of Nebraska (Lee), 91–93
affirmation, Maryrose Allen, 89, 90–91
African American physical educators. *See also* Allen, Maryrose R.; Henderson, Edwin B.; Turner, Anita J.; Williams, Charles H.
backgrounds, 19, 20, 176
collegiate personnel, 7, 30, 185–86, 192, 194, 195
credentials and status, 6, 167, 185–86
desegregation, 181–82
facilities and resources, 36, 185
marriage and employment, 44
professional networks, 42
public schools, 29–30, 181–82. *See also* Washington, D.C., public schools
training, 21, 27–28, 177–80
views on womanhood, 89–90, 137, 140–41, 149–50, 170–72
African Americans
experiences in gym class, 5–6
historically black colleges and universities (HBCUs), 124–25
public education, 29
recreation and sports, 50, 52, 136
self-representations, women, 89–90
sports and racial uplift, 94, 136, 138, 168–70, 171–72
women and work, 20
Agnes Scott College, 105, 110, 174, 195
Ainsworth, Dorothy Sears, 17, 38, 110
Alabama State College, 136
Albright, Tenley, 241
Alden, Florence D., 55, 59
Allen, Maryrose R., 22f, 82f, 83f
affirmation, 89, 90–91
Beauty-Health philosophy, 87–91, 94–95, 99

biography, 19, 79–80
black womanhood, 88–91
decorporealization, 89–90
Howard University, 34, 78, 79
inequities at Howard, 93–96, 100–101
normalization, 89, 90
philosophy, 11–12, 80–81, 87–91
self-governance, 93–96
teaching and diluting democracy, 98–99
Amateur Athletic Union (AAU), 52, 70, 140, 142, 235
amenorrhea. *See also* exercise and reproductive health
athletic, 239, 246, 250
exercise-induced, 13, 242, 244, 336n143
Female Athlete Triad, 232, 239, 242–43, 245, 249, 251
secondary, 239–40, 241–42, 247, 250
American Academy of Pediatrics, 234
American Academy of Physical Education, 79
American Alliance for Health, Physical Education, Recreation and Dance (AAHPERD), 15, 79
American Association for Health, Physical Education, and Recreation (AAHPER), 80, 196, 203, 207, 209, 233
American Association for the Advancement of Physical Education (AAAPE), 15, 41, 42
American Association of University Women, 43
American Baptist Home Mission Society (ABHMS), 144
American College of Sports Medicine (ACSM), 203, 239, 243, 249
American culture, physical education, 3, 10
American Girl, 50, 56, 63, 73, 84
American Medical Association (AMA), 203, 232, 233
American Physical Education Association (APEA), 11, 41, 78
American Physical Education Review, 15
American Psychiatric Association, 198
anatomy, sex differences, 48, 53–54, 204, 207, 210, 216, 222
Anderson, William G., 156
Anderson Normal School, 21
Anglo-Americans, experiences in gym class, 5

anthropometry, 9
anti-gay climate, U. S., 186, 198–99
Applebee, Constance M. K., 115, 116f
Aristotle, nutritive theory of menstruation, 66
Armstrong, Samuel C., 125
Association for Intercollegiate Athletics for
    Women (AIAW), 187, 196, 219
Åstrand, P.-O., 237
Athletic Conference of American College
    Women (ACACW), 109, 113, 121
Athletic Federation of College Women (AFCW),
    109
Athletic Girl, 51
athletics. *See* competitive activities; extramural
    sports
athletics, Title IX, 188, 195–96
Atkins, Louise, 136
Atlanta Baptist Female Seminary, 143
Atlanta Compromise, 134, 139
awards
    Gulick Award, 79
    Women's Athletic Associations, 98, 99, 107–9,
        110–12

Baker, Gertrude M., 40, 265n23
Baker, Mary C., 129, 130
Ballard, Lula, 139
Baptists, Spelman College, 143, 144
Barnard College, 54
basketball
    extramural, 112, 114, 115, 117–18, 119, 135,
        139, 159
    intramural, Smith College, 111
    photographs, 55f, 120f, 169f
    race and class, 5, 52, 115, 136, 170, 229
    sex differences, 53, 54, 58, 116, 137, 204, 205,
        209, 210, 212, 213, 222, 235, 237
    women's recollections, 17, 85, 97, 110, 286n35
Bay Area Sports Day, 123
Bayh, Birch Evans, 158–59, 307n22
Beauty-Health philosophy, Allen, 87–91, 94–95,
    99
Beecher, Catharine, 14
Bell, Margaret, 18, 26, 277n28, 280n5
    menstruation, 64, 65, 68, 235, 280n6
    University of Michigan, 34, 38, 108
Beloit College, 79, 92
Bennett College, 99, 131
Berenson, Senda, 292n21
biological foundationalism, 263n28
biology. *See also* exercise and reproductive
        health; nature/nurture debate; science
    nature and nurture, 48–49
    reproductive health, 63–64, 66–67, 232–33,
        241–46

science of, 7–8, 47–49, 207, 215
biomedicine, menstruation, 67–68, 232–33
bioreductionism, 48–49, 207, 215
Birrell, Susan, 221
black institutions. *See* historically black colleges
        and universities (HBCUs)
black physical educators. *See* African American
        physical educators
black womanhood, 88–91, 124–25, 126–27,
        132–33, 137, 139, 142–43, 146, 147
Blue Blazer Girl, 112
Body Aesthetics, 99
body and identity, modern era, 254–55
Body Sculpture through Movement, 99
Boston Normal School of Gymnastics (BNSG),
        17, 19, 20, 21, 23, 27, 31, 79, 83, 84, 85, 97,
        125, 265n13
Boston University, 79
bourgeois womanhood, 49–51, 56–57
"Boy Problem," 161–62
Boy Scouts, 203
boys' gym classes, 3, 8
    cadet program, 160–61
    fitness testing, 163–65
    Washington, D.C., public schools, 159–60
Brevard College, 213
Brown University, 114
Brown v. Board of Education of Topeka, 4, 12,
        167, 201
Bryn Mawr College, 113, 114–17, 152
Bunting, Helen Masters, 119–22
Burchenal, Elizabeth, 18, 266n31

cadet program, Washington, D.C., 160–61
Cahn, Susan, 140
calisthenics, 14, 52, 106f, 127, 134, 145, 150
Carnegie Foundation, Tuskegee, 134
Carver, George Washington, 136
Central School of Hygiene and Physical
        Education, 31, 126, 129
Cheska, Alyce, 221, 223
civil rights movement, 12, 208
class, active womanhood, 49–53
coaches. *See also* physical educators and coaches
    collegiate personnel, 192–94, 196–97
    exercise and reproductive health, 251–52
    high school, female, 188–89
Coachman, Alice, 140, 141f
Coe College, 17, 79, 84, 86, 91–92
coed institutions
    departmental structure and power, 38–41,
        91–93, 94–96, 183–84, 191–92, 194–95
    facilities and equipment, 35–36, 184–85
coed physical education and sports
    difference and equity, 217–19

in 1950s, 205
Old Guard's view, 106
similarity and equality, 219–21
Title IX, 214
Cold War, 202, 206, 304n246
Coleman, Mary Channing, 18, 23, 24f, 37, 70, 107
collective syndrome, Female Athlete Triad, 232, 239, 242–43, 245, 249, 251
College Man, archetypal, 104
colleges and universities. *See also* historically black colleges and universities (HBCUs)
black institutions, 124–25
curricular debates, 103–4
debates over women's sports, 102–5, 150–52
enrollments, 103
extramural sports, female, 113–23, 135–36, 140–43
female physical educators, 32–41, 182–86, 191–97
menstruation and exercise, rules, 70–72, 74–75, 282n46, 283n56
student behavior, 104
Colored Intercollegiate Athletic Association (CIAA), 94, 129
Commission on Intercollegiate Athletics for Women (CIAW), 187
competitive activities. *See also* extracurricular activities; extramural sports
Bryn Mawr, 114–17
colleges and universities, 102–5, 150–52
high school girls, 171–72
Old Guard's philosophy, 105–9
Stanford University, 117–23
student pressure for, 109–13
Tuskegee, 134–38
women, competition, and difference, 150–52
Coope, Jessie, 126
Crafts, Virginia, 210
Creative Dance Group, Hampton, 131–33
credentials, female physical educators, 176–80, 185–86, 190
Cromwell, Amelia M. (Roberts), 134–35, 136
Cummings, Mabel, 70
curricular debates, colleges and universities, 103–4

dance programs, 264n41
Creative Dance Group at Hampton, 131–33
Hampton Institute, 126, 131–33
Howard University, 90, 99
May Day festivals, 110, 115, 126, 127, 130, 149
Spelman College, 149–50
University of Nebraska, 97
Darnell, Kathryn E., 59

Darwin, traits in humans, 47
decorporealization, Allen, 89–90
Delsarte, François, 156
democracy
Allen, 98–99
Lee, 96–98
recreation, 61
Denham, Julia R. S., 149
department organization. *See* administrative structure and power
Didrikson, Babe, 86
dietary intake, energy availability, 248–51
differences. *See also* race; sex differences
and bodies, 254–55
binary dualities, 48, 51, 61, 88, 100, 206–9, 212–13, 222, 257
physical education, central tenet, 7, 10, 13, 253–54, 257
science of, 7–8, 47–49, 89, 206, 207, 215, 225–26, 254, 255
Western notions of, 7–8, 254
discrimination. *See also* inequity
female recreation, 52–53
gym class, 5–6, 8
physical education's complicity, 8
Division for Girls and Women's Sports (DGWS), 209, 218, 235, 237, 238
Division I, II, III, collegiate personnel, 192–97
Drinkwater, Barbara, 216, 240, 246, 247
Du Bois, W. E. B., 99, 124, 128
Dudley, Gertrude, 54, 72
Duke University, 33, 36, 38, 42–43, 107, 184
DuQuin, Mary E., 221
Durkee, J. Stanley, 94
Dyment, Bertha Sabin Stuart, 122
dysmenorrhea, 65, 67, 74, 235, 238, 280n6

Earlham College, 18
eating disorders
energy availability, 248–51
Female Athlete Triad, 232, 239, 242–43, 245, 249, 251
economics, school equipment budgets, 5
education degrees, 6, 15, 19–21, 177–80, 190–92, 262n17, 312nn6–8
Educational Amendments Act of 1972, 4, 6, 187–88, 201. *See also* Title IX
Eisenhower, Dwight D., 202
employment
combining marriage and, 43–45, 180–81
demand for teachers, 15–16, 19, 29, 32, 76, 85, 174
hiring, 28–32, 176–77
types of jobs, 28–29, 174, 181

energy deficit theory, exercise and reproductive health, 248–51
environmentalists, nature/nurture debate, 48–49
equipment, women's gyms, 34–36, 92, 195
Equity in Athletics Disclosure Act (EADA), Title IV, 318n109
Erdelyi, Gyula J., 237, 238
Espenschade, Anna S., 204, 237
ethnicity. *See* race
exercise
    health and fitness, 202–3, 320n24
    health-related, 207, 214–15
    physical activity and health, 224–26
exercise and reproductive health, 63–64, 232–33.
    See also amenorrhea; menstruation
    body fat theory, 239
    doctors' views, 66–67, 233–34, 239–40
    endocrinological paradigm, 234, 239–40, 242–43
    energy deficit theory, 248–51
    Female Athlete Triad, 232, 239, 242–43, 245, 249, 251, 333n93
    metaphors, 233, 238, 242–43
    physical education (1940s–1950s), 235–36
    physical education (1960s), 236–38
    physical education (1970s), 240–41
    physical education (1980–95), 246–48
    physical education (1995–2005), 251–52
    research on males, 247–48
    scientific disputes (1980–95), 241–46
    subclinical disorders, 241–42
extracurricular activities, women's. *See also* competitive activities; extramural sports, women's
    Agnes Scott College, 110
    conservative programs, 105–9
    Hampton Institute, 126, 130–31
    Milwaukee-Downer, 111–13
    Smith College, 111
    Spelman College, 145, 148–49
    Stanford University, 117–23
    Women's Athletic Associations (WAAs), 108–9, 113
extramural sports, women's. *See also* competitive activities
    Bryn Mawr, 114–17
    competition for women, 102–5, 150–52
    Hampton, 130
    Spelman, 148–49
    Stanford, 117–23
    Tuskegee, 135, 140–43
    white institutions, 113–23

facilities, women's programs, 34–36, 91–92, 184–85, 195

Faculty Athletic Committee (FAC), 118
Faculty Committee on Athletics (FCA), 119
Faculty Committee on Women's Athletics (FCWA), Stanford, 119, 121
fairness in the gym. *See also* philosophy, female physical educators
    Allen at Howard, 100–101
    Lee at University of Nebraska, 93, 100–101
    physical, 201–2, 205–6, 211–12
    sex differences, 57–58, 253–54
    Title IX, 4, 6, 180, 187–88
Farmville State Normal School for Women (Virginia), 18, 114
Favia v. Indiana University of Pennsylvania, 196
Felshin, Jan, 221
Female Athlete Triad
    debates, 241–43, 245–46, 250–51
    energy availability theory, 248–49
    naming of, 232, 239, 242–43
female bodies
    athletic, perspectives on, 244–46, 249–51
    bourgeois ideal, 50
    prejudice and liberation, 255–56
    science of, 48, 66, 203, 207, 215
femininity
    black, 151–52
    bourgeois ideals, 49–51
    Hampton, 126–27, 130
    heterosexual norms, white teachers, 23–28, 55–58, 61–62, 105–6, 151
    Mabel Lee, 85–87
    Maryrose R. Allen, 87–88, 90–91
    physical education trainees, 23–28, 187
    Spelman, 146, 149–50
    Tuskegee, 137–38, 140–43
    Washington, D.C., public schools, 170–72
feminism, 12, 201–2, 207–8, 215
    "difference dilemma," 62, 100–101, 230–31, 254
    diversity and equity, 227
    essentialism, 61–62, 100, 208, 219
    gender equality, 12, 58, 152, 206, 220
    gender equity, 4, 12, 58, 206, 226, 227, 247
    liberal, 207–8, 215, 220, 221
    questioning dualities, 221, 227
    radical, 208, 215, 219
    suffragists, 58
    women's athleticism, 123, 152, 207–8, 214–15
    "Women's Lib" and physical education, 215–16
field days, 107, 111, 126, 145
fitness
    American preoccupation, 9, 49
    concepts of, 1950s, 202–3
    research, 203, 207, 214, 225–26

fitness tests
    performance and identity, 8–9
    sex-based ability, 5
    Washington, D.C., public schools, 163–65, 169
    Youth Fitness Test, AAHPER, 207
flappers of 1920s, 50, 51
Florida, public schools, 29
Founders Day, Spelman, 145, 148
Frisch, Rose, 239
Frymir, Alice W., 54, 59, 66

Galen, plethora theory of menstruation, 66,
    68, 72
gays and lesbians. *See also* sexual orientation
    female teachers and coaches, 45, 187, 197–99
    in United States, 51, 186, 198–99
    physical education, 186–87, 197–98
gender. *See also* femininity; masculinity; race
    binaries of sex and, 7–8, 48, 50–51, 207–8,
        215, 221, 254
    "Boy Problem," 161–62
    experiences in gym class, 4–6, 8
    ideals in 1920s, 49–51
    questioning dualities, 221, 227
    "Woman Question," 161–62
    women, competition, and difference, 150–52
gender equality, 12. *See also* feminism
    feminism, 12, 13, 58, 152, 206, 220
    physical education, 256
gender equity, 12. *See also* feminism
    diversity and, 227, 228
    feminism, 12, 13, 58, 206, 226, 227, 247
    Lee and Allen, 100–101
    sex differences and, 12, 13
    suffragists, 58
    Tuskegee, 137, 140–41, 142
General Education Board, 134, 144, 149
Gibson girl, 50
Giles, Harriet E., 143
"girl nature," Mabel Lee and, 81–87
Girl Scouts, 28, 203
Girls' Athletic Association. *See also* Women's
        Athletic Association (WAA)
    female gym teachers, 181
    Hampton Institute, 126
girls' gym classes. *See also* physical education
    cadet program, 160–61
    high schools, Washington, D.C., 159, 161–62
    sex segregation, 3–4, 154
golf, University of Michigan, 56f
Grange, Red, 77
Great Depression, 16, 37, 93, 139
Great White Mothers, 102, 151
    programs, 105–9
    student resistance, 109–13

Trilling, 106, 108
Greendorfer, Susan, 221
Gregg, James Edgar, 128
Griffin, Pat, 221
Grout, Julia R., 33f
    background, 16–17
    personal life, 42–43
    Woman's College of Duke University, 33–34,
        36, 38
Gulick Award, 79
gym class. *See* physical education
gym teachers. *See* physical educators and
        coaches
gynecologists, opinions on exercise, 66,
    234, 239

Hampton Institute, 299n136
    Allen, 79
    black femininity, 126–27
    black masculinity and sexuality, 132
    competitive sports, boys, 126, 129–30
    Creative Dance Group, 131–33
    department structure, 128, 183
    extracurricular activities, girls, 126, 127,
        130–31
    governance, 125, 129, 144
    hiring process, 30–31
    Moton, Charlotte, 31, 129, 131
    nature/nurture debate, 126–27
    physical activities, 126, 129
    physical education staff, 31, 125–26,
        128–29
    physical education trainees, 22f
    teacher training, 21
    Thomas, Azalie, 19
    Williams, Charles H., 128–32
Hampton Model, black education, 125, 133
Hampton University, 183
Hanna, Delphine, 18, 24, 35
Harper's Bazaar, athletics and motherhood,
    232
Harris, Dorothy V., 215–16, 218, 221–24, 240,
    246–47
Harvard Summer School for Physical Education,
    19
Harvard University, 21, 37, 114, 239
Hazelton, Helen W., 58
health
    concepts, 1950s, 202–3
    concepts, 1960s, 206–7
    concepts, 1970s–1980s, 214
    concepts, 1990–2005, 224–26
    physical educators' ideas, 9
Health Crusade, 164–65, 170
health education, 264n41

health, physical education and recreation
(HPER)
careers for women, 174, 175, 191, 196–97
collegiate personnel, 191–92
female physical educators, 175, 179, 197–99,
251–52
inequality, 6–7, 256
health professionals, menstruation advice, 67,
233, 239, 243
Healthy People 2010, 225
Heimbach, Althea, 35, 111
Henderson, Edwin B., 159, 166, 167, 168–70,
171–72, 173
civil rights and NAACP, 307n25
gender and race, 171–72
photograph with basketball team, 169f
heterosexuality
American attitudes, 50–51, 186
female teachers and coaches, 45, 198
Hampton's dance program, 132
Tuskegee's female athletes, 137–38
undergraduate women, 104, 109
high schools. *See also* public education
black activism, 168
enrollments, 28–29
female physical educators, 29–30, 180–82,
188–90
graduation rates, 103
physical education and sports, 3, 4, 162, 165
reforms, 161–62
Hirschland, Ruth, 202
Hiss, Anna, 18, 265n26
historically black colleges and universities
(HBCUs), 124–25, 128. *See also* colleges
and universities
Atlanta Compromise, 134, 139
competitive activities, women's, 105, 124–25,
151–52
enrollments, 124
facilities and resources, 94–95, 185
female teachers and coaches, 30, 185–86, 192,
193
governance, 128, 139
Hampton Institute, 125–33
hiring process, 30–32
Spelman College, 125, 143–50
teacher training programs and graduates, 21,
177–80, 181–82
Tuskegee Institute, 125, 133–42
Homans, Amy Morris, 23, 27, 31, 85
homophobia, 5, 7, 25, 50–51, 57, 86, 132,
186–87, 197–99, 224, 230, 292n22
homosexuality
American attitudes, 50–51, 186, 198–99
class and race, 51, 86, 132

female physical educators, 45, 187, 197–98
Hampton's dance program, 132
teachers' attitudes, 25, 45–46, 86, 106, 187,
221, 224, 230–31, 292n22
hormones
menstruation, 66–67
reproductive, 234, 239–40, 242–43
Howard University
Allen, 11, 19, 34, 78, 79–80, 100–101
gender inequities, 94–96, 100–101
men's sports, 78, 93–94, 95
Slowe, 128
teacher training, 21
tennis class, 89f
women's program, 94–96, 98–99, 150, 152
Women's Sports Day, 99, 131
Howe, Arthur, 130
Huelster, Laura J., 34, 201, 209–10
human nature, scientific theories, 48–50, 206–7,
215, 226
Hunter College, 114

Indiana University of Pennsylvania (IUP), 196
individuality, as principle
Allen, 98–99, 100
Lee, 96–98, 100
inequity. *See also* gender equity; racial inequities
difference and, 7–8, 13, 254, 255
difference and, public schools, 159–61, 165–68,
172–73
difference and, women's competition, 150–52
infertility, menstrual problem, 65
intercollegiate sports, men's, 36, 37, 77–78, 93,
94, 96–97, 100–101, 102, 119, 129, 135, 140,
185, 195–96
intercollegiate sports, women's. *See also*
competitive activities; extramural sports,
women's; Play Days
black institutions, 136
Bryn Mawr, 114–17
female personnel in, 191–97
Hampton, 130
Smith College, 110–11
Spelman, 148–49
Sports Days, 80, 99, 103, 107, 113, 121, 124,
131
Stanford, 117–23
Title IX, 187–88
Tuskegee, 135, 140–43
white institutions, 113–14
Inter-Scholastic Athletic Association (ISAA),
169–70
interscholastic sports, girls, 188–89
intramural activities, girls and women
Agnes Scott, 110

Great White Mothers, 107–8
Hampton, 126, 127, 130
Milwaukee-Downer, 111–13
Smith, 110–11
Spelman, 145, 148
Tuskegee, 134–35
Washington, D.C., public schools, 159, 164

Jackson, Nell C., 36, 140, 195, 213
James Madison University, 114
Jim Crow laws, 51, 143
jobs. *See* employment
John F. Slater Fund, 134, 144
Johns Hopkins University, 119
Johnson, Mordecai Wyatt, 94
Jokl, Ernst, 237
Journal of the American Medical Association
    (JAMA), 232
Junior Red Cross, 164
justice
    physical education, 253–57
    social, in physical education, 227, 229–30

Kellor, Frances A., 55
Kennard, Beulah, 59
Kent State University, 238
Kinsey, Albert, 186
Kraus, Hans, 202

Lee, Mabel, 80f, 81f
    biography, 11–12, 17, 78–79
    critique of men's programs, 96–97
    female body and exercise, 83–85
    femininity, 85–87
    "girl nature," 81–87
    instructional program, Nebraska, 97–98
    jobs and problems, 91–93
    manuscript collection, 284n2, 284n3, 288n99
    menstruation, 83, 84
    philosophy, 80–81, 98
    physical sex differences, 53, 81–82
    preaching and betraying democracy, 96–98
    psychosocial sex differences, 85
    racial attitudes, 86–87
    self-governance, 91, 93
    sexuality, 83, 84, 86
    teacher education, 23–24
    University of Nebraska, 23–24, 77, 78, 81f, 87,
        100–101
lesbianism. *See also* homosexuality; sexual
        orientation
    female teachers and coaches, 45, 186–87, 197–99
    student behavior, 25, 104
    teachers' attitudes, 25, 46, 86, 106, 187, 198,
        224, 292n22

    unmarried teachers, 45
Levinson, Ruth D., 268n66
Lewis, Dioclesian, 14, 18
Longwood College, 114

McCarthy, Senator Joseph, 186
McCue, Betty, 237
McKemie, Kate, 174
McKinstry, Helen, 54, 56, 64
Marble, Alice, 86
marriage, physical educators, 43–45, 180–81
Martin, Emily, 256
masculinity
    "Boy Problem," 161–62
    Hampton, 132
    norms in 1920s, 50
    Stanford, 118
maverick teachers, 212–14, 221–24, 227, 229–30,
    257
May Day Festival
    Agnes Scott, 110
    Hampton, 126, 127, 130
    Spelman, 149
menarche, delayed, 234, 239–40, 241–42, 245
men's programs
    criticized by Lee, 96–97
    Howard, 78, 93, 95–96
    Nebraska, 77, 93
    Stanford, 118, 119, 122
    Tuskegee, 134, 135, 142
menstrual dysfunction. *See also* exercise and
        reproductive health
    delayed menarche, 234, 239–40, 241–42
    dysmenorrhea, 65, 67, 74, 235, 238, 280n6
    energy deficit theory, 248–51
    Female Athlete Triad, 232, 239, 242–43, 245,
        249, 251
    infertility, 65, 245–46
    menstrual variations, 64, 245–46, 247–48
    secondary amenorrhea, 239–40, 241–42, 247
menstruation
    administrative systems, colleges, 74–75
    Aristotle's nutritive theory, 66
    class attendance, 70–71, 72, 283n56
    exercise and, 63–64, 69–70, 232–34, 235–38
    Galen's plethora theory, 66
    Mabel Lee, 83, 84
    menstrual health and problems, 64–66
    paradigms and authority, 66–68, 75–76,
        232–33
    research on cycle's effects, 283n64
    Smith College policies, 71–72, 73
    statements and regulations, 69–71
    teachers' views, 64–66, 69–70, 72–74
    tracking college policies, 282n46

Michigan State University, 195, 237
military training, Washington, D.C., 160–61
Mills College, 105, 121, 122, 123
Milwaukee-Downer College, 105, 112f
    facilities, 34–35
    Heimbach, 111
    intramural competition, 107, 111
    Women's Athletic Association (WAA),
        111–13
Mind and Body, 15
Miner Normal School, 19
monthly periods. *See* menstruation
Mosher, Clelia Duel, 18, 64, 119–21, 282n34
Moton, Charlotte, 31, 129, 131
Moton, Robert R., 129, 135, 136, 138–39
Moulton, Gertrude, 17–18, 24, 25f, 34, 35, 38

National Amateur Athletic Federation, 42, 78,
    120
National Association for Girls and Women in
    Sport (NAGWS), 41, 196
National Association for the Advancement of
    Colored People (NAACP), 154
National Association of Physical Education for
    College Women (NAPECW), 42, 80
National Center for Education Statistics,
    degrees, 312n8, 315n60
National Collegiate Athletic Association
    (NCAA), 187–88, 249
National Council for Accreditation of Teacher
    Education (NCATE), 177
National Education Association, 15, 233
National Physical Education Association
    (NPEA), 42
National Physical Education Service (NPES), 16
National Section on Women's Athletics (NSWA),
    41, 42, 235
National Tuberculosis Association, 164
Native Americans, physical education, 3, 52
nature/nurture debate, 47–49, 202, 206, 207, 215,
    226
    Hampton Institute, 127
    Lee's views, 81–82, 85, 87
    nonconformists' ideas, 212–13, 224
    teachers' views, 58–60, 203–5, 209–11, 216–17,
        218, 219, 230
Neal, Patsy, 213–14
New Deal, 93
New Negro, 131, 138, 147, 150
New Woman
    calisthenics, 106f
    female icon, 50, 51, 56–57, 84, 105
    formal schooling, 49–50, 63
    monthly cycle, 73–74
New York City, 5, 169

Central School of Hygiene and Physical
    Education, 31, 126, 129
    Hunter College, 114
No Child Left Behind Act of 2001, 189
Normal Institute for Physical Education, 14
normalization, Allen, 89, 90
Norris, J. Anna, 17, 40, 72, 102
North Carolina College for Women
    (Greensboro), 23, 37, 70, 107, 283n56

Oberlin College, 21, 24, 28, 34, 35, 38
Oglesby, Carole, 221
Ohio State University, 35, 109
Old Guard
    curricular programs, 105–6
    extracurricular programs, 107–9
    student resistance, 109–13
Olympic Games, 52, 86, 140, 171, 234
Olympic Trials, 142
Oregon Agricultural College, Lee, 79, 92, 97
osteopenia, active women, 250
osteoporosis, Female Athlete Triad, 232, 239,
    242–43, 245, 249, 251

Packard, Sophia B., 143, 144
Park, Marion Edwards, 117
Patterson, Frederick D., 139, 142
Patterson, Inez, 19
Pembroke College, 114, 283n56
Perrin, Ethel, 17, 57–58, 69
Peters, Roumania, 140
Petty, Christine Evans, 136, 139–40
philosophy, female physical educators. *See also*
        fairness in the gym
    Allen and "Beauty-Health," 87–91, 98–99
    difference and equity, 57–58, 206, 209–12,
        217–19
    diversity and equity, 226–27, 228
    fairness, 57–58, 201–2, 205–6, 230–31
    mavericks, 212–14, 221–24, 231
    similarity and equality, 57–58, 206, 209–12,
        219–21
    social justice, 227, 229–30
"Phy Ed-iquette," female majors, 23, 46
physical ability, fitness tests, 8–9
physical activity. *See also* exercise
    binary thinking, 7–8
    concepts of, U.S., 202–3, 207, 214, 224–26
    women, competition, and difference, 150–52
physical education
    compulsory, college-level, 4, 30, 36–37, 182,
        191
    compulsory, public schools, 3, 4–5, 29, 181,
        189
    credibility gap, 9, 36–38, 174, 182–83, 190

critiques, 264n40
difference and fairness, 7–8, 10, 100–101, 230–31, 255, 257
"difference" as central tenet, 7, 10, 13, 253–54, 257
differentiation from sports, 10, 264n41
"diversity" in gym, 1990–2005, 226–27
division of labor, 5–7, 29–30, 154–55
fitness crusade, 1950s, 203
history of, as profession, 14–16, 41–42, 174–75, 176–77, 187–88, 191, 201–2
homophobia, 7, 186–87, 197–99, 224, 230
science, 9–10, 59–60, 337n8
status of black personnel, 6, 7, 45–46, 167, 181–82, 185–86, 200
status of female personnel, 5–7, 38, 45–46, 181, 185, 188–90, 192–96, 199–200
student experiences, 3–6, 190
Title IX, 180, 187–88, 214
training and employment opportunities, 20–23, 28–30, 174, 176–80, 181, 188–90
physical educators and coaches
advanced training, 177–80
certification, 20, 177, 190
gender inequities, 5–7, 38, 45–46, 181, 185, 188–90, 192–97, 199–200
racial inequities, 6, 7, 45–46, 181–82, 185–86, 192, 193, 194, 199–200. *See also* African American physical educators
training and employment, 6–7, 14–15, 20–23, 28–30, 174, 176–80, 181, 188–90
physical educators and coaches, female
active womanhood, ideals, 23–28, 55–57, 105–8, 137, 141, 146, 149–52, 187
backgrounds, 16–20, 176, 265n13, 312n3
battles over department structure, 38–41, 91–93, 94–96, 183–84
collegiate personnel, 30, 182–86, 191–97
credentials, 176–80, 190
defending requirements, 36–37, 182
difference and equity, 57–58, 206, 209–12, 217–19
diversity and equity, 227, 228
football debate, 208–9
grades K–12 personnel, 29–30, 180–82, 188–90
Great White Mothers, 102, 105–9
hiring process, 30–32
homosexuality, views on, 7, 25, 86, 187, 197–99, 224, 230
intercollegiate sports personnel, 192–95
job opportunities, 6–7, 28–30, 181, 188–90, 191
marital status, 43–45, 180–81
mavericks and progressives, 212–14, 221–24, 227, 229–30, 257

menstruation, ideas and policies. *See* menstruation
multiple responsibilities, 34, 181, 185–86, 190, 192
nature/nurture debate, 58–60, 204–6, 209–11, 216–17
personal lives, 42–45
political valence, 60–62
professional networks and organizations, 41–42, 187, 196
questioning dualities, 212–14, 221–24
salaries, 181, 185–86, 188–89, 192–94
seeking respect, 36–38, 182–83
settling into jobs, 32–34
sex differences, ideas, 53–56, 58–62, 156, 204–5, 209–12, 215–17
similarity and equality, 56–58, 206, 209–12, 219–21
social justice, 224, 227, 229–30
training, 20–28, 176–80
Play Days, 102, 150
Allen at Howard, 99
historically black colleges and universities (HBCUs), 124
Lee at Nebraska, 97
North Carolina College for Women (Greensboro), 107
Spelman College, 149
Stanford University, 121
University of Minnesota, 102
University of Wisconsin, 108f
Washington, D.C., public schools, 159
Woman's College of Duke, 107
Women's Sports Day Association, 80, 99, 131
Plessy v. Ferguson, Supreme Court, 51
plethora theory, menstruation, 66, 68
Plowman, Sharon A., 246
Posse Gymnasium, 21
Posse School, 31
Prairie View A&M, 136
Pratt, Hazel H., 59
Pratt, Lucy, 126
Pratt Institute, 54
President's Council on Physical Fitness (PCPF), 207
President's Council on Youth Fitness (PCYF), 202
professional organizations
guidelines on menstruation, 69, 235–36, 237–38
position on athletics, 187–88, 217–18, 219
women's, 41–42, 196

public education. *See also* Washington, D.C.,
     public schools
     enrollments, 28–29
     female personnel, 29–30, 180–82, 188–90
     segregated structure, 29, 154–55, 168
     social changes and reforms, 161–62
Public School Athletic League (PSAL), 169, 170
Purdue University, 194
Purdy, Bonnie J., 217

race
     constructing "whiteness," 49–51, 55–57, 86–87,
          151
     gender and, Howard University, 87–91, 95–96
     gender and, Spelman, 146–50
     gender and, Tuskegee, 137, 140–43
     gender and sexuality, Hampton, 130–33
race differences
     black teachers' views, 87–91, 99, 131–33, 137,
          140–43, 168–72
     experiences in gym class, 4–6
     white teachers' views of blacks, 7, 27–28,
          86–87, 125–27, 145–46, 149–50
     women, competition, and difference, 150–52
race relations, U.S., 51, 52
race suicide, birth rates, 63
racial inequities. *See also* African American
          physical educators
     collegiate personnel, 7, 185–86, 192–95
     degree recipients, 177–80
     personnel in grades K–12, 181–82
     public schools, Washington, D.C., 165–72
Radcliffe College, 37, 114, 283n56
Rally Day, Smith, 111
Read, Florence M., 146, 147, 149, 304n262
Rehabilitation Act of 1973, Section 504, 4, 201
reproductive health. *See* menstruation; exercise
          and reproductive health
Research Quarterly, 15
Rockefeller, John D., 144
Rockne, Knute, 77
Rowell, Olive, 127
Rynda, Eleanor, 210

St. Denis, Ruth, 131
Sanborn, Charlotte Feicht, 246
Sargent, Dudley Allen, 18, 19, 156
Sargent School, 17, 18, 19, 21, 27, 31, 79
schoolteachers, female physical educators, 29–30,
          180–82, 188–90
science. *See also* nature/nurture debate; sex
          differences
     health and exercise, 203, 207, 214, 224–26
     human nature and differences, 7–8, 47–49, 89,
          206–7, 215, 226, 254, 255

menstruation, 66–67. *See also* exercise and
     reproductive health
physical education, 9–10, 59–60, 207
sex differences, 7–8, 48, 207, 215, 278n32
sexuality, 50–51, 186, 198
Scott, M. Gladys, 22
Scott, Phebe, 210
Sears, Eleonora, 50
Section 504, Rehabilitation Act, 4, 201
segregation
     Allen's views, 88, 95
     physical activity, by sex, 3–4, 29, 52
     racial, 27, 51, 52, 140, 170, 173, 181–82
     Tuskegee, 134, 139, 140, 141–42
     Washington, D.C., public schools, 154–55,
          165, 168
     Young Women's Christian Association, 4, 6,
          50, 261n3
self-governance, 38–41, 91–96, 183–84, 194–95.
     See also administrative structure and power
Seven Sister schools, 105, 124, 144
sex differences. *See also* philosophy, female
          physical educators
     Allen, 87–88, 100–101
     fairness and, 7–8, 10, 230–31, 253–54, 257
     Lee, 81–83, 85, 100–101
     science of, 7–8, 47–49, 81–83, 207–9, 215,
          278n32
     teachers' views, 11, 53–56, 58–60, 60–62, 156,
          204–5, 209–12, 215–17, 255
sexuality. *See also* homosexuality
     Allen's views, 89–90
     dance program, Hampton, 132–33
     female college students, 104, 109
     Lee's views, 84, 86
sexual orientation
     experiences in gym class, 5, 8
     female teachers, 45, 187, 197–98
     stigmas in physical education, 7, 187, 197–98
Shawn, Ted, 131
sick period, term, 64
Simon, Marguerite, 148, 271n118
Slowe, Lucy, 128
Smith, Helen, 58
Smith College, 105, 109
     Ainsworth, 17, 38, 110
     competition, 110–11
     department structure, 40–41, 75
     menstruation policies, 71–72, 73, 238
     Rally Day, 111
social justice, physical education, 227, 229–30
Somers, Florence, 54
Spelman College
     academic identity, 144, 146–47
     black womanhood, 143, 146, 147, 149–50

dance, 145, 149
extracurricular activities, 145, 148–49
facilities, 35, 149
governance, 144, 147
hiring process, 31–32
missionary philosophy, 143, 145
physical education, 145, 147–48
student body, 143, 147
white teachers, 145–46
Spelman Messenger, 148
sports. *See also* competitive activities; extramural
   sports, women's
   black girls and women, 50, 52, 136, 140
   bourgeois women, 49–51
   menstruation, 65–66. *See also* Female Athlete
   Triad
   working–class women, 51–53
Sports Days, 80, 99, 103, 107, 113, 121, 123,
   124, 131
The Sportswoman, 115
Springfield College, YMCA International
   Training School, 20, 21, 128, 289n114
Stanford, Jane, 118
Stanford, Leland, 117
Stanford University
   academic identity and reforms, 117, 118, 119,
      121–22
   Bunting, 119–22
   evaluation of majors, 26
   Faculty Athletic Committee (FAC), 118
   menstrual absences, 68, 236, 283n56
   Mosher, 18, 64, 119–21
   sports and gender, 118, 119, 123
   Triangle Sports Day (TSD), 121–23
   Women's Athletic Association (WAA), 117,
      119, 122–23
   women's physical education staff, 183f
   women's sports, 117–23
State Normal and Industrial School for Women
   (Virginia), 114
Stoneroad, Rebecca, 154, 156, 158, 163, 164,
   306n9
suffragists, 58
Supreme Court
   Brown v. Board of Education of Topeka, 4, 12,
      167, 201
   Plessy v. Ferguson, 51
Swarthmore College, 114

Tapley, Lucy Hale, 145
Taylor, Mrs. Charles I., 184–85
teacher education. *See* training programs
teachers. *See* physical educators and coaches;
   physical educators and coaches, female
Teachers College of Columbia University, 21

Temple University, 19, 21
Tennessee Agricultural and Industrial State
   Normal School, 136, 142
Thelin, John, 104, 122
Thomas, Azalie, 19, 134
Thomas, M. Carey, 114–17
Title IV, Equity in Athletics Disclosure Act
   (EADA), 318n109
Title IX (Educational Amendments Act of 1972)
   collegiate personnel, 7, 191, 192–97
   compliance, 195–96
   enactment and scope, 180, 188, 191, 318n109
   gym class, 4, 188, 201, 214
   intercollegiate sports, 191, 195–96
   physical educators' views, 187–88, 214, 218–19,
      227, 240, 241, 252
   secondary school personnel, 6–7, 188–90
Title VII, 192
Towne, Alice (Deweese), 22
track and field
   black participation, 136, 140
   Spelman, 148
   Tuskegee, 135–36, 139–43
   Tuskegee Relays, 135–36, 138
   white teachers' attitudes, 53, 59, 65–66
training programs
   assessment of majors, 25–28
   development, 14–15, 176–77
   information sheet, University of Illinois, 178f
   majors, University of Wisconsin, 179f
   opportunities and disparities, 6, 20–23, 177–80
   requirements and curricula, 21–23, 176–77
   standards of femininity, 23–28
   surveys of alumnae, 27, 43–44, 180–81, 269n87
Triangle Conference, 121, 122
Triangle Sports Day (TSD), 121–23
Trilling, Blanche M., 18–19, 26f, 33, 54
   Great White Mothers, 102, 106, 108, 109
   University of Wisconsin, 23, 25–26, 27, 35–36,
      39–40
Turner, Anita J., 19, 154, 157, 165, 167, 170–71,
   173
Tuskegee Institute, 19, 21
   Abbott, Cleve, 136–37, 139, 142
   Abbott, Jessie H. (Scott), 19, 136, 138, 142
   black womanhood, 137, 140–43
   educational system, 133–34, 138–39
   gender icons, 136, 302n215
   governance and funding, 133, 134, 138–39, 142
   Jackson, Nell, 36, 140, 195
   physical activities, 134, 135, 137
   physical education staff, 19, 134–35, 136, 139–40
   physical education students, 135f
   Washington, Booker T., 31, 129, 133–34
   women's sports, 135, 139–43

Tuskegee Messenger, 136
Tuskegee Relays, 135–36, 138, 140, 148
Tuskegee State Normal School, 133

United States Field Hockey Association, 115
University of California, Berkeley, 117, 118, 119,
    121, 122, 123
University of Chicago, 72
University of Illinois
    assessment of black alumna, 27–28
    Grange, 77
    Huelster, 34, 201, 209–10
    information sheet for physical education
        majors, 178f
    Jackson, Nell, 195
    physical education alumnae, survey, 180–81
University of Kansas, 59
University of Michigan, 283n56
    Bell, 18, 34, 38, 108
    photographs, 55f, 56f, 193f
    physical education majors, 26–27, 43–44
    swimming pool, 35
University of Minnesota
    debate over gym requirement, 37–38
    department structure, 40
    menstrual excuses, 72
    Norris, 17, 40, 72, 102
    physical education alumnae, survey, 43
    Play Day, 102
    Women's Athletic Association (WAA), 36, 109
University of Nebraska, 39, 77, 87, 93, 268n66
    debate over gym requirement, 182
    facilities, 92, 184–85
    Lee, 23–24, 77, 78, 79, 92–93
    menstrual policy, 84, 283n56
    Physical Education Club, 97
    physical education majors, 22, 23
    Women's Athletic Association, 81f, 97–98
    women's physical activities, 97–98
University of Oregon, 236
University of Texas, 195
University of Wisconsin, 69, 283n56
    department structure, 39–40
    facilities, 35–36
    photographs, 106f, 108f, 179f
    physical education alumnae, surveys, 27, 43
    Trilling, 23, 25–26, 26f, 35–36, 39–40
U.S. Census Bureau, education degrees, 262n17
U.S. Olympic Development Committee, 209

Van Hagen, Winifred, 14, 20
Virginia State College, 131

Warwick, Florence, 149
Washington, Booker T., 31, 129, 133, 134

Washington, D.C., public schools, 12, 19, 79, 90
    athletics and male privilege, 156–62
    black initiatives, 168–72
    black teachers, on race and gender, 170–72
    "Boy Problem," 161–62
    cadet program, 160–61
    difference and inequity, 155, 172–73
    Dunbar High School basketball team, 169f
    fitness tests, 163–64, 165, 169
    football game between Central and Tech,
        157f
    fund allocation, 166
    gender and race, 170–72
    gender inequities, 157–59, 161
    health education, 164–65
    physical education programs, 153, 159–60,
        163
    physical educators, 154–55, 156, 158–59, 160,
        167
    racial inequities, 165–72
    racial segregation, 154–55, 168–69
    separate-but-equal rhetoric, 172–73
    sports and racial uplift, 168–70, 171–72
    Western High School fencers, 160f
    "Woman Question," 161–62
Wayman, Agnes, 54, 55, 65, 102
Wellesley College, 107, 108
    Boston Normal School of Gymnastics
        (BNSG), 17, 19, 20, 21, 23, 27, 31, 39, 82,
        84, 85, 125, 265n13
    Hygiene and Physical Education program,
        21–22
    menstrual period, 64, 283n56
Wells, Christine, 221, 223, 240, 246, 247
Wells, Katharine, 64
Westcott, Edith C., 160
Whittier Training School (Hampton), 125, 126
Willard, Frances E., 255–57
Williams, Charles H., 128–32
Wills, Helen, 86
Wilson, Edward C., 163
Wilson, Emory M., 163
Wolters, Raymond, 128, 138
womanhood. *See also* femininity
    active, 49–53, 255–57
    black, concepts of, 89–91, 124–25, 126–27,
        132–33, 139, 142–43, 145, 147, 149–50,
        170–72
    bourgeois, 49–51, 115–16
    working-class, 51–53
Woman's American Baptist Home Mission
    Society (WABHMS), 143
Woman's College of Duke University, 33–34, 36,
    38, 42–43, 107
Women's Athletic Association (WAA)

disputes with teachers, 110–13
Duke, Women's Recreation Association, 36
Hampton Institute, 126, 131
Howard University, 99
Milwaukee-Downer, 111–13
Ohio State University, 109
points and awards systems, 107–9
Stanford University, 117, 119, 121–23
University of California, Berkeley, 117, 122
University of Minnesota, 36, 109
University of Nebraska, 81f, 97, 98
Women's Health Equity Act of 1993, 243
women's movement. *See* feminism

Women's Sports Day Association (WSDA), 80, 99, 131
Women's Sports Foundation, 199
Wood, Grace C., 129
Wright, Elizabeth, 37

YMCA International Training School, 20, 21, 128, 289n114
Young Women's Christian Association, 4, 6, 28, 50, 52, 69, 103, 135, 145, 261n3
Young Women's Hebrew Association, 4, 50, 261n3
Youth Fitness Test, AAHPER, 207

CPSIA information can be obtained
at www.ICGtesting.com
Printed in the USA
BVOW11s1956040617

485954BV00003B/9/P